W0050568

Contemporary Perspectives in Neurosurgery

Series Editor: Robert N.N. Holtzman

Robert N.N. Holtzman   Bennett M. Stein
Editors

Surgery of the Spinal Cord

Potential for Regeneration and Recovery

With 141 Figures in 229 Parts

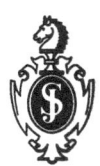

Springer-Verlag
New York Berlin Heidelberg London Paris
Tokyo Hong Kong Barcelona Budapest

ROBERT N.N. HOLTZMAN, MD
Assistant Clinical Professor of Neurological Surgery, College of Physicians and Surgeons of Columbia University; Adjunct Neurosurgeon, Lenox Hill Hospital, New York, NY 10021, USA

BENNETT M. STEIN, MD
Byron Stookey Professor of Neurological Surgery, College of Physicians and Surgeons of Columbia University; Chairman of the Department of Neurological Surgery, The New York Neurological Institute, New York, NY 10032, USA

Library of Congress Cataloging-in-Publication Data
Surgery of the spinal cord: potential for regeneration and
  recovery/Robert N.N. Holtzman, Bennett M. Stein,
  editors.—1st ed.
        p.   cm.—(Contemporary perspectives in neurosurgery)
    Includes bibliographical references and index.
    1. Spinal cord—Regeneration.   2. Spinal cord—Surgery.
  I. Holtzman, Robert N.N.   II. Stein, Bennett M.
  III. Series.
    [DNLM: 1. Nerve Regeneration.   2. Spinal Cord—surgery. WL 400
  S961]
  RD594.3.S94   1991
  617.4'82059—dc20   91-4877

Printed on acid-free paper.

© 1992 Springer-Verlag New York, Inc.
Softcover reprint of the hardcover 1st edition   1992

All rights reserved. This work may not be translated or copied in whole or in part without the written permission of the publisher (Springer-Verlag New York, Inc., 175 Fifth Avenue, New York, NY 10010, USA), except for brief excerpts in connection with reviews of scholarly analysis. Use in connection with any form of information storage and retrieval, electronic adaptation, computer software, or by similar or dissimilar methodology now known or hereafter developed is forbidden.
The use of general descriptive names, trade names, trademarks, etc., in this publication, even if the former are not especially identified, is not to be taken as a sign that such names, as understood by the Trade Marks and Merchandise Marks Act, may accordingly be used freely by anyone.
While the advice and information in this book is believed to be true and accurate at the date of going to press, neither the authors nor the editors nor the publisher can accept any legal responsibility for any errors or omissions that may be made. The publisher makes no warranty, express or implied, with respect to the material contained herein.

Production managed by Martha Kürzl; manufacturing supervised by Rhea Talbert.
Typeset by Asco Trade Typesetting Ltd., Hong Kong.

9 8 7 6 5 4 3 2 1

ISBN-13:978-1-4612-7675-3   e-ISBN-13:978-1-4612-2798-4
DOI: 10.1007/978-1-4612-2798-4

This volume is dedicated to

Sidney and Filia Holtzman
for their nurturing and sense of discipline
without which this series could not have been created
—RNNH—

the memory of my parents Walter C. and Marjorie C. Stein
for their devotion and love
—BMS—

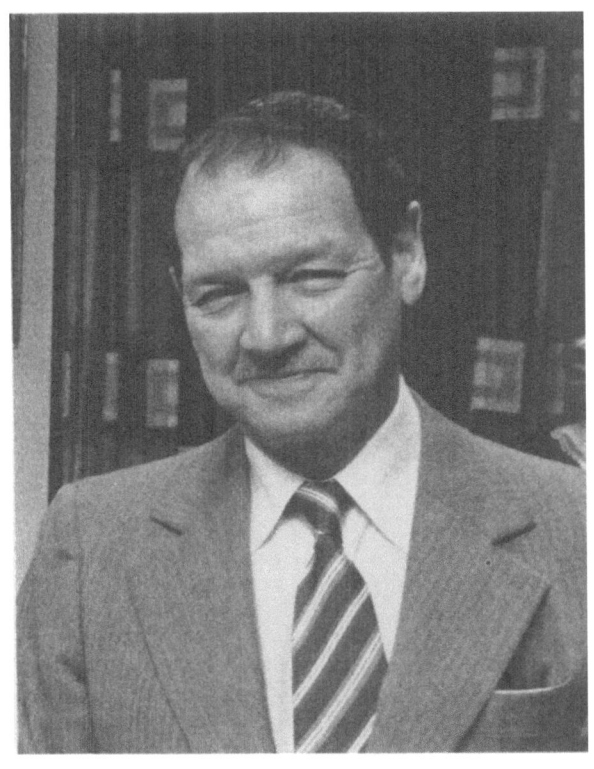

Guest of Honor:

Edward B. Schlesinger, MD
Byron Stookey Professor of Neurological Surgery Emeritus
and Former Chairman of the Department of Neurosurgery
New York Neurological Institute

Foreword

By the time of publication of this volume the Eighth Stonwin Medical Conference will have been held. Each successive year has brought together a group of scientists, physicians and surgeons who have contributed their knowledge, experience and expertise to the roundtable discussions. The resulting publications are a testimony to these stimulating and often controversial presentations and debates.

The Exchange Program consisting of Ronald H. Winston Travelling Fellows is well on its way. Both Dale M. Swift, MD and Stephen T. Onesti, MD of the Department of Neurosurgery of the New York Neurological Institute spent six weeks each in the Soviet Union and their counterparts Sergei Obukhov, MD, Shalva S. Eliava, MD, Igor Kachkov, MD and Georgii Shchekutiev of the N.N. Burdenko Neurosurgical Institute spent equivalent time here in the United States. Similarly, Luan Wenzhong, MD of the People's Hospital in Beijing was here as a Ronald H. Winston Travelling Fellow in May of 1988.

For the Stonwin Conference and the Exchange Program all of us are immensely grateful to the longstanding inspiration of Harry Winston and his wife Edna who passed on their energy and enthusiasm to their son and our great friend Ronald.

HENRY B. ROBERTS, JR.
Publishing and Editorial Consultant
Stonwin Medical Conference

Preface

In the past several years the possibility of spinal cord regeneration and concomitant recovery of neurological function has been the subject of intense scientific investigation worldwide. This renewed interest stems in part from experimental evidence that points to: 1) both the natural and exogenously enhanced survival of traumatized neurons; 2) the regeneration of axons and dendrites with collateral sprouting; 3) the unmasking of existing, but previously unrecognized pathways; 4) the *re*direction of neuronal process *re*growth by humeral growth factors modified by adhesive macromolecules and electrochemical channeling; 5) the recognition of molecules inhibiting the elongation of axons in the post-traumatic state and 6) a better understanding of the barrier to regrowth caused by gliotic scar formation.

To explore and discuss these advances a group of internationally prominent scientists, bioengineers, neurosurgeons and radiologists was assembled at the Sixth Annual Stonwin Medical Conference. It was readily apparent that the problems posed and discussed by this group continue to be among the most difficult facing clinicians and investigators alike. Recent data on spinal cord regeneration is being amassed and analyzed and the reader will recognize that some of the relevant material presented in this volume was based upon experimental data derived from studies elsewhere in the nervous system.

This text also addresses matters of the architecture, physiology and electro-chemistry which are relevant to the problem of spinal cord integrity and recovery from injury. Certainly the patterns of vascular irrigation and drainage of the segments and the dynamics of anterograde and retrograde flow as well as venous stasis represent critical areas of study. Other questions are more difficult to answer and include an understanding of the fusion of embryonic segments and the function of the central grey reticular system as concerns the function of individual segments and the spinal cord as a whole.

Recently some inroads have been made in an attempt to encourage regrowth in areas of neuronal injury. These include: 1) transplantation of fetal neuronal tissue into damaged areas; 2) the use of peripheral nerve grafts and biomechanical guidance systems such as the millipore implants coated with astrocytes; and 3) bioengineered neural networks that may in the future provide adaptive nerve splice implants and auxilliary memory devices to assist in the restoration of neurological function.

Neuroradiologists can now supply highly specific information about the gross anatomical integrity of the spinal cord using high field magnetic resonance imaging (MRI). Neuroimaging can begin to address functional anatomy with MR angiography, MR spectroscopy in addition to PET and SPECT imaging. The advent of these technologies has provided great enthusiasm, but their ability to predict spinal cord recovery or the full extent of a given injury has not yet been achieved.

Neurosurgeons continue to deal with mechanically deforming processes with steadily improving microtechnology including laser coagulation and ultrasonic aspiration for intramedullary lesions. The decompression of syringomyelic cavities and the excision of arteriovenous malformations have as well been managed with highly refined microtechnology, but the neurosurgeon's ability to predict partial or complete restoration of neurological function based upon operative findings has not yet been achieved in all instances.

It is well recognized that a spinal cord deformed by a slowly progressing mass such as a neurofibroma or meningoma may not recover its normal contour after tumor excision, yet the neurological deficits may dramatically resolve despite the post-operative radiographic appearance of focal atrophy. At the same time clinicians are encountering cases of focal and diffuse spinal cord atrophy. Some of the instances of focal atrophy due to compression are accompanied by neurological deficits which partially remit or plateau after surgical decompression. It is suspected that years later further atrophic changes occur with a progressive and irreversible neurological deterioration.

This small volume is a testimony to the pioneering investigative work that is proceeding in the face of what was considered, a decade ago, a hopeless and impossible task.

New York   ROBERT N.N. HOLTZMAN, MD
                                        BENNETT M. STEIN, MD

Acknowledgments

The Stonwin Medical Conference has taken place over the past six years with the generous help of a number of individuals whose concern with its success has taken precedence over other matters of importance. Their names are mentioned with great respect and appreciation.

Dr. Sanford P. Antin, MD consultant neuroradiologist
Mrs. Laura Boccaletti, photographer
Dr. Joseph Bossum, scientific consultant
Mrs. Ophelia Davidova, coordinator of the Exchange Program and all matters relating to the Stonwin Conference at the N.N. Burdenko Neurosurgical Institute
Mr. Alan Fields, Director of Restaurants, Harvard Club of New York
Dr. Thomas Q. Garvey III, archivist
Ms. Nancy A. McMenemy, coordinator of all matters pertaining to the Stonwin Conference through my private office
Mr. Henry B. Roberts, Jr. publishing and editorial consultant
Mrs. Evelyn Smith, coordinator of all matters pertaining to the Exchange Program and the Stonwin Conference at the Department of Neurosurgery New York Neurological Institute
Professor Lionel Tsao, Department of Chinese Studies, Hunter College, New York
Mrs. Susan Weiler, transcriber of the manuscript
Mrs. Ruth Winston, coordinator of all the travel arrangements
Leonid A. Yudin, MD PhD Deputy Rector, Sechenov Medical Academy, Moscow, USSR

Contents

Contributors

J. Lobo Antunes, MD
Professor and Chairman, Department of Neurosurgery, Universidade de Lisboa, Faculdade de Medicina, Neurocirurgia, Hospital de Santa Maria, Lisboa, 1699 Codex, Portugal

Jacqueline A. Bello, MD
Director, Division of Neuroradiology, Department of Radiology, Montefiore Medical Center, Bronx, NY 10467, USA

Zhang Cheng, MD
Professor of Neurosurgery, Director of the Neurosurgical Department, Affiliated Hospital of Shandong Medical University, Jinan, 250012, P.R. China

Wu Cheng-Yuan, MD
Associate Professor of Neurosurgery, Deputy Director of the Neurosurgical Department, Affiliated Hospital of Shandong Medical University, Jinan, 250012, P.R. China

George V. DiGiacinto, MD
Associate Attending Division of Neurosurgery, St Luke's–Roosevelt Hospital Center, New York, NY 10025, USA

S.S. Eliava, MD
Attending Neurosurgeon, N.N. Burdenko Neurosurgical Institute, AMS, Moscow 125047, USSR

Y.M. Filatov, MD
Chief of Neurosurgical Division–Vascular Pathology, N.N. Burdenko Neurosurgical Institute, AMS, Moscow 125047, USSR

EMILY D. FRIEDMAN, MD
Assistant Professor of Neurosurgery, Department of Neurosurgery, University of Pennsylvania Hospital, Philadelphia, PA 19104, USA

JAMES E.O. HUGHES, MD
Assistant Clinical Professor, College of Physicians and Surgeons of Columbia University; Associate Attending Neurosurgeon, Division of Neurosurgery, St. Luke's Roosevelt Hospital Center, New York, NY 10025, USA

ROBERT HECHT-NIELSEN, PHD
Chair of the Board, HNC Inc., San Diego, CA 92121, USA

ROBERT N.N. HOLTZMAN, MD
Assistant Clinical Professor of Neurological Surgery, College of Physicians and Surgeons of Columbia University; Adjunct Neurosurgeon, Lenox Hill Hospital, New York, NY 10021, USA

MICHEL KLIOT, MD
Assistent Professor, Department of Neurosurgery, University of Washington, Seattle VA Medical Center, Seattle, WA 98195, USA

GUY LAZORTHES, MD
Professor of Neurosurgery, Department of Neurosurgery, Rangueil Hospital, Faculty of Medicine, University of Toulouse, Toulouse, France 31052

NORMAN E. LEEDS, MD
Head, Section of Neuroradiology, The University of Texas M.D. Anderson Cancer Center, Houston TX 77030, USA

ARCADY V. LIVSHITS, MD
Professor and Chief, All-Union Center of Spinal Cord Neurosurgery and Electrostimulation of Organs, Moscow 125047, USSR

MIGUEL MARIN-PADILLA, MD
Professor of Pathology, Professor of Maternal and Child Health, Department of Pathology, Dartmouth Medical School, Hanover, New Hampshire 03756, USA

PAUL C. McCORMICK, MD
Assistant Professor of Clinical Neurological Surgery, College of Physicians and Surgeons of Columbia University; Professor of Neurosurgery, Columbia Presbyterian Medical Center, New York Neurological Institute, New York, NY 10032, USA

EDWARD H. OLDFIELD, MD
Chief, Surgical Neurology Branch NINCDS, National Institute of Health, Bethesda, MD 20892, USA

ZHANG QING-LIN, MD
Associate Professor of Neurosurgery, Affiliated Hospital of Shandong Medical University, Jinan, 250012 P.R. China

EDWARD B. SCHLESINGER, MD
Byron Stookey Professor of Neurological Surgery Emeritus, College of Physicians and Surgeons of Columbia University; Former Chairman of the Department of neurosurgery, The New York Neurological Institute, New York, NY 10032, USA

JOEL SIEGAL, MD CANDIDATE
Center of Neuroscience, Case Western Reserve University, School of Medicine, Cleveland, OH 44106, USA

JERRY SILVER, PHD
Professor, Center of Neuroscience, Case Western Reserve University, School of Medicine, Cleveland, OH 44106, USA

GEORGE M. SMITH, PHD
Professor, Center for Neuroscience, Case Western Reserve University, School of Medicine, Cleveland, OH 44106, USA

BENNETT M. STEIN, MD
Byron Stookey Professor of Neurological Surgery, College of Physicians and Surgeons of Columbia University; Chairman of the Department of Neurological Surgery, The New York Neurological Institute, New York, NY 10032, USA

NARAYAN SUNDARESAN, MD
Associate Professor of Neurosurgery, Mt. Sinai School of Medicine; Associate Attending Division of Neurosurgery, St. Luke's–Roosevelt Hospital Center; Chief of Neurosurgery, Beth Israel North Hospital, New York, NY 10128, USA

T.P. TISSEN, MD
Division of Neuroradiology, N.N. Burdenko Neurosurgical Institue, AMS, Moscow 125047, USSR

SOPHIE TYRRELL, MD/PHD CANDIDATE
Center for Neuroscience, Case Western Reserve University, School of Medicine, Cleveland, OH 44106, USA

WEN C. YANG, MD
Associate Professor of Radiology, Mt. Sinai School of Medicine, Attending Radiologist; Department of Radiology, Beth Israel Medical Center, New York, NY 10003, USA

BAO XIU-FENG, MD
Associate Professor of Neurosurgery, Affiliated Hospital of Shandong Medical University, Jinan, 250012 P.R. China

I. INTRODUCTION

A Historical Note and Perspective

Edward B. Schlesinger

From the middle of the 19th century when neurologists first became vitally interested in animal experimentation, great dissension persisted regarding the nature of the activity in the isolated segment of the spinal cord after injury in man. Experiments had revealed the major reflex phenomena that supervened in lower mammalians after transection, and it was deduced by some that similar phenomena occurred in man. In 1884, Brian Bramwell suggested as much and in 1886, Gowers, with his wonderful descriptive skill, sketched the clinical phenomena graphically. Nonetheless, when Bastian published his paper "On the Symptomatology of Total Transverse Lesions of the Spinal Cord," his influence blindly reversed the maturing doctrine. His findings unfortunately were reinforced by other men of excellent reputation, such as Bruns in Germany and Thorburn in Britain. Gordon Holmes, in his Goulstonian lectures in 1915, on "Spinal Injuries of Warfare" did not clarify the issue. It was not until George Riddoch's monumental "The Reflex Functions of the Completely Divided Spinal Cord in Man" meticulously described the changes after transection that the true course of the clinical syndrome was definitively presented. He noted in his treatise that "The clinical picture of complete cord transection alters so much at a later stage than that at which Holmes made his observations in France that many of his suggestions cannot be accepted." Riddoch's work, of course, was carried out in London at the Empire Hospital for Injuries of the Nervous System, where he had obviously observed his patients later in recovery than had Holmes. It has been said that all great progress comes from the destruction of dogmas. Riddoch effectively performed that mission!

There is little before the 20th century of more than historical interest concerning the responses of the spinal cord to injury. The studies of Adamkiewicz in 1882 and subsequently those of Kadyi in 1886 on the anatomy of its vascular supply were, however, landmarks. Yet, the unique nature of the blood supply was not fully recognized until tragic complications occurred in early attempts to occlude aneurysms of the thoracic aorta. The actual clinical course of patients sustaining irreversible cord injuries was slow to become defined. An inkling into the nature of regenerative processes has been even longer in establishing itself. For many years there continued to be sporadic reports describing functional recovery after complete severance of the spinal cord—cases in which the cord was diligently approximated and sutured. In the experimental animal, the basis of these reports is somewhat easier to comprehend. The experimenters just did not know their quadruped neurophysiology!

It would be wasteful here to take your time for a detailed historical narrative of the birth and development of our knowledge of microscopic cord structure and function. I must, however, mention Marshall Hall who, in 1841, introduced the term "spinal shock" to epitomize the transient loss of function distal to the level of transection, and Sherrington for his seminal contributions to the basic neurophysiology of the cord. His work set the stage for the modern era of knowledge concerning the nature and function of neural connections.

In 1916, sample lecture titles at the American Neurological meeting were: "The Effect of Laminectomy and Simple Exposure of the Cord Upon the Reflexes" by Dr. Pearce Bailey and Charles A. Elsberg, "A Case of Complete Division of the Spinal Cord in the Lower Dorsal Region with Conservation of Spinal Reflexes below the Level of the Lesion" by Dr. Walter F. Schaller. Even as Riddoch was carrying out his important studies in London, an unusual American neurologist with an abiding interest in spinal cord function was responding to an urge to serve the cause of liberty against German aggression. When a reserve officer training camp was organized at Plattsburgh, New York, he was among the first to attend and was commissioned a first lieutenant in the Reserve. On the declaration of war he went overseas as a major in the 314th United States infantry, and arrived in France in July, 1918, as a field officer. It was a misfortune for all of us that he died in battle on September 30th, 1918.

Why take valuable time from this gathering of experts to dwell upon this individual? First, because he has been largely unsung. An experimental worker who in the early part of the century devised a method of evaluating graded wounds to the spinal cord in experimental animals, he was the first to study reproducible injury to the mammalian spinal cord and its recovery potential. Incidentally, he actually suspected that a chemical toxic factor was responsible for some of the destructive changes that followed injury to the cord. All of his work was ignored until the renewed interest in spinal cord injury of recent decades. Alfred Reginald Allen was a remarkable individual. Born in 1876, he was a descendant of English Quakers. He attended Lehigh University and obtained his medical degree in 1898 from the University of Pennsylvania. He became a personal assistant to S. Weir Mitchell, who undoubtedly reinforced his interest in neurology. After research in pathology at Pennsylvania, he was appointed to the neurological staff. He had unique gifts as a musician and student of harmony, and was an early enthusiast in the photography of pathology specimens and of

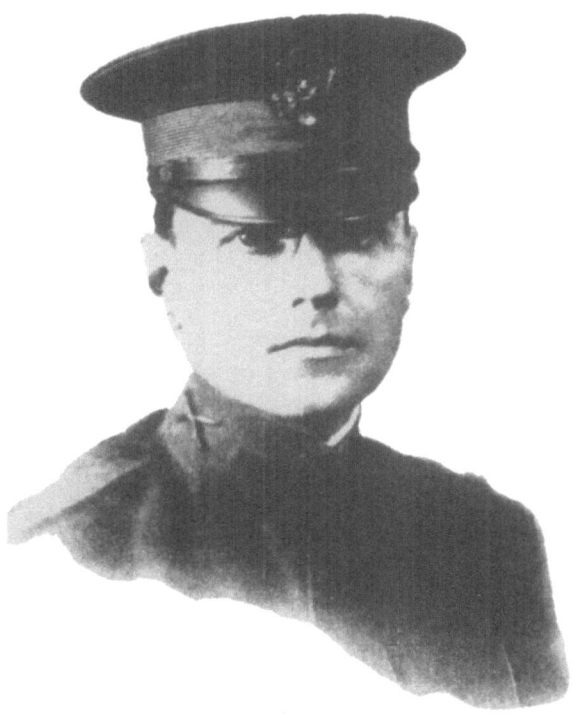

Major Alfred Reginald Allen, U.S.A.
1876–1918

photomicrographology. Some of these illustrated his landmark paper "Injuries of the Spinal Cord" in the Medical Bulletin of the University of Pennsylvania in 1908. While very young, he composed an opera and wrote many songs and even an overture. He organized the Savoy Opera Company of Philadelphia for the amateur production of Gilbert and Sullivan operas. He not only trained the cast and chorus but also conducted the orchestra. The papers of this talented individual reveal a rare combination of neurological insight and deductive skills. There is little question that if he had lived his name would be included in the pantheon of neurological greats.

The accepted dictum of Bastian was that the spinal cord injured patient, with rare exception, died with flaccid paraplegia within a year. That observation was valid, up to a point. We now know that the patient remained in spinal shock with flaccid paralysis because of his toxic infections, poor metabolic support, and anemia. However, our early record in the

Second World War was not praiseworthy, due to a continuing low level of basic knowledge and, frankly, a lack of deep interest. It was not until 1943–1944 that a combination of medical concern and political pressure led to a crash Armed Forces program in the care and study of the spinal cord injured patient. A revolutionary change in emphasis and concern, it was carried out by the medical corps in exemplary fashion. A great deal of clinical value was learned or retained after the designation of special centers and the assignment to them of appropriate personnel including psychiatrists, urologists, neurosurgeons, and internists, along with experts in rehabilitation and, most importantly, a dedicated nursing staff. It is not my purpose to go into detail in describing this effort but it deserves more attention in the literature. For present purposes it is chiefly background.

This new emphasis led to a great stir of activity, with the urologists making major contributions in the neurology of the urogenital system, the psychiatrists recognizing the importance of the individual's sense of belonging, and the physiatrists the essential need of a measure of independence to the crippled. After the war few of the pioneering groups persisted, but fortunately uniquely gifted urologists and physiatrists moved into the veterans hospitals, a repository for many injured spinal cord patients. The physical medicine community, with an abundance of enthusiasm created by high voltage personalities, held sway while most other experts drifted back into their civilian patterns. Perhaps early on the rehabilitation people carried their enthusiasm too far in neglecting a realistic evaluation of patient goals and their biological limitations but eventually came around to a more medically oriented position.

Surprisingly, the neurological and neurosurgical management of problems intrinsic to paraplegics was never a high priority for research. Attempts were made to ameliorate spasticity by physical therapy and various drugs. The drugs still available today are moderately helpful but the side effect of muscle weakness continues to be a problem. At intervals, stimulation of the muscles of ambulation by computer control to permit paraplegics to walk hits the news media with great fanfare and then drifts into its proper perspective as premature.

The management of peripheral nerve injuries is a parallel story of enormous wartime interest, rapidly disappearing in peacetime. Ripples of interest appear in the neurosurgical group with improvement in surgical technique but few breakthroughs in clinical success.

The lesson to be learned is clear. It requires the cooperation of the biochemical, biophysical, neurophysiological, and neuropathological communities to begin to unravel the complexities of regeneration. Both World Wars gave transient impetus to its study, but brought us only fractionally closer to understanding cord and root pathophysiology.

Clinical experience and neuropathological studies have taught our generation that the human spinal cord and its connections have a restricted ability to regenerate efficiently. It was felt that when partial or complete recovery of deficits occurs, either the initial injury was not anatomically complete or the organism used alternative routes or substitutes for the function of the damaged area. The damaged fibers, in spite of attempts to regenerate, obviously become enmeshed in glial scar. Decades of experimental studies demonstrated that damage to long tracts in mammals was followed by abortive and anatomically distorted regeneration. Even when regenerative capacity was somehow prolonged (Windle), functional restoration after transection never seemed to occur. The absence of the neurilemma of the peripheral nerve (a simpler model) in the central nervous system was considered an important factor militating against tract regeneration.

The critical problem for the clinician has always been when and whether to explore versus expectant or so-called conservative treatment. Guttmann, at Stoke–Mandeville, has been the most experienced and effective advocate of conservative treatment. The orthopedic community generally has looked with disfavor on the neurosurgical approach favoring extensive bony decompression, and incidentally creating subsequent complications due to instability. Many orthopedists felt that many cases would have responded better to traction and eventual stabilization. Most neurosurgeons rely on certain principles: Briefly, if the patient demonstrates a total physiological transection of the cord over significant time, with no evidence of early recovery, decompression is not considered worthwhile. If the patient has good function with progressive deterioration, decompression is entertained. With any significant impingement on the cord and evidence of residual function, operation is considered advisable. It is recognized that the cauda equina area requires different judgmental decisions from the thoracic and cervical regions. The importance of stabilization is increasingly taken into account, and this has improved rehabilitation opportunities and reduced chronic cephalad progression of cord damage. The role of acute cervical disc extrusion is recognized. The halo, anterior discectomy, and anterior stabilization have been introduced, adding to the clinical armamentarium of valid treatment measures.

Over the post-war years various modes of therapy obtained wide publicity, as in the use of hypothermia by ice water irrigation of the exposed cord over long periods of time. The practicality of such heroic treatment is obviously questionable. Osterholm's 1972 papers "Altered Norepinephrine Metabolism following Experimental Spinal Cord Injury" and "Protection Against Traumatic Spinal Cord Hemorrhagic Necrosis by Norepinephrine Synthesis Blockade with Alpha-Methyl-Tyrosine" introduced the concept of prophylactic neutralization of potential toxic factors contributing to cord damage. As biochemical research, his reports proved vulnerable. As would be anticipated, many other workers picked up the thread. All suffer the same fate as Osterholm's work, namely, conceptual importance but marginal clinical value.

It was as short a time ago as 1973 that Guttmann stated "It is not denied that regenerating nerve fibers may penetrate the glial and fibrous scar barriers under favorable conditions; it is clear that one of the tasks for future research on anatomical aspects of nerve fiber outgrowth is to attempt to ascertain more precisely what are these 'favorable conditions'". There is scant difference in our charge today but we are on somewhat firmer ground in our insights into regeneration. As I see it, there are three discrete areas to pursue. The first concerns methods of preventing progressive damage to neural structure after injury. The second relates to attempts at aborting local changes blocking the purposeful migration of axons across the zone of injury, and the third, to means of directing their growth to meaningful connections.

Growth, either developmental or regenerative, we now know is controlled by inborn genetic information and cell to cell interaction. Both are precisely programmed. The major difference between developmental growth and regenerative growth is that the former occurs spontaneously whereas the latter is induced by stimulative signals after injury or cell loss. Regeneration is thus a partial renaissance of the developmental process. Success depends on how closely the appropriate embryological environment can be restored.

If I may transport you back to a more primitive decade of neurophysiological research I would like to describe a study I did many years ago. I attempted to find an agent with a relaxant effect capable of reducing spasticity and so permit rehabilitation. Several intriguing findings linger in my memory. One is that, contrary to published reports, certain drugs capable of reducing spasticity acted differently depending on the degree of residual neural central control. For example, although Mephenesin given intravenously in 2% supersaturated solution was reported in the literature as having no effect on spasticity after complete or subtotal cord section, I found that in much higher concentrations it was effective but not toxic, as one might anticipate. The ability to wiggle a single toe almost imperceptibly made a dramatic difference in the dose response. This finding, which was reproducible, made me an early convert to the concept that there was a biochemical dimension to the environment of the isolated segment not accessible to my crude resources. Since those were the heydays of the Eccles versus Nachmanson debates regarding the electrical versus chemical signs of nerve activity, the eyes of most experimenters were on another ball. Looked at from the standpoint of the molecular biologist and physicochemist today, the isolated cord segment and its altered pharmacological responses continues to be a fruitful area of study.

The experiments of Hamburger and Levi-Montalcini eventuated in the discovery of nerve growth factor, target-derived neurotrophic substances that promote the survival of developing neurons in vivo. Their revolutionary finding opened a new universe of thinking and experimental approaches. It was inevitable that focused research efforts would turn up other control mechanisms in the central nervous system, and this has proven to be an exciting and revealing odyssey.

We have come to understand that the seemingly permanently immutable nervous system we were taught not long ago actually is undergoing constant change, with myriad cells in transitional function and in response to biochemical mediators moving purposefully in organized patterns. These newly acquired insights have directed workers into rewarding studies about the mechanisms of cell differentiation and their migrations, and to the concise role of biochemical control factors and their genetic substrata. The latter include organizers, growth factors, and even inhibitory factors. Some appear to be intrinsic and central whereas others arise in peripheral end organs in the act of fashioning their maturing requirements. Some stream directly through nervous tissues; some are delivered by the blood and perhaps other channels. This bombardment of constantly accruing information about development and regeneration in the nervous system is a never-ending delight, and radically alters our perceptions.

The complexity of the problems we contemplate today appears overwhelming. The questions to be asked are clear but the problem will consist in unraveling such mysteries as: what determines axonal growth and its eventual synaptic connection? We have a great deal to learn about the nature of the substances that direct or inhibit growth or promote cell metamorphosis into special forms with special missions. We are far from an awareness of all of the biochemical activators and their origins. Is there enough specificity in the system so that we may eventually be able to plug into the right connections in the spinal cord, after having mastered the problems of breaking through glial barriers and avoiding inappropriate synaptic connections? The slow, methodical attack on the human genome, with its mustering of many talents in many disciplines, probably is a good model for research in the regenerative processes. In any event, these and many other questions will arise in your discussion over the ensuing days. I merely desire to mention some of the problems facing you as they are postulated in the neurophysiological community.

I would like to close on a cautionary note. It has become increasingly obvious over the last decades that our resources are limited, for a multitude of reasons. Science has been forced to adopt the techniques of the advertisers and merchandisers, and the public has become more skeptical of our sallies and retreats in retailing our achievements. The legislators are quick to join in with this increasingly cynical attitude since it affords them great public exposure at little risk; a veritable shell game in view of their known personal excesses. What I am trying to say is stated much more effectively by Sladek and Schoulson in a recent review in *Science* entitled "Neural Transplantations: A Call for Patience rather than Patients." They point to successful experiments in 1985 when Parkinson's disease in monkeys, induced by neurotoxins, was treated by grafting embryonic dopamine neurons from the substantia nigra. The monkeys presumably showed major improvements in tremor, motor, freezing, and other Parkinson features. It was a model worthy of consideration. The authors point out that the expectation would have been that further experimental surgery in humans should have proceeded on the lines of the African green monkey experiments, or with the use of autologous adrenal autografts in Parkinsonian monkeys and possibly later extension of these studies to fetal cells as in the monkey studies. Instead, the enthusiasm of the Mexican group led to a headlong rush to reproduce their findings. The results have been disillusioning. The authors point out that it seems timely to reassess our values and, I would add, husband our resources. To that end, I would suggest that editors be more critical and fearless, that senior investigators devote more time as models for their neophytes, and that we all adopt a little more humility in evaluating the limits of our competence.

This essay, a truncated historical perspective of changing concepts and the direction of research in regeneration in the spinal cord, leans heavily on the literature and does not represent personal research by the author, except where noted. Among many studies that contributed to this review, H. Mei Liu's "Biology and Pathology of Nerve Growth" proved to be a major source of information and references.

II-A. BASIC SCIENCE

CHAPTER 1

Central Nervous System: Structure versus Injury and Regeneration versus Recovery

Miguel Marin-Padilla

Since classical times, the structural complexity of the mammalian central nervous system (CNS) has often been claimed to be one of the main obstacles for achieving adequate or clinically useful functional recovery after damage. The reconstruction of a CNS injured region will be aborted by failure in the reorganization of one or another of its multiple fiber–neuronal pathways and hence a complete functional recovery is unattainable. In other words, the CNS of high order animals has lost its regenerating ability, an ability otherwise retained by their peripheral nervous system. However, in recent years, the rigidity of this conception has been softened by an increasing awareness of the extraordinary plasticity of the CNS.[1–3] Recent observations indicate that some degree of rearrangement and/or remodeling at both structural and functional levels does occur normally in the CNS, particularly during late prenatal and early postnatal developments.[4] Furthermore, the process of learning new tasks implies a CNS capacity to rearrange and/or to modify its basic circuitries in response to environmental influences.[5] Therefore, CNS neurons and fibers seem to be able to rearrange the distribution of their different synaptic arrays and thereby to modify their functional activity and spatial interrelationships.

"Collateral sprouting" appears to represent one of the basic mechanisms by which the CNS is able to carry out some of the above-mentioned abilities.[6–8] When a single neuron (or a group of them) loses some of its afferent fibers, collateral sprouts from nearby preserved fibers invade the deprived area and start to occupy "vacated" synaptic sites.[9–11] The occupation of vacated synaptic sites appears to be selective and depends on critical and mutually receptive periods among the surviving neurons and fibers of the damaged region.[12] Consequently, the recovery of a lost specific function may not always be achievable after damage. On the other hand, collateral sprouting could be affected by a variety of local factors (necrosis, hemorrhages, gliosis) and be misdirected, causing anomalies in the rewiring of the damaged region. The establishment of anomalous connections among the surviving neuronal and fibrillar elements of a damaged region could result in functional dysfunctions.[13] The establishment of anomalous connections represents a form of CNS aberrant regeneration that could probably result in functional anomalies. Are postinjury local anomalous interneuronal connections able to survive, to undergo further modifications, and to influence eventually other distant regions of the CNS? These are crucial questions not yet adequately answered. The idea that some functional disturbances (mental retardation, epilepsy, dyslexia) that often follow CNS injury could reflect the presence of anomalous interneuronal connections has been inadequately explored with appropriate neurohistological techniques such as the rapid Golgi method.

Another mechanism often mentioned in the functional recovery of CNS injury is the "unmasking" of existing but unrecognized pathways.[14] It appears that in the course of CNS development many more pathways are laid down and tested than those that eventually will be used. The reactivation of such alternate pathways could explain some of the functional recovery that follows CNS injury. Further studies with appropriate methods are also needed to understand fully the location and structural organization of these unmasked pathways. A clear understanding of the basic mechanisms underlying the development of the structural and functional anomalies that often follow brain injury is indeed a great challenge to all of us, scientists and clinicians alike.

In this chapter, anomalies in the neuronal circuitry observed in some cases of encephaloclastic porencephaly will be explored using the rapid Golgi method. This type of CNS disorder includes a variety of cortical malformations (cystic formation, pial–marginal heterotopias, brain warts) believed to be caused by ischemic or vascular injuries that occur late in prenatal development when neuronal migration has either ended or is nearly completed.[15,16] The study of these cortical anomalies is of a crucial scientific and clinical importance because epilepsy and other forms of functional anomalies are common sequelae of this disorder. These cortical anomalies represent a type of structural reorganization of a prenatal brain injury. Therefore, they are a unique opportunity to study postinjury brain recovery, sprout regeneration, and the establishment of normal or anomalous connections. The scientific and clinical relevance of these types of studies cannot be overemphasized and they should be encouraged. The main focus of this chapter is to emphasize both the structural organization of the CNS and the importance of its study.

Before proceeding to the presentation of the data, it is essential to analyze the normal structural organization of the human cerebral cortex around the time of birth. It is also essential to recognize some of its basic neuronal and fiber systems and establish their spatial interrelationships. Needless to say, our present understanding of the structural organization of the human cerebral cortex (and CNS as a whole) still is rather incomplete. This lack of fundamental knowledge undoubtedly explains our poor understanding of the underlying mechanisms causing such clinical disorders as mental retardation, epilepsy, dyslexia, autism, and cerebral palsy, to mention only a few of the most prominent and less understood ones.

Furthermore, it is important to recognize that many of these clinical disorders are probably the result of CNS injury and that some form of sprouting regeneration and rewiring may be involved in their causation.

Structural Organization of the Human Cerebral Cortex

At the time of birth, the human cerebral cortex is relatively well developed and its horizontal layers (I, II, III, IV, V, VI, and VII) are all recognizable.[17] Most of its basic neuronal types, their size, location, interrelationships, and distribution can readily be studied with appropriate techniques. A mosaic reconstruction (from rapid Golgi preparations) of the cytoarchitecture of the motor cortex of a healthy newborn infant is reproduced herein (Fig. 1.1). It represents a section of the motor cortex perpendicular to the pial surface and to the long axis of the precentral gyrus. It illustrates the morphology of its basic neuronal types, their size, location, distribution, and spatial interrelationships, but not their number, which undoubtedly is much greater than reproduced in this model. The mosaic neither reproduces the distribution of the various corticipetal fibers systems (specific and nonspecific thalamic, interhemispheric or callosal, and cortico-cortical fibers) that have already arrived at the cortex by the time of birth. The addition of these fibers to the mosaic will unnecessarily complicate its structure and its comprehension will be jeopardized. All neurons of the mosaic are reproduced at the same magnification to facilitate their comparative analysis. Information of this kind is quite useful to understand better the normal architecture of the brain, and is invaluable in the study of the structural anomalies associated with neurological diseases.

The full comprehension of this mosaic is not easy even for the experienced eye, although it represents an oversimplification of the actual structural organization of the cerebral cortex. Even the simple description of its various elements and that of their interrelationships will be lengthy and much complicated and will not serve the educational purpose of this chapter. Let us use it as a basic reference to which we could come back when necessary, and consider it as a simple scheme of the cortical organization. For the purpose of this chapter, let us reduce this mosaic to only one of its basic components and explore how this particular element receives, handles, and sends neural information. Having a clear understanding even of a simple cortical neuron could significantly contribute to a better comprehension of the whole.

The Layer V Giant Pyramidal Neuron

Let us select the Betz cell—the layer V giant pyramidal neuron—of the motor cortex and analyze its structure and function. It is the most important projective neuron of the motor cortex and participates in the control

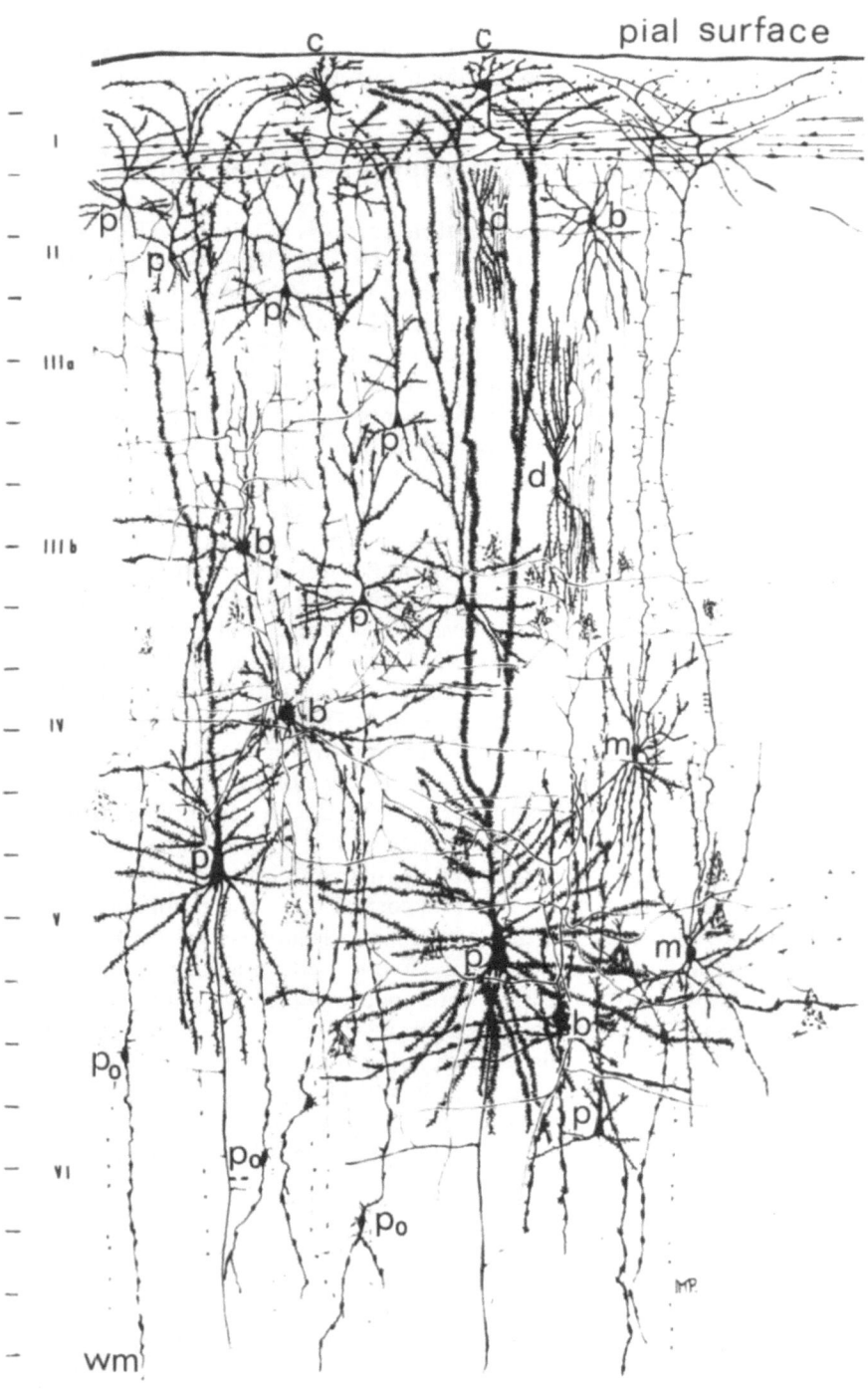

of voluntary motor activity.[19] Its prenatal development has been well studied, and it is among the first neurons of the cortical plate to achieve both structural and functional maturities.[17-19] It is the largest neuron of the cerebral cortex (Figs. 1.1–1.3). Its body is located in layer V and its apical dendrite reaches layer I where it fans out in a terminal dendritic bouquet. It has several long basal dendrites distributed almost exclusively within layers V and VI (Figs. 1.2, 1.3). It also has a few collateral dendritic branches arising at various levels of its apical dendrite. How this cortical neuron receives, handles, and sends information could be explored by analyzing its receptive surface, its associated short-circuit interneurons, and its axonic distribution, respectively.

Layer V Pyramidal Neuron Receptive Surface

Almost the entire surface of this neuron is covered by dendritic spines.[20] Each spine is a postsynaptic structure and together they constitute the most important receptive system of neural information of this neuron.[20] The number of dendritic spines per neuron ranges from 2000 to 2500, of which about one half are found in the surface of the apical dendrite. The great majority of the axospinodendritic synapses are excitatory in nature. The dendritic shaft between the spines also represents a receptive surface and the axodendritic synapses established at this level are mostly inhibitory in nature.[21]

The fact that the apical dendrite of this neuron crosses the entire thickness of cerebral cortex explains why it has received more scientific attention than any other region of the neuron.[22,23] The spine distribution along the apical dendrite of layer V pyramidal neuron (Fig. 1.2) follows a specific

◁——

Figure 1.1. Mosaic reconstruction of camera lucida drawings of the cerebral cortex of a newborn infant illustrating its basic neuronal types, their size, laminar location, distribution, and spatial relationships. The mosaic represents a section of the motor cortex (area 4) perpendicular to the pial surface and the long axis of the precentral gyrus. To facilitate their comparative analysis all neurons are reproduced at the same magnification. The different cortical laminations and a 100-μm scale are depicted at the left side of the mosaic. The following neurons are shown: pyramidal neurons (p) of layers II, IIIa, IIIb, IV, V, and VI; basket cells (b) of layers II, III, IV, and V; Martinotti cells (m) of layers IV and V; polymorphous neurons (po) of layers VI and VII; and Cajal–Retzius cells (c) of layer I. To avoid confusion none of the afferent fiber systems reaching this cortical area by the time of birth are illustrated. Camera lucida reconstructions of this type are invaluable in the study of the normal as well as the abnormal structure of the brain. Reconstructions of this type should be available from each one of the cortical regions of the human brain. Also illustrated are the pial surface and the white matter (wm) for orientation. (Modified from Marin-Padilla M. *The Rapid Golgi Method. Encyclopedia of Neurosciences.* vol I. Boston: Birkhauser Boston Inc; 1987.)

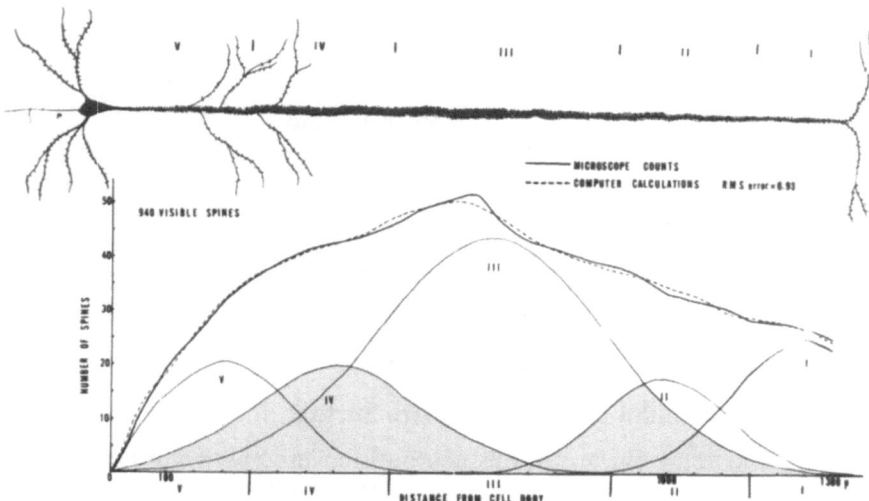

Figure 1.2. Graphic representation of the spine distribution curve along the apical dendrite of layer V pyramidal neurons of the human motor cortex. Visible spines are those located to each side of the dendrite and hence visible to microscopic observation. Those located in front or back of the dendrite are invisible for obvious reasons. The apical dendrite is divided into 50-μm segments starting at the neuronal body; the number of visible spines of each segment is recorded in the ordinate, and the distance (in micrometers) of each segment from the neuronal body in the abscissa. The apical spine distribution curve is quite characteristic and similar in many mammals. A computer analysis of it has indicated that it may be the summation of five different populations of spines, each one with a distinct distribution and cortical location. The spine distribution curve of neurons is invaluable in the study of clinical disorders as well as experimental models. (From Marin-Padilla M, et al. *Brain Res.* 1969;12:493–496, with permission.)

type of curve that is similar to all mammals studied,[22,23] including man.[20,24] This spine distribution curve reflects that of the excitatory axospinodendritic synapses through layers I to V. The computer evaluation of this curve has indicated that it could represent the summation of five different curves.[24] This model proposes the existence of five overlapping but distinct populations of spines distributed along the apical dendrite. Each population of spines, represented in the model by a distinct gaussian curve, makes synaptic contacts with a different afferent system of fibers and is associated with a distinct cortical lamination (Fig. 1.2). During the ascending maturation of the cortex, synapses are established at different levels of the apical dendrite of layer V pyramidal neurons by different afferent fiber systems. Nonspecific thalamic fibers will establish synaptic contacts preferentially with the apical dendritic segment crossing layer V; specific thalamic fibers with that crossing layer IV; callosal fibers with that crossing layer III;

cortico-cortical fibers with that crossing layer II; and, primitive corticipetal fibers with that at the level of layer I (Fig. 1.2). Hence, practically all information reaching the cerebral cortex could at one or another level (layers I, II, III, IV, and V) establish direct contact with the apical dendrite of the layer V pyramidal neuron (Fig. 1.2). Injury to any one of the afferent fiber systems reaching the cortex could result in specific synaptic and/or spine deprivation along apical dendrite of the pyramidal neuron and hence in recognizable structural anomalies. Abnormalities in the spine distribution curve along the apical dendrite of layer V pyramidal neurons have been demonstrated in some clinical chromosomal trisomies[25,26] as well as in experimental denervation studies.[27,28] Therefore, spine distribution curves provide indices that could be used in the study of cortical anomalies underlying neurological disorders. They could also be used in the study of reinnervation of vacated synaptic sites by collateral sprouting (sprouting regeneration) after CNS injury.[27]

Layer V Pyramidal Neuron Associate Short-Circuit Neurons

How the information received by the layer V pyramidal neuron is handled, selected, and eventually discharged remains poorly understood. The fact that its apical dendrite may receive more than 1000 bits of information through its dendritic spines alone represents an extraordinary amount of input that must be selectively handled. The collaboration of specific short-circuit inhibitory interneurons may be required for this task. Perhaps selective segmental dendritic inhibition and lateral cortical inhibition are roles played by the interneurons in the overall functional organization of the cerebral cortex. Four short-circuit neurons with distinct structural–functional association with layer V pyramidal neurons so far have been recognized (Fig. 1.3). They are the Martinotti cell, the Cajal double-tufted cell, the cortical basket cell, and the chandelier cell (Fig. 1.3). Each one of these associated interneurons is characterized by a specific type of axonic contact and by functional inhibition of a distinct portion of the layer V pyramidal neuron. These interneurons receive information from afferent fibers running through the level of their cortical location and therefore share the same information reaching the segment of the pyramidal neuron at the same level.

The Martinotti Cell

The Martinotti cell (Fig. 1.3M) is a stellate cell located in layer V, with spiny dendrites distributed within this lamination.[17] Afferent fibers reaching this neuron are those distributed predominantly within layer V where it is located. This neuron has an ascending axon that reaches layer I where it fans out in a way that mimics that of the terminal apical dendritic bouquet of the pyramidal neuron.[17] Its terminal axonic branches establish

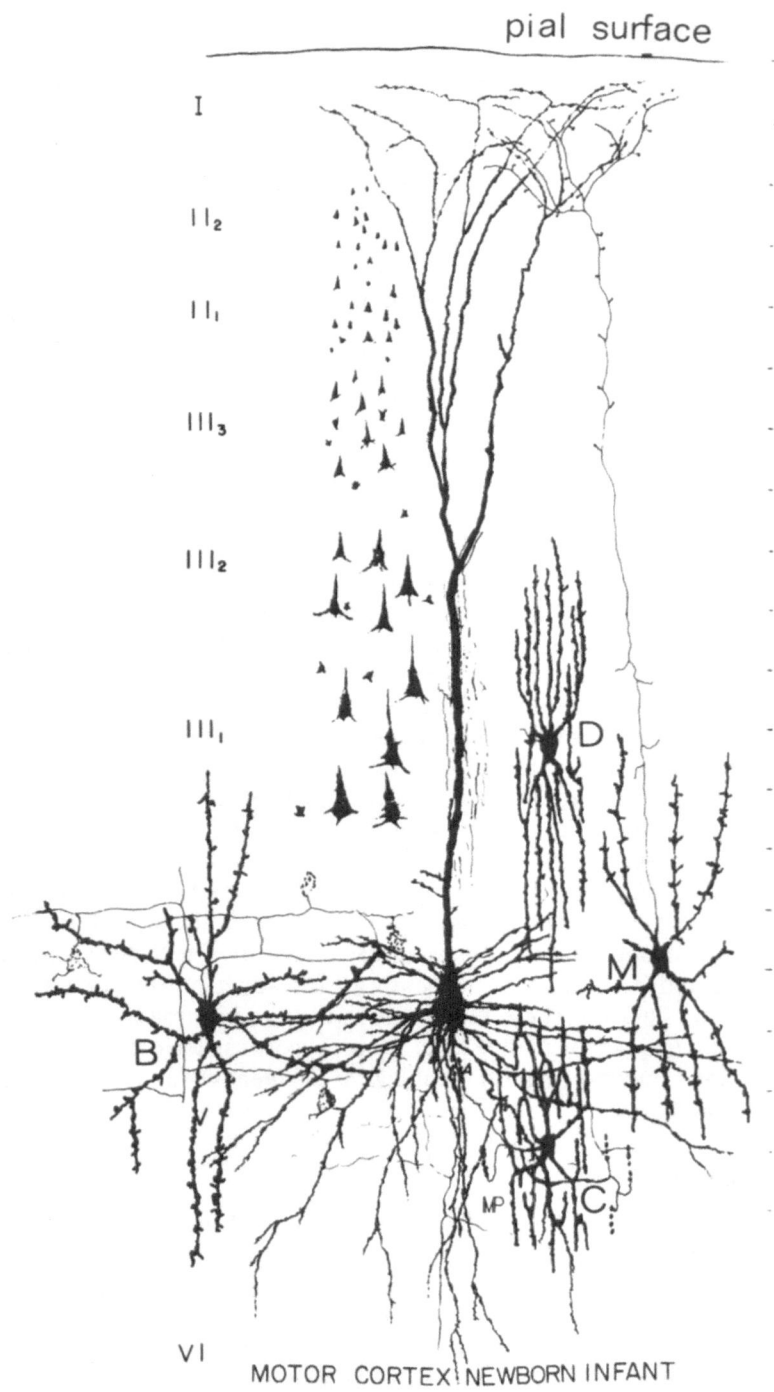

MOTOR CORTEX NEWBORN INFANT

axodendritic synapses with the terminal dendritic branches of the pyramidal neuron. These contacts are believed to be inhibitory in nature.[17] Hence, excitatory input received by the pyramidal neuron throughout the spines of its terminal apical dendritic bouquet may be handled by the Martinotti cell's axon segmental dendritic inhibition.

The Cajal Double-Tufted Cell

The Cajal double-tufted cell (Fig. 1.3D) is a fusiform neuron with ascending and descending varicose and spineless dendrites located throughout layers II and III.[29] It receives input from afferent fibers running through layers II and III, and its axonic termination is quite characteristic. It branches into several fine and quite long ascending and descending terminals that run parallel and in close proximity to the apical dendrites of the pyramidal neurons. They establish axodendritic contacts with the apical dendritic shaft of pyramidal neurons believed to be inhibitory in nature.[30] Hence, excitatory inputs received by the spines of the apical dendrite of layer V pyramidal neurons crossing layers II and III may be handled by the double-tufted cell's axon segmental dendritic inhibition.

The Cortical Basket Cell

The cortical basket cell (Fig. 1.3B) is a GABAergic stellate cell with long dendrites with few spines distributed through layers II to V.[19,31] They can be classified according to size and location into giant (layer V), large (lower layer III), medium (upper layer III), and small (layer II) neurons.[19,32] Each type receives information from afferent fibers through its cortical location. The axon of these interneurons divides into ascending and descending branches from which several long horizontal collaterals arise.

Figure 1.3. Schematic reproduction of a layer V pyramidal neuron of the human cortex with four of its associated inhibitory interneurons illustrating their structure, relative size, cortical location, distribution, and spatial interrelationships. The following neurons are illustrated: the giant pyramidal cell of layer V with its apical dendrite reaching and branching within layer I; the Martinotti cell (M) of layer V with its ascending axon (a) reaching and making contact with the terminal dendritic bouquet of the pyramidal cell; the double-tufted cell of Cajal (D) with its axon (a) distributed around the apical dendrite of the pyramidal cell and making inhibitory axodendritic contacts with it; a basket cell of layer V (B) with its axon (a) reaching and making inhibitory axosomatic (pericellular nest or basket) contact with the pyramidal cell body; and the chandelier cell (C) with its axon (a) making arrays of inhibitory axo-axonic contact ("candles") with the first portion of the pyramidal cell axon. The mutual collaboration among these neurons is essential for the normal functional activity of the pyramidal neuron. Furthermore, congenital or acquired alterations involving any of these interneurons could result in functional alterations and hence in clinical neurological disorders. Scale = 100 μm.

From these horizontal collaterals finer terminals arise that establish axo-somatic contacts with the pyramidal cell body. When several axonic terminals arrive at the same neuronal body a distinct pericellular nest or basket is formed around it. The cell received its name from these peculiar and often complex perisomatic axonic baskets.[31] These axosomatic contacts are inhibitory in nature. Each basket cell is a spatially oriented flat neuron distributed within a narrow rectangular territory that is perpendicular to the pial surface and to the long axis of the precentral gyrus. Hence, lateral and spatially oriented inhibition within the cerebral cortex may be possible through the activity of this type of interneuron.[31,32] The massive input received by a layer V pyramidal neuron could also be selectively handled by the basket cell's axon somatic inhibition.

The Chandelier Cell

The chandelier cell (Fig. 1.3C) is a relatively small GABAergic stellate interneuron with short and recurrent dendrites with few spines located predominantly through layers III, IV and V.[33,34] The axonic distribution of this neuron is its most distinctive feature from which it has received its colorful name. Its axon divides into several ascending and descending branches from which many shorter terminals arise that establish axo-axonic contacts with the first portion of the pyramidal cell's axon. These terminals (the "candles" of the chandelier) represent arrays of presynaptic boutons that embrace the pyramidal cell's axon and establish with it axo-axonic inhibitory contacts.[35] Therefore, the massive input received by the layer V pyramidal neuron could also be selectively handled by the chandelier cell's axon-specific axonic inhibition.

It should be emphasized that our knowledge concerning how the layer V pyramidal cell functions and mutually collaborates with its associated interneurons is insignificant and at best preliminary. Furthermore, some of the above statements concerning the functional roles of these inhibitory interneurons need to be studied and corroborated further. However, one can state that selective injury to any of these associated short-circuit neurons will most certainly result in layer V pyramidal cell structural as well as functional alterations and consequently in disease processes. In this context, it should be pointed out that a reduction in the number of GABAergic basket cells has been described in some types of epilepsy.[36] In addition, preliminary observations have indicated the short-circuit inhibitory neurons may be poorly developed in Down syndrome (trisomy 21).[37] The possible relationships between these observations and the type of mental retardation that characterizes this syndrome are currently under investigation.

Layer V Pyramidal Neuron Axonic Distribution

The axon of this neuron has an enormous expanse.[5] Before leaving the cortex as part of the pyramidal tract it gives off a variety of collaterals,

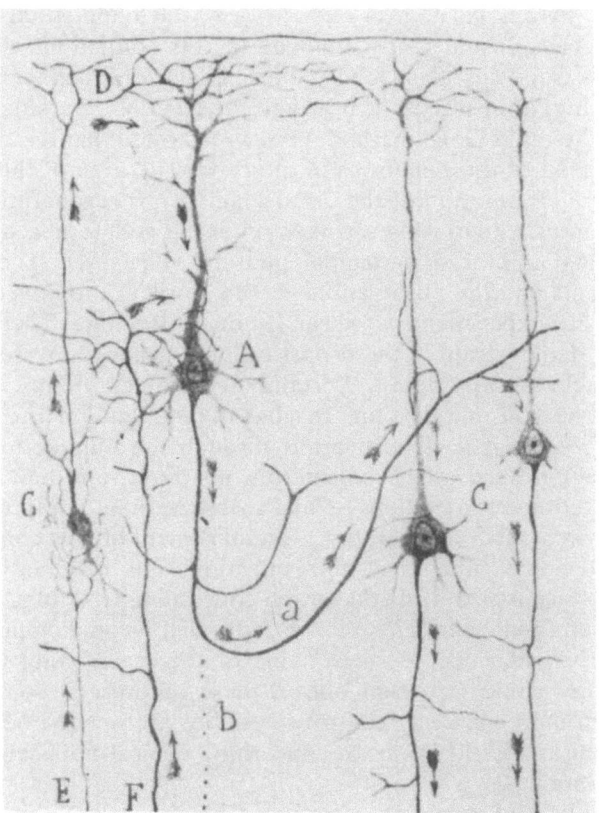

Figure 1.4. Reproduction of one of Cajal's original drawings illustrating the axonic collateral sprouting that follows a traumatic injury to the distal portion (b) of a pyramidal cell (A) axon. He pointed out that the collateral sprouts regeneration (a) could reach neighboring uninjured neurons and establish contacts with them. He further illustrates, with his now famous arrows, that the information reaching the mutilated neuron could be channeled through nearby uninjured pyramidal neurons (C) and thus the functional activity could be diverted. The mutilated pyramidal cell (A) could receive information directly from afferents (F), or indirectly at its terminal dendritic bouquet (D) through the collaboration of Martinotti cells (G). (From Cajal S Ramón y. *Degeneration and Regeneration*. London: Hafner Publishing Co; 1968, with permission.)

including short ones that are locally distributed and long ones that reach distant cortical regions and terminate within spatially oriented vertical territories.[38] As an important component of the pyramidal tract it also reaches bulbar and spinal centers. Generally speaking, injury to this tract results in a large variety of well studied clinical disorders whose description herein is beyond the scope of this chapter. Contrarily, intracortical injury to the layer V pyramidal neuron axon is less well understood and un-doubtedly has been insufficiently studied. In this context, it should be pointed out that Cajal described long ago proximal axonic collateral regen-eration (sprouting) after traumatic injury to the layer V pyramidal neuron axon.[39] Using the rapid Golgi method, he demonstrated that the traumatic section of the axon of these neurons in the cerebral cortex of the cat was followed by: a) degeneration of the distal segment, b) regeneration of its proximal collaterals, and c) what seems to represent collateral connections with neighboring uninjured pyramidal neurons (Fig. 1.4). These were acute experiments and the observations were recorded 2 to 3 weeks after injury. No chronic experiments were carried out at the time. Therefore he was unable to demonstrate if these posttraumatic changes were able to persist. Nonetheless, Cajal stated "Certainly the projection fibre is not re-paired; but the nervous impulse that reaches the mutilated neurone is not absolutely lost, since it is now diverted through the enlarged channels of the collaterals, toward other congenerous neurones, and may increase the energy of the motor reaction." Cajal's observations imply collateral sprouting (a form of CNS regeneration), establishment of new connections (rewiring), and some functional reorganization. His observations and statement introduce a powerful conception concerning CNS plasticity and imply unforeseen (and essentially unexplored) scientific and clinical possi-bilities of great significance. Perhaps some of the recent fetal CNS im-plantation studies could represent one of these unforeseen possibilities. However, much more carefully controlled studies are needed before any definitive conclusion could be made concerning clinical applicabilities of CNS transplantation.

Obviously, collateral sprouting, a form of CNS regeneration, the subse-quent establishment of new and unpredicted connections, and some func-tional reorganization seems to occur after cortical injury. These changes imply modifications of the local circuitry that in time could result in func-tional alterations. However, important and crucial questions remain to be scientifically answered. Are such acquired structural modifications able to persist? Are they able to establish functionally active contacts? Are they able to undergo further modifications? Are they the cause of eventual func-tional disorders? Are they able to influence distant neural centers? These are some among the many important questions that remain poorly under-stood and need to be answered.

Encephaloclastic Porencephaly

Encephaloclastic porencephaly, a congenital CNS disorder, is the result of an ischemic or a vascular cortical injury that occurs late in prenatal cortical development when neuronal migration is either ended or is nearly com-pleted.[15,16] At birth the affected infant shows cystic destruction of some

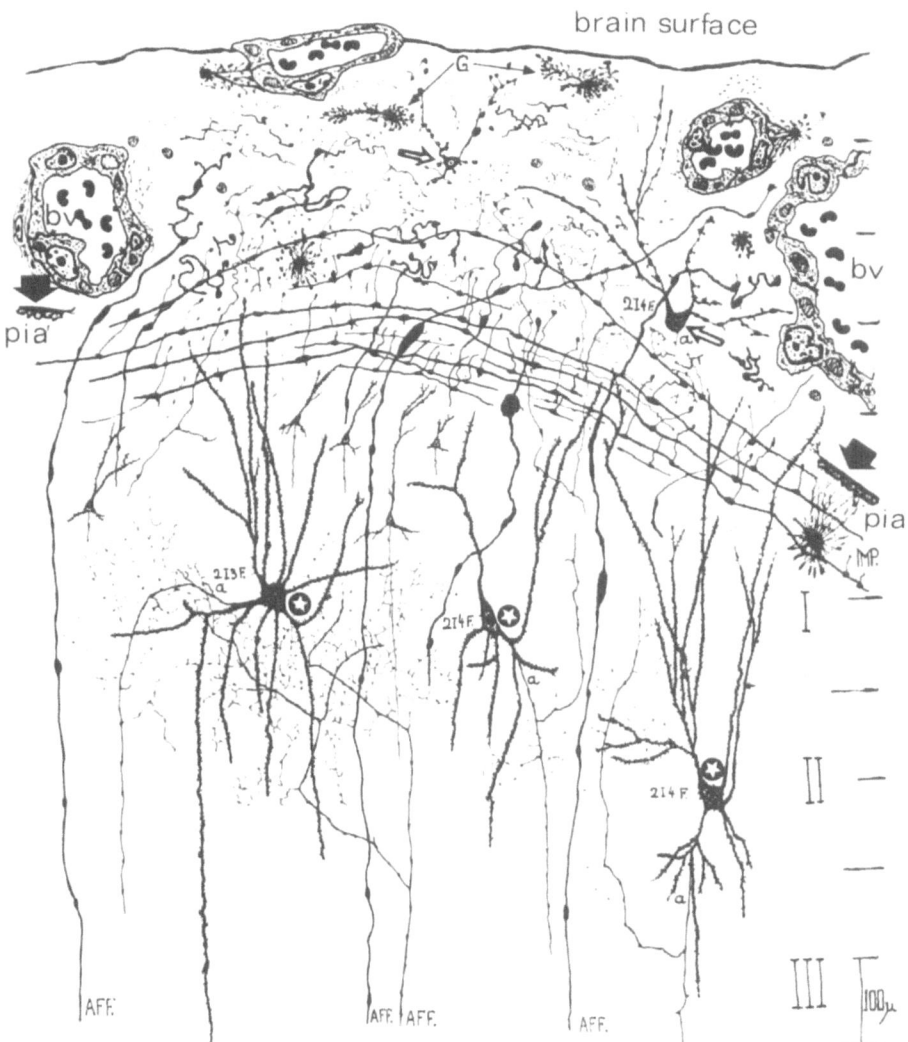

Figure 1.5. Mosaic reconstruction of camera lucida drawings of rapid Golgi preparations of a pial–marginal heterotopia overlying a cortical porencephalic cyst from a 4-week-old infant. It illustrates the destruction of the pial–external CNS basal lamina complex (between *thick arrows*), the disorganization of the components of layer I and II, the penetration of neurons (*white arrows*), fibers and glial cells (G) into the leptomeningeal space, the presence of large meganeurons (starts), and the anomalous distribution of some afferent fibers (AFF). The severe dislocation of the normal cortical architecture, the development of meganeurons, and the anomalous distribution of some afferent fibers are considered to represent acquired alterations resulting from a prenatal cortical injury. The potential of postinjury structural alterations of this type to eventually cause functional disturbances, such as epilepsy, cannot be ignored and should be evaluated further and studied with appropriate methods. Also illustrated are blood vessels (bv) within the leptomeningeal scar, the cortical layers I, II, and III, and a 100-μm scale.

25

areas of the brain alternating with unaffected ones. The cortical destruction varies significantly from case to case and could range from small to quite large cysts. Cortical pial–marginal heterotopias, meningeal glial–neuronal scars, brain warts, and anomalies of neuronal migration are commonly found in areas with cyst formation. Children with this disorder who survive often develop epilepsy and/or mental retardation. With this type of disorder nature provides us with an excellent opportunity to study (with appropriate methods) the structural recovery of the cerebral cortex after a prenatal injury. In addition, such a study could shed some light on the reason why this type of cortical damage and subsequent recovery so often results in epilepsy.

Rapid Golgi studies of the cortical pial–marginal heterotopias found in children born with this congenital disorder have shown significant structural alterations (Fig. 1.5). These alterations are considered to represent an abortive and/or aberrant type of postinjury structural recovery that shows both fiber sprout regeneration and anomalies among surviving and possible targeted neurons. Layer II of the cortex and its surroundings have been the main focus of this study. Under the heterotopic area this lamina is disorganized, it shows an abnormal amount of terminating fibers that cover a large area, and more importantly the presence of large meganeurons (Fig. 1.5). Most of these meganeurons are stellate cells that have undergone an extraordinary enlargement of the size of their soma and in the length and number of their dendrites. These modified neurons (meganeurons) have also considerably increased their receptive surface and their long dendrites are covered by numerous spines. In some Golgi preparations the numerous fiber terminals and the meganeurons share the same spatial distribution (Fig. 1.5). This could indicate a possible relationship that must be further explored. Although these are still preliminary studies, the following working hypotheses are advanced: the numerous terminating fibers found in layer II probably represent regenerating sprouts, and the meganeurons represent acquired modifications of targeted neurons. The possible structural-functional interrelationship between these two alterations is under study. Furthermore, the relationship of these alterations (especially of the meganeurons with epilepsy) is also under careful study. The presence of large neurons often has been described in this devastating convulsive disorder although their nature remains unknown.[40]

Conclusions

First, postinjury collateral sprouting as a form of CNS regeneration in high order mammals should not be ignored any longer. It must be investigated further, in both clinical and experimental settings, using appropriate techniques including the rapid Golgi method. Second, recent observations that indicate that neurons could also undergo significant modifications after

CNS injury, including dendritic and somatic enlargement with an increase in their receptive surface, should also be investigated and corroborated. Third, the survival time of the above-mentioned fibrillar and neuronal alterations must be investigated as well as the possibility of their undergoing either further structural modifications or eventual degeneration. Fourth, both the collateral sprouting and the neuronal changes could represent aberrant forms of CNS regeneration and, hence, they could be responsible for functional disorders. Fifth, the possible relationship between the fibrillar and neuronal alterations that follow CNS injury and the occurrence of clinical disorders such as epilepsy, dyslexia, and mental retardation must be explored in both clinical and experimental situations. Sixth, it should be emphasized that a basic understanding of the structure of the CNS is *a sine qua non* for understanding its normal as well as its abnormal function; and, that the CNS structure must be studied with adequate neurohistological methods capable of demonstrating its basic neuronal and fiber systems and their spatial interrelationships.

Acknowledgment. Study supported in part by the National Institute of Neurological Diseases and Stroke grant £NS-22897, NIH.

References

1. Eidelberg E, Stein DG. Functional recovery after lesions of the nervous system. *Neurosci Res Prog Bull*. 1974;12:189–303.
2. Stein DG, Rosen JJ, Butters N. *Plasticity and Recovery of Function in the Central Nervous System*. New York: Academic Press; 1974.
3. Finger S. *Recovery from Brain Damage, Research and Theory*. New York: Plenum Press; 1978.
4. Gaze RM, Keating MJ. Development and regeneration in the nervous system. *Br Med Bull*. 1974;30:105–189.
5. Brodal A. *Neurological Anatomy, in Relation to Clinical Medicine*. Oxford: Oxford University Press; 1981:38–45.
6. Liu C-N, Chambers WW. Intraspinal sprouting of dorsal root axons. *Arch Neurol Psychiatry*. 1958;79:46–61.
7. Murray M, Goldberger ME. Restitution of function and collateral sprouting in the cat spinal cord: partially hemisected animal. *J Comp Neurol*. 1974;158:19–36.
8. Illis LS. Experimental model of regeneration in the central nervous system. I. Synaptic changes. *Brain*. 1973;96:47–60.
9. Zimmer J. Long term synaptic reorganization in rat fascia dentata deafferented at adolescent and adult stages: observations with the Timm method. *Brain Res*. 1974;76:336–342.
10. Lynch GB, Stanfield B, Parks T, Cotman CW. Evidence for selected axonal growth in the dentate gyrus of the rat. *Brain Res*. 1974;69:1–11.
11. Raisman G, Field PM. A qualitative investigation of the development of collateral reinnervation after partial deafferentation of the septal nuclei. *Brain Res*. 1973;50:241–264.
12. Isaacson RL. Experimental brain lesions and memory. In: Rosenzweig, Bennet EL, eds. *Neural Mechanisms of Learning and Memory*. Cambridge, Boston: MIT Press; 1976:521–543.
13. Blacemore C. Development of functional connections in the mammalian visual system. *Br Med Bull*. 1974;30:152–156.
14. Wall PD. Mechanisms of plasticity of connections following damage to the adult mammalian nervous system. In: Bach-y-Rita P, ed. *Recovery of Function. Theoretical Considerations for Brain Injury Rehabilitation*. Huber: Bern; 1980:91–105.
15. Gross HM, Simanyi M. Porencephaly. Congenital malformations of the Brain and the Skull. In: Vinken PS, Bruyn GW, eds. *Handbook of Clinical Neurology*. Elsevier, North Holland Publ; 1977:337–361.
16. Barth PG. Disorders of neuronal migration. *Can J Neurol Sci*. 1987;14:1–16.
17. Marin-Padilla M. Prenatal and early postnatal ontogenesis of the human motor cortex. A Golgi study. I. The sequential development of the cortical layers. *Brain Res*. 1970;23:167–183.
18. Brodal A. *Neurological Anatomy in Relation to Clinical Medicine*. 3rd ed. Oxford: Oxford University Press; 1981:817–845.
19. Marin-Padilla M. Prenatal and early postnatal ontogenesis of the human motor cortex. A Golgi study. II. The Basket-Pyramidal system. *Brain Res*. 1970; 23:185–191.

20. Marin-Padilla M. Number and distribution of the apical dendritic spines of layer V pyramidal neurons in man. *J Comp Neurol.* 1967;131:475–490.
21. Somogyi P, Cowey A. Double bouquet cells. In: Peter A, Jones EG, eds. *Cerebral Cortex.* vol I. New York: Plenum Press; 1984:337–361.
22. Valverde F. Apical dendritic spines of the visual cortex and light deprivation in the mouse. *Exp. Brain Res.* 1968;3:337–352. Structural changes in the area striata of the mouse after enucleation. *Exp. Brain Res.* 1968;5:274–292.
23. Globus A, Scheibel AB. Loss of dendritic spines as an index of pre-synaptic terminal patterns. *Nature.* 1966;212:463–465.
24. Marin-Padilla M, Stibitz GR, Almy CP, Brown HN. Spine distribution of the layer V pyramidal cell in man: a cortical model. *Brain Res.* 1969;12:493–496.
25. Marin-Padilla M. Structural abnormalities of the cerebral cortex in human chromosomal aberrations. A Golgi study. *Brain Res.* 1972;44:625–629.
26. Marin-Padilla M. Structural organization of the cerebral cortex (motor area) in human chromosomal aberrations. A Golgi study. I. D (13–15) trisomy, Patau syndrome. *Brain Res.* 1974;66:375–391.
27. Valverde F, Esteban ME. Peristriate cortex of the mouse: Location and effects of enucleation. *Brain Res.* 1968;9:145–148.
28. Globus A, Scheibel AB. The effects of visual deprivation on cortical neurons. A Golgi study. *Exp Neurol.* 1967;19:331–345.
29. Cajal S Ramón y. *Histologie du Systeme Nerveux de L'Homme et des Vertebres.* Paris: Maloine; 1911:519–598.
30. Peters A, Proskaner CC, Ribak CE. Chandelier cells in the visual cortex. *J Comp Neurol.* 1982;206:397–416.
31. Marin-Padilla M. Origin of the pericellular baskets of the pyramidal cells of the human motor cortex. *Brain Res.* 1969;14:633–646.
32. Marin-Padilla M, Stibitz G. Three-dimensional reconstruction of the baskets of the human motor cortex. *Brain Res.* 1974;70:511–514.
33. Marin-Padilla M. The chandelier cell of the human visual cortex: a Golgi study. *J Comp Neurol.* 1987;256:61–70.
34. Somogyi P, Freund TF, Cowey A. The axo-axonic interneurons in the cerebral cortex of the cat, rat, and monkey. *Neuroscience.* 1982;7:2577–2607.
35. Peters A. Chandelier cells. In: Peters A, Jones EG, eds. *Cerebral Cortex.* vol. I. New York: Plenum Press; 1984:361–380.
36. Riback CE. Morphological, biochemical and immunocytochemical changes of the cortical GABAergic system in epileptic foci. In: Ward AA, Penry JK, Purpura D, eds. *Epilepsy.* New York: Raven Press; 1983:103–130.
37. Marin-Padilla M. Unpublished personal observation.
38. Feldman ML. Morphology of the neocortical pyramidal neurons. In: Peters A, Jones EG, eds. *Cerebral Cortex.* vol. I. New York: Plenum Press; 1984:123–201.
39. Cajal S Ramón y; May RM, trans. *Degeneration and Regeneration of the Nervous System.* London: Hafner Publishing Co; 1968:631–677.
40. Meldrum BS, Corsellis JAN. Epilepsy. In: Huma Adams J, Corsellis JAN, eds. *Greenfield's Neuropathology.* New York: John Wiley and Sons; 1984:921–950.

Discussion

Thalamic Interaction with the Primary Motor Cortex and the Nature of the Corticospinal Tract

Dr. Hecht-Nielsen suggested that the thalamus is responsible for the release of motor commands and that the cortex is responsible for the formulation of motor commands. Dr. Marin-Padilla agreed saying that layer IV was primarily implicated, but that interhemispheric information, such as is involved with coordination of movements of the hands will involve layer III. Thalamic output will target the pyramidal cells and the inhibitory neurons surrounding them. The corpus callosum comprises one of the "extrapyramidal" systems. The corticospinal pyramidal system descends to the centers of the brain stem, interacts with the cerebellar systems, and then proceeds into the spinal cord.

At the microscopic level we know very little about the organization of the spinal cord. The anterior horn cells have a certain similarity to the Betz cells. The problem is that the Betz cell is vertically oriented and if a proper vertical section is made the entire nerve can be visualized. In order to see the entire neuron in the spinal cord 100 or more sections are required. Dr. Holtzman inquired as to the existence of an "apical dendrite" for the anterior horn cell. Dr. Marin-Padilla responded that it is a stellate or multipolar cell that extends in all directions, making it difficult to study. It has many apical dendrites that are oriented in a complex three-dimensional arrangement. In order to reconstruct the cell, following each dendrite, hundreds of sections are required—this is a very difficult task. That is why we know so little. However, it is not simply that it is a difficult task. We all have computers that can help us with the reconstruction. The problem is to present to the computer a correct picture of the anterior horn cell derived from the thousands of sections necessary to obtain it. We need to know the definite structure before the computer can analyze it. We need a computer to read the thousands of microscopic sections.

Collateral Sprouting in Amyotrophic Lateral Sclerosis (ALS)

Dr. Oldfield inquired, given that resprouting occurs horizontally from pyramidal cells of the motor cortex, is there any evidence in amyotrophic lateral sclerosis (ALS) of longitudinal regrowth of the long fiber tracts in the spinal cord. Dr. Marin-Padilla indicated that Cajal's work demonstrating collateral sprouting was done in the newborn cat and dog. Dr. Friedman added that by inference she would believe since ALS is a disease of adulthood that there might be a considerable astrocytic response, but not much collateral sprouting.

Dr. Livshits raised the question of the projection of glial tissue as an initial event into areas of prospective regeneration after neural injury and the possible modifications of the regenerative process by various drugs.

Dr. Marin-Padilla continued . . . the point about making a lesion in the cerebral cortex remote from the gray matter: leaving the gray matter intact permits the study of regrowth and projection of axons. I do not know how to study this in the spinal cord because you must study areas remote from the level of injury or lesioning.

Dr. Oldfield inquired as to the existence of any evidence in the cortex of increased numbers of processes from degenerated pyramidal cells or adjacent residual cells in an area of damage.

Dr. Marin-Padilla said that he did not know the answer and was not certain that that had ever been studied. You will have to make a very clean lesion in a neonate and a mature dog. You will have to be extremely careful to avoid bleeding, edema, and other local problems. In the case of a cerebral infarct you may have an immediate recovery that is modified by other factors such as edema. Thereafter, a slow progression of recovery may ensue that takes years. The only way to explain the slow recovery is by sprouting in areas in which there was no permanent damage.

Dr. Kliot added that there is no doubt that different areas of the brain show different propensities for sprouting in the adult organism. For instance, in the hippocampus there is some work that shows the capacity of sprouting from local neurons and from projection neurons that are cholinergic and catecholaminergic. Dr. Marin-Padilla pointed out that enucleation of an eye in an adult has resulted in a modification of the lamination of the lateral geniculate body. Among other questions that must be answered is the question of whether local regeneration is beneficial or harmful to a functioning organism.

Collateral Sprouting in Alzheimer's Disease

Dr. Antunes mentioned a study from the group at NIH demonstrating the presence of collateral regeneration in the hippocampus in patients with Alzheimer's disease. In other words, collateral sprouting is a capability of the nervous system that is preserved even in elderly individuals.

Besides the anatomical considerations raised by Dr. Kliot, there are also phylogenetic considerations. For example, there are catacholaminergic fiber systems in all species from amphibians up to mammals with a stronger ability to regenerate and they are constant. These fibers are unmyelinated and phylogenetically old. The same phenomenon seems to occur in some neuroendocrine systems that we have studied, in particular the projections of the paraventricular and supraoptic nuclei that have a tremendous ability to regenerate. There are common features that are constant in all species from the lowest to the highest. That may represent another clue in the understanding of why some fiber systems regenerate. The only existing pathological entity where collateral regeneration has been demonstrated in man is Alzheimer's disease.

Questions Regarding the Organization of the Spinal Cord and Their Bearing as Regards Regeneration

In an effort to provoke controversy and give impetus to discussion, Dr. Holtzman raised the question of the disposition of gray matter and white matter in the spinal cord. Why should the gray matter be contained within a ring of white matter? Why do neuronal systems decussate in the spinal cord? Why is the corticospinal tract split into three parts, one crossed and two uncrossed? In order to build a structure one has to know its component parts intimately. We seem to know these structures quite well anatomically yet we are unable to rebuild these systems when they are disrupted. Furthermore, what happens to the Betz cells when the spinal cord is damaged? Do they undergo irreversible chomatolysis? What really occurs in terms of Wallerian degeneration distal to an area of injury? Can those tracts ever recover even if the damaged segment of spinal cord is repaired, bypassed, or replaced? Has the Betz cell the ability to recover and function normally again?

I wonder if any thought has been given to these questions. We have assembled here to assess the possibility of reconstructing the damaged spinal cord, but is there physiological or anatomical evidence to suggest that even if we work at the damaged segments, spend 100 years studying the structure of each segment, and artificially reproduce its function, will factors remote from that segment preclude functional recovery?

Dr. Marin-Padilla noted that studying the spinal cord of primitive animals demonstrated that portions of the cord could survive, indicating that they do not have the dependence on cortical influences that mammals have. We must inquire what is the basic nature of the spinal cord before it has been dominated by higher centers. If I were to conduct such an investigation I would try to go up the evolutionary scale, sacrificing different animals and studying the spinal connections to cortex to observe how the segments behave until a law of behavior could be established. Then I would know at which evolutionary level this law applies. But we do not have a basic organizational understanding of the spinal cord. We do not know the basic structure of the cord. White matter may surround the gray simply because it is the easiest path from an ontogenetic standpoint. Another possible explanation may be based on the fact that all neuroblasts migrate from the ependyma and they will move toward the surface in search of fiber tracts. Therefore, it is possible that the white matter is always outside the gray matter because this represents a big channel into which neuroblasts incorporate as they migrate outward from the ependyma.

As concerns the cerebral cortex, everybody says that the white matter is inside the gray. That is a misconception because when you study the cerebral cortex early in development, the white matter is also outside and the first neurons that migrate toward this original white matter and occupy it give rise to layer I. Then there is incorporation of the cortical plate with internalization of part of the white matter. In the early human embryo the first thing in the cerebral cortex is external white matter exactly like that of the spinal cord. Thereafter there is interposition of the cortical plate with internalization of the most recently added white matter, but the most primitive white matter remains outside (layer I).

Dr. Kliot added that these questions posed by Dr. Holtzman are intriguing, but at the moment you almost have to go to church to come up with an answer to some of them. I think we also have to realize that there is an enormous amount of basic research going on directed at understanding many of these issues, namely, how things form and develop. Dr. Marin-Padilla has beautifully pointed out how complex the mammalian central nervous system is and, as he has indicated, researchers are going back to study much simpler systems such as that of the grasshopper to analyze and study these basic issues. I believe everyone in this conference realizes that the answers will be slow in coming and that research at the low animal life level will be crucial.

Ethical Questions Concerning the Study of Human Fetuses

Dr. Marin-Padilla noted that we now have access to human fetuses and have observed that there is a time in development when movements of the arms and legs are present before the cortex is formed. We may ask what is the basic structure of the spinal cord at that time and how does it change during ontogeny before the formation of the cerebral cortex?

Since we have access to these fetuses we have a unique opportunity to study the different stages of spinal cord ontogeny before the complexity of that structure is such that deciphering it becomes extremely difficult. It is the use of a human child in such studies that creates an enormous ethical problem. We scientists and physicians may circumvent that if our protocol is well organized and if we can demonstrate sufficient charity and compassion for those fetuses who have died in utero. This requires close and supportive relationships with the involved families.

This communication with parents is critical because they must understand that the brain and spinal cord must be preserved immediately after the infant's death. Within 2 hours all the anatomical structures have lost their integrity and cannot be studied. Last, I do not completely agree with Dr. Kliot. To answer these questions we must ask the NIH to fund clinical studies on human fetuses—not only on the grasshopper.

Engineering and Regeneration

Dr. Hecht-Nielsen mentioned that to his knowledge there has never been a demonstration of any cellular type, whether it be a neuron or any other cell, that is incapable of regeneration to some degree. He continued, "I believe that there are instances both clinically and experimentally of Betz cell axon regeneration of some degree. No one, I think, can state explicitly what is possible, but certainly some amount of regeneration has been noted and so I think that there is definitely hope and reason to pursue these issues vigorously. Furthermore, I think it is important to realize and to remember constantly that biology is limited to what biochemistry can produce. Look at the eye. The eye is a very poor design. No engineer in the world would put the photoreceptors behind all the wiring and all the piping as the eye is built. I mean that as a design it makes little sense from the engineering standpoint; however, the chances are good that biologically it is not feasible to put the photoreceptors on the front for various mechanical and phylogenetic reasons.

In biology we often see things that appear backward and illogical from the engineering standpoint and I think the architecture of the spinal cord is one. No engineer in his right mind would put the gray matter in the center and all of the tracts around it, but there are probably very good reasons both in terms of evolutionary progression and in terms of embryological development for having it that way.

Spinal Cord Autonomy during Embryogenesis

Dr. Holtzman inquired how long in the embryo is the spinal cord autonomous from cortical control?

Dr. Marin-Padilla responded: The cortex begins to have what appear to be synapses in layers V and VI at about 15 to 16 weeks of gestation. The spinal cord is completely developed by 10 weeks of gestation with all structures present, for example, metameric segmentation, nerves, dorsal root ganglia, ventral and dorsal roots, but not necessarily the long tracts such as the pyramidal tracts conveying cortical influences. In the cerebellum climbing fibers will begin to reach the Purkinje cells at 31 weeks of gestation. There is no cerebellum to speak of before 31 weeks. Therefore, at that time many portions of the spinal cord are independent of supraspinal influences.

Dr. Holtzman then asked if an embryo at that time would develop spasticity if the spinal cord were transected? Dr. Marin-Padilla answered perhaps not. Since the cord is not dependent on supraspinal centers it is able to reorganize itself. That is my contention. Dr. Holtzman asked if there was any literature referring to spinal lesions in fetuses. Dr. Marin-Padilla responded No, but the work could probably be done in chimpanzees. A chimpanzee is the only animal that it is feasible to remove a fetus from the uterus surgically and put it back and it will continue to mature to term. Any other animal will spontaneously abort the fetus.

Dr. Kliot mentioned that Kay Kalo performed a study in which lesions were placed in rat fetuses and they survived into postnatal life. There was a point where regeneration can occur and a point at which that capacity was lost within the first week or two. Another pertinent point is the fact that interneurons that can be inhibitory are made later than some of the others. Therefore, the entire physiology of the spinal cord may be different in the embryo. It is well known that researchers have taken fetal material and performed in vitro electrophysiological studies. This was done with the visual system and synapses were demonstrated in midgestation in the cat. No one knows if spasticity will develop in a cord lesion, but there are well documented examples of regeneration occurring during development.

Dr. Friedman suggested that a suitable model to study the embryology of the central nervous system is the marsupial because this animal is born in an embryological condition. The opossum has been studied in terms of its corticospinal tract development. It is conceivable that when the animals are born, before they are in the pouch, the spinal lesions could be made and studied at successive later intervals. Dr. Marin-Padilla agreed and noted that the marsupial is a primitive animal with a relatively simple cortex and spinal cord. This would be an ideal model.

The Transplantation of Fetal Tissue

Dr. Livshitz raised the question of the validity of transplanting fetal cerebellar tissue and spinal tissue. Dr. Marin-Padilla responded that Sotelo in France has done elegant work concerning the transplantation of cerebellar tissue. He chose an animal in which, for genetic reasons, the Purkinje cells would degenerate and disappear within several months of birth, leaving the animal completely ataxic. He then transplanted fetal cerebellum from animals not so affected genetically into the abnormal cerebellum and the transplanted fetus was born without ataxia. That was an extraordinary piece of work.

The only problem that everyone faces dealing with fetal tissue transplants is how long will they last. It appears that they do not last that long. Nature takes over and destroys the cells. But, for a while one could actually identify Purkinje cells that were introduced and demonstrate that the entire cerebellum comprised Purkinje cells belonging to another species. Furthermore, climbing fibers coming from the medulla were able to establish contact with the foreign Purkinje cells.

CHAPTER 2

Reconstructive Neurosurgery: Novel Strategies Promoting the Regeneration of Injured Dorsal Root Sensory Fibers into the Adult Mammalian Spinal Cord

Michel Kliot, George M. Smith, Joel Siegal, Sophie Tyrrell, and Jerry Silver

The surgical repair of peripheral nerve injuries is possible through the ability of neurons to regenerate axons successfully within the environment of the peripheral nervous system (PNS).[1] Unfortunately in humans as well as other mammals, the mature central nervous system (CNS) demonstrates only a limited capacity for regeneration.[1] Thus, surgical attempts to reconstruct pathways within the mammalian CNS have so far met with little, if any, success.

Since the time of Cajal,[1] the failure of the adult mammalian CNS to regenerate has been attributed to a number of factors in the immediate environment of the injured axon. One factor emphasized repeatedly over the years is the formation of a mechanical barrier in the form of a glial or connective tissue scar at the site of axonal injury.[2] Another factor, identified more recently, is the presence of a molecular environment inhibitory to axonal growth. For example, molecules have been isolated from the white matter of the adult mammalian CNS that inhibit the elongation of axons.[3]

A number of different strategies have been devised to overcome these mechanical and biochemical obstacles to CNS regeneration. Segments of peripheral nerve have successfully promoted the axonal growth of CNS neurons.[4] In addition, implants coated with embryonic nerve cells have been shown to reduce scar formation and promote the growth of lesioned axons within the adult mammalian CNS.[5,6] Unfortunately, to date axonal growth beyond either the "peripheral nerve bridges" or cell-coated implants has been minimal.

We have been developing new methods of promoting central nerve regeneration using a dorsal root injury model: application of a crush injury to the central process of a dorsal root (see Methods). This model offers several distinct advantages for studying regeneration. First, the distance that regenerating fibers must traverse from the PNS to their central target, the dorsal horn, is small. Second, the amount of intervening white matter is relatively small. Third, the superficial position of the involved neural pathways facilitates their surgical manipulation. And fourth, the function of the injured and recovering dorsal root fibers can be assessed through sensory testing of the animal's behavior.

The limited capacity of adult mammalian neurons to regenerate is clearly demonstrated by injured dorsal root sensory fibers.[7-9,10] These fibers can grow successfully beyond either a crushed or cut lesion within the PNS. However, at the PNS/CNS interface [i.e., dorsal root entry zone (DREZ)], most of these regenerating axons either reverse direction and grow back toward the periphery or make stable presynapticlike endings on the reactive astrocytes within the DREZ. Although a distance of less than 1 mm separates the DREZ from the dorsal horn, only rarely do fibers penetrate the DREZ and reach the spinal gray matter.[8]

Several hypotheses have been advanced to explain the failure of sensory axons to regenerate past the DREZ to any significant extent. One explanation involves the astrocyte population within the DREZ. These astrocytes undergo reactive changes (gliosis), including hyperplasia and proliferation, in response to degenerating axons.[10] These changes are thought to establish a permanent barrier to the passage of regenerating sensory fibers.[2] An additional explanation is suggested by recent evidence demonstrating that protein components of adult myelin, made by the oligodendroglia, are a potent inhibitor of axon elongation.[3] Therefore, the white matter of the dorsal columns as well as the Tract of Lissauer may constitute additional hurdles in the path of regenerating fibers.

In striking contrast to the situation in adult mammals, the crushed dorsal root fibers of newborn rats have been shown to regenerate successfully into the spinal cord and form terminal arbors within their appropriate target regions.[11] In an attempt to restore this regenerative potential to the adult mammal, we have employed specially designed Millipore implants, coated with embryonic astrocytes, to serve as a substrate for directing regenerating dorsal root fibers to their target. This strategy arose from the recognition of the important and changing role that the astrocyte plays during development.[6] Whereas in the adult, astrocytes are a major participant in scar formation, in the embryo they have been shown to promote the growth and guidance of axonal pathways.[12] We have therefore used implants coated with embryonic astrocytes to reestablish conditions conducive to axonal growth in the adult CNS.

Methods

Anesthetized adult male and female albino rats (250–400 g) underwent bilateral laminectomies to expose the caudal part of the spinal cord and nerve roots of the cauda equina. The fifth lumbar root (L5) on one side was isolated and loosely knotted with fine suture for future identification. This root was then crushed, exerting maximal force three times for 10

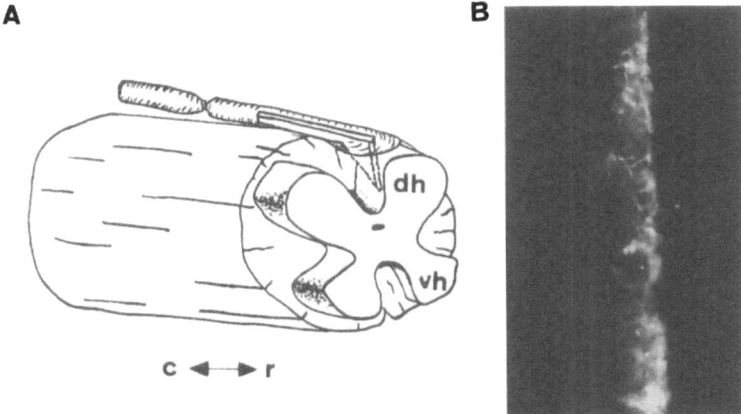

Figure 2.1. A, Schematic representation of the 5th lumbar root and spinal cord illustrating the placement of the pennant shaped implant. **B,** A fluorescent photomicrograph of a cross-section of the implant showing GFAP staining of the astrocytes coating the surface. c, caudal; r, rostral; dh, dorsal horn; vh, ventral horn.

seconds each, approximately 2 to 3 mm from its DREZ. In most animals the adjacent one or two roots rostral and caudal to the crushed root were transected and removed to prevent spurious labeling with anatomical tracer.

Animals were then divided into several experimental groups. One group (n = 6) was simply closed and allowed to recover after the nerve crush. The other groups were implanted with a Millipore structure in the shape of a pennant. As shown in Fig. 2.1A, the flag portion was inserted through the medial aspect of the L5 DREZ with the pole portion lying just medial and adjacent to the nerve root. A second group of animals (n = 4) received "naked" Millipore pennants that had not been coated with any cells. A third group (n = 26) received implants coated with a purified population of astrocytes isolated from the spinal cords of embryonic 16- or 18-day-old rat fetuses using the method described by Smith and Silver.[13] Glial fibrillary acidic protein (GFAP) staining revealed 95% purity and almost total coverage of the implant surface with astrocytes (Fig. 2.1B).

After a recovery period of 3 to 4 weeks, the animals were reanesthetized and the suture tagged L5 root reisolated. This root was cut 5 to 6 mm distal to its DREZ and a highly concentrated solution of horseradish peroxidase (HRP) was applied to its proximal end for 1 to 2 hours. After 24 hours the animals were anesthetized, perfused with fixative, and the L5 root-cord was removed en bloc and sectioned for HRP histochemistry. A control group of animals (n = 4) underwent HRP labeling of an intact L5 root.

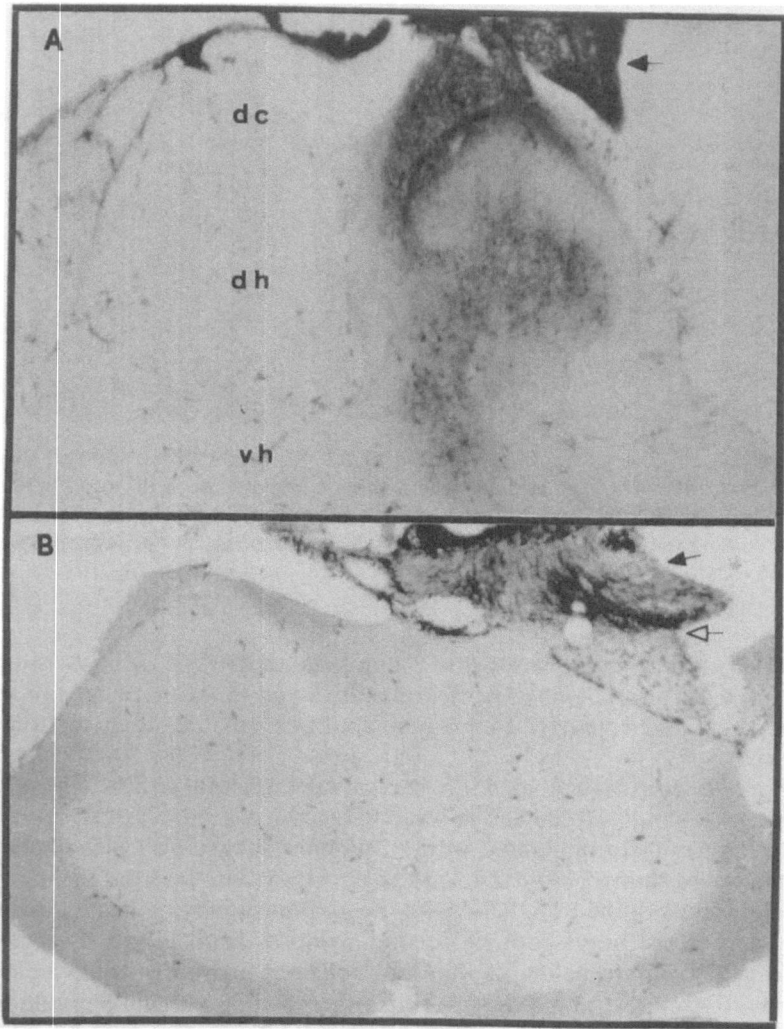

Figure 2.2. A, Pattern of HRP labeling for an intact L5 root. This photomicrograph shows darkly staining fibers in the root (*dark arrow*), dorsal columns (dc), dorsal (dh), and ventral (vh) horn. **B,** HRP labeling of a root crushed 3 weeks previously. Labeled fibers in the root (*dark arrow*) stop short of the spinal cord (*open arrow*) in a pattern suggestive of the PNS/CNS interface.

Results

The pattern of HRP labeling of an intact L5 root is illustrated in Fig. 2.2A The root is filled with darkly staining fibers that enter the spinal cord. Many of the large caliber fibers travel rostrally within the dorsal columns. Numerous fibers also densely innervate extensive portions of the dorsal horn. A smaller number of labeled fibers pass into the ventral horn and a few extend across to the contralateral side. This pattern of HRP labeling for an intact dorsal root is reproducible and similar to that shown by others.[14]

The pattern of labeling for an L5 dorsal root that was crushed 3 weeks previously is strikingly different (Fig. 2.2B). Although a substantial number of fibers regenerate past the crush site, almost all stop short of the cord surface in a pattern consistent with the boundary demarcated by peripheral and central glia.[10] Only rarely do axons penetrate beyond the DREZ, and these end superficially within the spinal cord after traveling for only a short distance. Axons with extensive terminal arbors are not found within the dorsal horn gray matter.

The insertion of an uncoated Millipore implant, in addition to crushing the L5 root, incites an injury response that varies in severity. At the very least, a moderate amount of scar tissue accumulates between Millipore and spinal cord. In some animals a severe reaction develops consisting of an intense inflammatory response surrounded by areas of recurrent hemorrhage and cavitation (Fig. 2.3A). These animals show no growth of axons past the DREZ.

Coating the implant with embryonic spinal cord astrocytes dramatically reduces the injury response. As illustrated in Figure 2.3B, the coated implant becomes well integrated with the parenchyma of the spinal cord and there is little, if any, surrounding hemorrhage and cavitation. Of great interest is the presence, in several animals, of HRP-labeled axons penetrating the spinal cord surface. In 11 out of 26 animals, labeled fibers extended into the white matter of the spinal card. In 6 out of 26 animals, labeled fibers extended into the gray matter of the spinal cord with the degree of ingrowth varying significantly. In our most successful example of regeneration, the pennant-shaped implant is positioned at the interface of dorsal columns medially and the tract of Lissauer laterally (Fig. 2.4). The flag portion of the implant actually replaces a part of the dorsal columns and the pole segment indents the surface of the cord. Camera lucida reconstruction at multiple levels reveals the vast majority of axons entering the spinal cord immediately adjacent to the Millipore implant (Fig. 2.5). Of particular interest is the finding that where fibers enter the spinal cord the tissue appears to be loosely organized and infiltrated with numerous phagocytic cells often containing yellow pigment (Fig. 2.5B). This association of a limited inflammatory response with successful fiber regeneration is a consistent finding. The resultant pattern of fiber ingrowth is different from

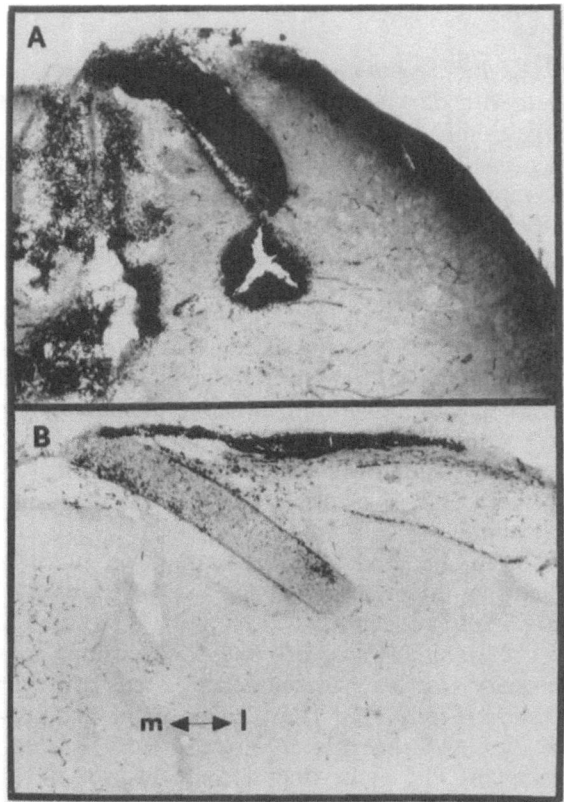

Figure 2.3. A, Cross-section of the cord in an animal with an uncoated implant. Note the surrounding regions of chronic hemorrhage and cavitation, particularly along the inferior aspect of the implant and in the dorsal columns. **B,** Cross-section through the cord of an animal with an implant coated with embryonic astrocytes. Note the markedly reduced inflammatory response and the integration of the implant with the surrounding parenchyma. m, medial; l, lateral.

that of an intact L5 root. In this particular animal, the rostrocaudal extent of fiber ingrowth is expanded and the medial–lateral extent compressed compared to the DREZ of an intact L5 root.

Fibers regenerating past the DREZ into the spinal cord can take one of several paths. As illustrated in Figure 2.6, numerous labeled fibers innervate extensive portions of the dorsal horn with normal-appearing terminals containing boutons. A separate group of fibers (*open arrow*) course laterally and superficially to the dorsal horn and end in a variety of bizarrely shaped clusters of densely packed terminal boutons (*black arrow*). Such abnormal terminals are present in only one of our animals and have not

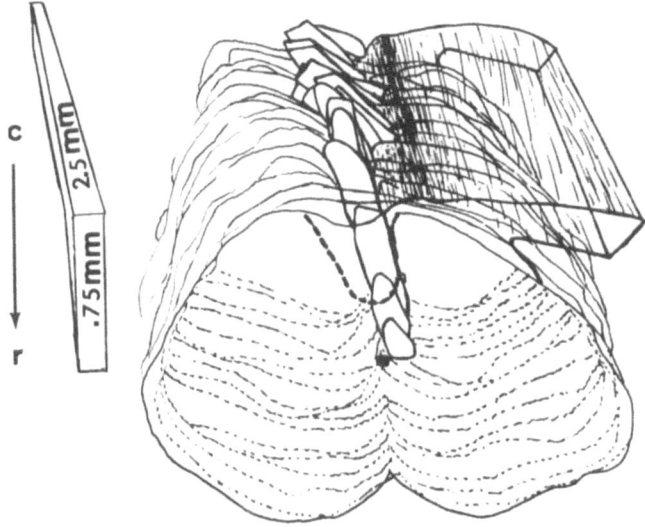

Figure 2.4. A three-dimensional camera lucida reconstruction of serial sections taken through the full extent of the spinal cord, L5 root, and implant. This reconstruction demonstrates the exact position of the implant within the cord in relation to the dorsal columns (*dashed lines*), central canal (*black dot*), and DREZ. c, caudal; r, rostral.

been identified before.[14] Other fibers enter the myelinated territory of the dorsal columns and extend only for short distances before ending in either tight spirals or sterile clubs. Finally, a small number of fibers actually grow into the Millipore implant itself (Fig. 2.7).

Discussion

Our results demonstrate that Millipore implants coated with embryonic astrocytes can reduce scar formation and, in some instances, induce the growth of lesioned adult dorsal root fibers across the DREZ into the mammalian spinal cord. Evidence that these fibers truly regenerated includes the following: a) the close association of ingrowing fibers with the implant surface that alters the normal configuration of the DREZ, b) the presence of abnormal terminal arbors not found in normal control animals, and c) the presence of fiber ingrowth directly into the implant itself. In addition, we do not think these examples of regeneration represent spared fibers surviving the crush injury for the following reasons: a) the absence of spared fibers in our control crush animals and b) the absence of labeled fibers within the dorsal columns rostral to the implant.

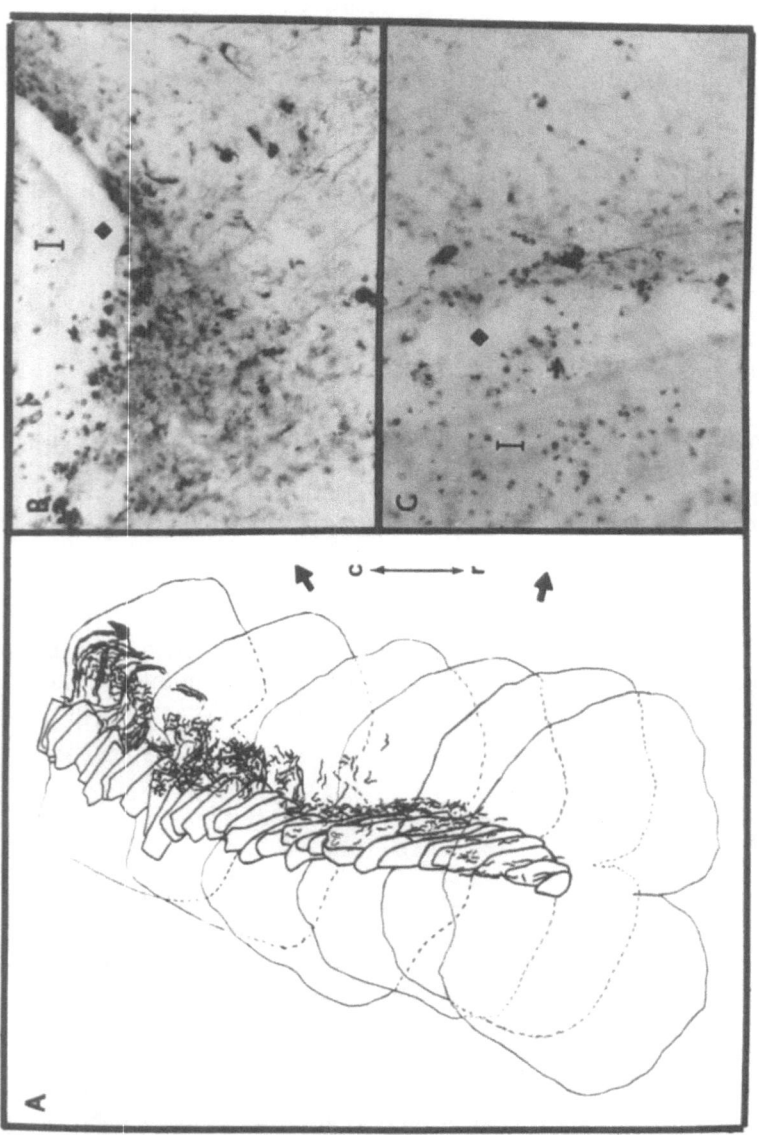

Figure 2.5. **A,** A three-dimensional camera lucida reconstruction of an animal with an embryonic astrocyte coated implant. Note the close association of ingrowing HRP-labeled fibers (*drawn in black*) with the implant surface. **B,C,** High power photomicrographs showing individual labeled axons at two levels. **B** is taken from a caudal section and **C** from a rostral section. Labeled fibers enter the cord within a narrow band of tissue immediately adjacent to the surface of the implant coated with embryonic astrocytes. Note the numerous phagocytes (*dark round cells*) present in **B**. The separation (*black diamond*) between the implant (I) and tissue is artifactual. c, caudal; r, rostral.

One of our most striking findings is the ability of regenerating fibers to form terminals within the gray matter of the adult mammalian spinal cord. These terminals possess boutons suggesting the presence of synapses. Our preliminary behavioral observations (unpublished) indicate that the regenerated root may indeed subserve sensory function. In several animals regained sensory function was reduced after transection of the root for HRP application. Although these results suggest that the boutons seen at the light level may represent functional synapses, confirmatory EM-HRP and electrophysiologic studies need to be done. Nevertheless, this remarkable capacity for reinnervation is supportive of work demonstrating ongoing as well as lesion-induced synaptic plasticity in the adult mammalian spinal cord.[15,16]

Many of the regenerated fibers form normal-appearing terminals within grossly appropriate regions of the spinal gray matter. However, a small population form unique terminal arbors with extremely abnormal morphology. The presence of aberrant terminals indicates that conditions during regeneration are not identical to those present initially during development. Potential explanations for these abnormal terminal fields include: a) a mismatch between axon and target and b) a change in the receptivity of target neurons, possibly induced by denervation.

Not all of the regenerating fibers entering the spinal cord form terminals. There are numerous examples of axons entering the dorsal column white matter and then traveling for only a short distance before ending in either a tight spiral or sterile club. These examples of abortive regeneration support the experimental results of Caroni and Schwab[3] demonstrating an inhibitory effect of adult myelin on axon elongation.

In this study there is a great deal of variability in the occurrence and extent of dorsal root regeneration. Only about 23% of the animals with embryonic astrocyte-coated implants demonstrate terminals within the gray matter of the spinal cord. There are several possible explanations for this variability. First, the condition of the astrocytes may vary considerably from animal to animal. Studies are currently underway using labeled astrocytes to correlate their viability and extent of migration with the degree of regeneration observed. Second, subtle changes in the placement of the implant could influence regeneration by varying the degree of exposure of ingrowing fibers to white and gray matter. Third, the amount of inflammation varies considerably from animal to animal. A limited inflammatory response is almost always associated with successful axon regeneration. It is therefore possible that the degree and extent of inflammation may be an important determinant of axon regeneration. Interestingly, inflammatory cells, particularly the macrophage, are known to secrete factors that can promote the growth of axons. Conceivably, embryonic astrocytes may be modulating the inflammatory response since interactions between astrocytes and cells of the immune system have been demonstrated.[17,18] Finally, Schwann cells may be participating in this intricate web of cellular interactions by serving as a potential substrate for axonal ingrowth.[19]

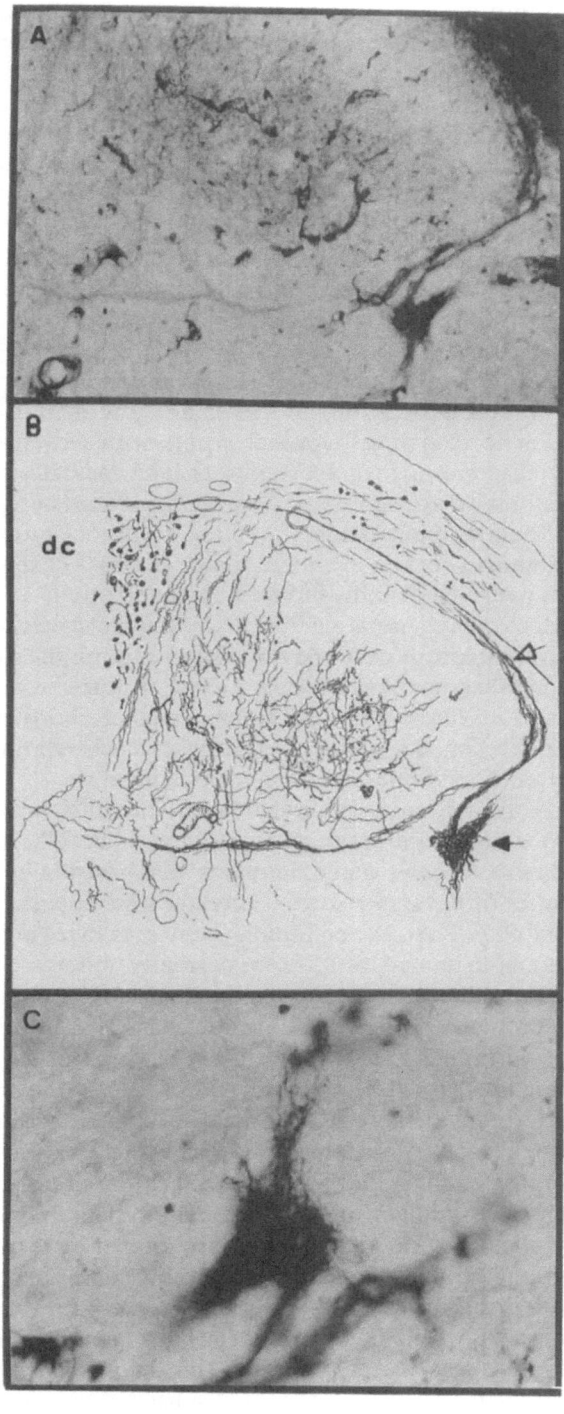

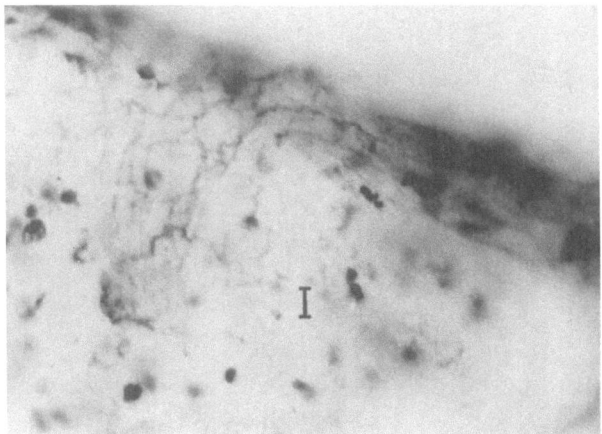

Figure 2.7. A high power photomicrograph of a fiber plexus deep within the implant (I) itself.

In summary, we have shown that under certain conditions injured dorsal root fibers can regenerate past the DREZ and form terminal arbors within the spinal gray matter of adult mammals. These results suggest that there is sufficient plasticity in the adult mammalian CNS to allow for the establishment of new synaptic connections. The association of a limited inflammatory response with examples of successful axon regeneration suggests the possibility that the adult CNS possesses a limited capacity for self-repair that is normally insufficient to give rise to axon regeneration. Our findings, however, suggest several strategies for promoting axon regeneration in the adult mammalian CNS: a) transplanting into the adult elements of the embryonic environment conducive to axon growth, b) minimizing axonal contact with the white matter, and c) modulating the inflammatory response. These results point to new approaches that may one day prove useful in the treatment of injuries to the human CNS (Fig. 2.8).

◁

Figure 2.6. A high magnification photomicrograph (**A**) and camera lucida drawing (**B**) of a single caudal section shown in Fig. 2.5A. After entering the cord, ingrowing labeled fibers take one of three courses: 1) Many fibers enter the dorsal columns (dc) medially but course only for short distances and end in sterile clubs. 2) Other fibers grow directly into the dorsal horn gray matter and form extensive terminal arbors. 3) A small group of fibers turns laterally and travels circumferentially around the dorsal horn (*open arrow*). Some of these fibers then turn medially and either arborize in the deep layers of the dorsal horn or continue on across the midline. Of particular interest are a few that end in bizarrely shaped dense clusters of terminals (*dark arrow*). **C**, Higher power photomicrograph of the abnormal terminal cluster.

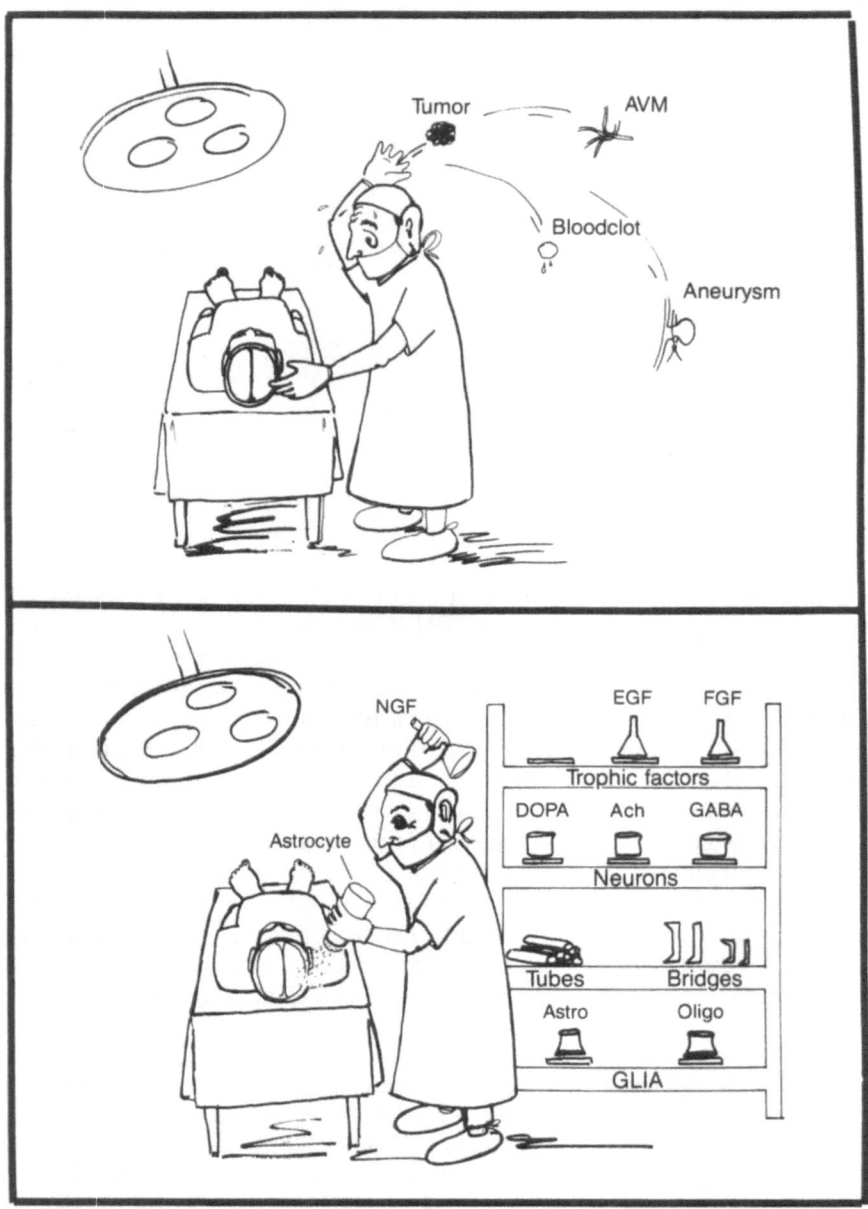

Figure 2.8. Caricature of neurosurgeon of today (*top*) and of tomorrow (*bottom*).

References

1. Cajal SRY. *Degeneration and Regeneration in the Nervous System*. New York: Haffner; 1928.
2. Reier PJ, Houle JD. The glial scar: Its bearing on axonal elongation and transplantation approaches to CNS repair. In: Waxman SG, ed. *Advances in Neurology, Vol. 47: Functional Recovery in Neurological Disease*. New York: Raven Press; 1988:87.
3. Caroni P, Schwab ME. Two membrane protein fractions from rat central myelin with inhibitory properties for neurite growth and fibroblast spreading. *J Cell Biol*. 1988;106:1281.
4. David S, Aguayo AJ. Axonal elongation into peripheral nervous system "bridges" after central nervous system injury in adult rats. *Science*. 1981;214:931.
5. Silver J, Ogawa M. Postnatally induced formation of the corpus callosum in acallosal mice on glia-coated cellulose bridges. *Science*. 1983;220:1067.
6. Smith GM, Miller RH, Silver J. Changing role of forebrain astrocytes during development, regenerative failure, and induced regeneration upon transplantation. *J Comp Neurol*. 1986;251:23.
7. Perkins S, Carlstedt T, Mizuno K, Aguayo AJ. Failure of regenerating dorsal root axons to regrow into the spinal cord. *Can J Neurol Sci*. 1980;7:323.
8. Liuzzi FJ, Lasek RJ. Some dorsal root axons regenerate into the adult rat spinal cord. An HRP study. *Soc Neurosci Abstr*. 1987;13:395.
9. Liuzzi FJ, Lasek RJ. Astrocytes block axonal regeneration in mammals by activating the physiological stop pathway. *Science*. 1987;237:642.
10. Stensaas LJ, Partlow LM, Burgess PR, Horch KW. Inhibition of regeneration: The ultrastructure of reactive astrocytes and abortive axon terminals in the transition zone of the dorsal root. In: Seil FJ, Herbert E, Carlson BM, eds. *Neural Regeneration*. Amsterdam: Elsevier; 1987:457.
11. Carlstedt T, Dalsgaard CJ, Molander C. Regrowth of lesioned dorsal root nerve fibers into the spinal cord of neonatal rats. *Neurosci Letts*. 1987;74:14.
12. Silver J, Lorenz SE, Wahlsten D, Coughlin J. Axonal guidance during development of the great cerebral commissures: Descriptive and experimental studies in vivo on the role of preformed glial pathways. *J Comp Neurol*. 1982;210:10.
13. Smith GM, Silver J. Transplantation of immature and mature astrocytes and their effect on scar formation in the lesioned CNS. *Prog Brain Res*. 1989.
14. Smith C. The development and postnatal organization of primary afferent projections to the rat thoracic spinal cord. *J Comp Neurol*. 1983;220:29.
15. Liu CN, Chambers WW. Intraspinal sprouting of dorsal root axons. *Arch Neurol Psychiat*. 1958;79:46.
16. Goldberger ME, Murray M. Lack of sprouting and its presence after lesions of the cat spinal cord. *Brain Res*. 1982;241:227.
17. Giulian D, Baker TJ. Peptides released by ameboid microglia regulate astroglial proliferation. *J Cell Biol*. 1985;101:2411.
18. Fierz W, Fontana A. The role of astrocytes in the interaction between the immune and nervous system. In: Federoff S, Vernadakis A, eds. *Astrocytes Cell Biology and Pathology of Astrocytes*. Vol 3. Orlando: Academic Press; 1986:203.
19. Richardson PM, Ebendal T. Nerve growth activities in the rat peripheral nerve. *Brain Res*. 1982;246:57.

Discussion

Sham Operation

Dr. Stein asked what happens when you do a sham operation where you insert the flag without cutting any roots or if the flag is not coated with astrocytes. Dr. Kliot responded that if you just put a flag in by itself without cutting any roots the animals get a little worse for a day or two and then recover. If you cut the roots and put the uncoated flag in they do not regain function. That outcome is more certain if you cut more than one root.

Factors Related to Technique

Dr. Bossum noted that when a nerve root is cut there is a certain amount of centrifugal pressure caused by traction on the pia that may cause axonal injury and result in the appearance of sprouting. Dr. Kliot mentioned that the nerve initially retracts and then you get the club formation and actually a dying back phenomenon occurs. This in part is due to the extrusion of axoplasm. That is why we went to the "stuffed model." We try to cut the root right at the dorsal root entry zone, but as you know it splays out. It has a more conical appearance as opposed to the human where it appears heaped up. In any event, what we do is plug it right into the site and what we are hoping is that regeneration will occur in the face of the crush injury. It has been suggested that some of our failures may be due to the fact that nerve growth will not occur through a crush and therefore it may be preferable to cut the roots.

Factors Related to Horseradish Peroxidase and Nerve Conduction Studies

Dr. McCormick mentioned that one of the problems encountered with evaluating interneuron structure in the cat when we used HRP was that it was unclear what was actually transsynaptic and what was transneuronal. Do you believe that to be a problem? And second, have you used any electrophysiologic studies, particularly compound axon potentials, to try and determine whether there is actual regeneration occurring? Dr. Kliot responded that we were not using wheat germ HRP. We do see labeled neurons. That could represent transsynaptic spread. You have to get into the next neuron's cell body and then its axon would be labeled, and occasionally we see that. However, it is more likely with the survival times we are using of 24 days and the fact that most of the time we just used HRP, not wheat germ HRP. There are neurons in the spinal cord that go out the dorsal root, so we think we are just retrogradely labeling those fibers.

The second issue you have raised is really important. As of this moment we have not obtained electrophysiological studies on our animals, but our intention is to proceed with those studies. All we have used is behavior and the leg jerk when I go back in the second time.

Dr. Livshitz asked about the potential use of subthreshold electrical stimulation in relation to regeneration. Dr. Kliot responded that I know you have used that modality extensively and I know that Dr. Taylor in Toronto has been using that device. I have seen the presentation of his work and it is very good. What they are claiming is recovery, some recovery, not regeneration. They are working on the anatomy now, but they have not demonstrated regeneration. I do not know what is actually occurring with subthreshold stimulation. Are you stimulating nerves to regenerate or reducing the impact of the injury? At NYU they have been using large magnetic fields that are speculated to reduce neuronal injury by altering the ionic fluxes of potassium and calcium. These thoughts coincide with issues brought up earlier, namely, how can we reduce injury to restore function? How can we promote sprouting and how can we promote regeneration?

Electron Microscopy

Dr. Kliot mentioned that we have a lot of tissues pending for electron microscopy. We are saving sections in an attempt to document synapses. Whether or not they are functional is impossible to say. I believe they are functional because the animals seem to regain sensation when tested. Whether this represents a local response at the segment or ascending input via the dorsal columns or spinothalamics cannot be determined.

Alteration of Glial Phenotype

Dr. Oldfield asked if anyone could give evidence that the enhancing glial cells really do change their phenotype being an enhancer to an inhibitor or are there subclones of glial cells that might be pharmacologically enhanced?

Dr. Kliot responded that the whole issue of subtypes has been best worked out in Martin Raff's work in the optic nerve systems for type I and type II. In the spinal cord it is not that well defined and I do not think it is that clear. What has been shown is that axons grow better on cultures of young astrocytes than old astrocytes, but it is only by a percentage difference of 2 to 3 times better. In studying young astrocyte cultures different cells migrate at different rates. The fastest are the macrophages. Next are the endothelial cells and young astrocytes are definitely faster than old ones. It may be that part of their utility in injury is that they can wall off and prevent some connective tissue elements from coming in, thereby preventing scar formation. Also it has been shown that there are four antibodies that stain young and not old. That is getting at the issue of phenotypy. We are using a very crude extract of astrocytes. We have been using embryonic day 16 or 17 spinal cord. We remove the dura and trypsinize the cord. Astrocytes are very sticky. You can shake off the other neurons and obtain a 95% pure population of astrocytes. Clearly it is not totally pure and perhaps it includes macrophages and other cells, including subpopulations of astrocytes.

Future Implications

Dr. Antunes asked what are the future clinical implications because this indeed is an artificial model as far as clinical situations are concerned. The only thing that approximates it is a brachial plexus avulsion injury that, as a matter of fact, we have many of in Europe associated with motorcycle accidents.

Dr. Kliot responded that I believe this is the basis of reconstructive neurosurgery that I expect will become a reality. If not the basis then perhaps a springboard to understand better regenerative processes. This work will require a more solid foundation and certainly work on primates before it can have any anticipated clinical application to situations such as nerve root avulsions.

Up until now we have been doing peripheral to central connecting. One day we would like to do central to central. There are people using Millipore coated with embryonic astrocytes in optic nerve regeneration who have shown nerve fibers growing along the Millipore tubules. However, when they reach the other end they do not do well. The key is going to be getting them to their targets. My own feeling is that there is sufficient plasticity in the targets to allow this to occur. This may take the form of growth-associated proteins that facilitate neuronal growth. These proteins result from genes that are active during specific embryonic periods and possibly may be turned on again in animals such as amphibians when neuronal injury has occurred. Abortive regeneration may imply that these genes are no longer capable of being turned on.

What I would like to do is to assay dorsal root ganglia in our system for growth associated protein to see if they are turned back on. It has been shown that they are turned on if you cut a dorsal root ganglion or a peripheral axon and they are turned off when you get peripheral regeneration. What happens with central regeneration will be interesting to know about.

Dr. Marin-Padilla remarked that when you study any nerve development, and I am presently working on the olfactory nerve, it needs the association of other cells to grow. Olfactory nerve is unusual because it is primitive and retains its primitiveness even in adults. Dr. Kliot added that it is an exception in the nervous system because it is unmyelinated. It is conceiveable that glia from olfactory nerve could provide a growth stimulus for regeneration.

CHAPTER 3

The Exuberance of Youth: Application of the Kennard Principle to Studies on Spinal Cord Plasticity

Emily D. Friedman

Dr. Holtzman asked me to discuss neuroplasticity and why the pediatric spinal cord might recover from injury better than the adult cord. Dr. Padilla has given us a beautiful introduction to the study of neuroplasticity. Neuroplasticity is the potential for adaptation by the central nervous system, based on anatomical remodeling and reorganization. Put simply, it is the ability of the central nervous system (CNS) to adapt to change. Little is known about spinal cord plasticity. The cord, because of its small size and complex bony encasement, is not accessible to study as the brain, in which nearly all of the seminal work in neuronal plasticity has been done. (Important contributions by such leaders in the field as V. Hamburger and H. Huttenlocher will be discussed later.) Since there are no studies specifically on human spinal cord plasticity, we must extrapolate from evidence gleaned from animal studies. As a pediatric neurosurgeon, it is fitting that I focus this discussion on the developing or maturing spinal cord and indeed, nearly all of the mammalian evidence for neuroplasticity is found in the neonatal period. A direct outgrowth of this research is the exploitation of fetal sources of tissue for transplantation into the CNS. This makes sense. If embryonic tissue is inherently more adaptable, then it would be the ideal transplant substrate. This will pose ethical problems; therefore cultured cell lines, perhaps genetically engineered, will be our transplant source in the future. Headlines such as the following in *American Health Magazine*: "Painful Dilemmas, Harvesting the Unborn for Brain Cell Grafts" will become moot issues.

Why is neuroplasticity worthy of our attention and study? As we enter the "Decade of the Brain," no scientific frontier is as mystifying and challenging as the CNS. It is the new *last* frontier, the new Manifest Destiny. Refinement of more sophisticated scientific techniques enables us not only to describe anatomical tracts, but also to define how they interact and how they remodel with maturity or as a result of injury or disease. This is the challenge to the clinician-investigator: to apply concepts learned from studying the plasticity of the immature CNS to the mature CNS. Stated another way, can the exuberance of youth be prolonged?

Table 3.1. Factors in plasticity.

Shift in cortical map
Disinhibition
"Conditioning lesion" effect
Lesion size
Age at injury

The Exuberance of Youth: Application of the Kennard Principle to Studies on Spinal Cord Plasticity

Margaret A. Kennard was a physiologist working at Yale University in the 1930s and 1940s. She documented the capacity for reorganization of motor function in the CNS, following cortical ablation in Brodmann's Area 4 and 6.[1] This capacity or potential for plasticity, she found to be directly related to age. Monkeys surviving cortical ablations performed during the first 6 months of life recovered voluntary motor function and exhibited less spasticity than animals operated on as older "infants," in the second year of life. The ability to reorganize motor function persisted for 2 years, or half the time to maturity in the monkey (*Macaca mulatta*). Animals operated on earlier recovered better; adult animals were left with severe paresis and spasticity. She concluded that the recovery of motor function was due to reorganization in the remaining cortex, and the greatest reorganization occurred in the first 6 months of life. Her results were summed up with the following quote: "It is better to have your brain lesion early, that is, if you can arrange it!"[3a]

Plasticity has been attributed to many different factors (Table 3.1). A shift in the cortical map has been demonstrated in experiments by Michael Merzenich, who amputated digits of monkeys and found that the somatosensory cortex representation of the missing digit shrunk, while adjacent digits' cortical representation enlarged to occupy the amputated digit's territory.[2] This was proven in adult monkeys in fact, suggesting that cortical maps are dynamically maintained and are alterable by experience even in adults.

Disinhibition may play a role in recovery after CNS lesions. If newborn animals sustain cord transection, segmental reflexes are disinhibited and permit recovery of locomotion. These animals lack subtle aspects of locomotion, however. Animals higher on the evolutionary scale have more cortical control of their spinal cord, therefore, more primitive species tolerate loss of descending input better.

A "conditioning lesion" effect has been theorized to promote neural plasticity. The CNS response to a lesion is to generate growth and trophic factors that encourage repair.[3] This is why many transplantation experiments have found greater success with first making a CNS lesion and days later, implanting graft tissue.

Lesion size is a factor, but smaller lesions are not necessarily better. In fact, large lesions during the embryonic or newborn period may mean greater total reorganization of neural pathways. Hemispherectomies in children who have far less language and motor deficits than expected attest to this fact.[4] Homotopic contralateral cortex may assume some of the functions of the missing cortex.

Age at the time of injury is a crucial factor in recovery. Young animals do recover better and faster. (This is a gratifying aspect of pediatric neurosurgery.) There is much documented evidence in the pediatric neurology literature that there exists a broad critical time period for recovery of function after loss of language-related or motor-related cortex, with greater recovery early in childhood and less recovery later.[4]

A central concept in neurobiology is that early in development there is an overproduction of neurons, dendrites, and synapses, that are eliminated during the course of development. The cell death corresponds to the time of interaction of a group of cells or "nucleus" with its target. Thereafter, response to stimuli in the surviving neurons becomes more discrete, corresponding to the pruning of axonal arbors and synapse elimination. Cajal first recognized this in spinal motor neurons. Viktor Hamburger, one of the founding fathers of neural development, showed that 50% of chick spinal motor neurons die during development.[5] If a limb bud is cut, neuronal death increases. If an additional limb bud is grafted on, fewer neurons die since they are enlisted to innervate the additional limb.

The visual system provides examples in man, as well as in other species, of plasticity early in development. It is known that uncorrected strabismus from infancy results in a loss of acuity in the nonfixating eye. This is the syndrome of *amblyopia ex anopsia*. There is functional elimination of the cortical input of one eye to avoid confusion due to the diplopia. Profound structural changes in the synaptic organization of the visual system have been documented in experimental animal models of strabismus. Innocenti studied kitten visual cortex and callosal projections during development.[6] Before the kitten has good vision, there is a callosal connection between the two visual cortices. At the time when binocular vision develops, and the axons have grown back from the chiasm through the brain stem to reach the cortex, the callosal connection retracts. When they created kittens with surgical strabismus, there was an imbalance of information received by the visual cortex and the callosal connection persisted in order to correct the visual information. This example of redundant connections with subsequent elimination in the normal situation, is an inherent principle of our CNS and contributes to the ability of the system to adapt to change. The absence of oscillopsia in patients with congenital nystagmus is another example of plasticity in the human nervous system.

Peter Huttenlocher has published on the synaptic density in human frontal and visual cortex as it changes with age.[7] Synaptic density in the infant is 50% greater than in the adult. In Area 17 of striate cortex the newborn has 2.5×10^8 synapses/mm^3. At 4 to 5 months of age when binocular vision appears, synaptogenesis increases rapidly to a high of $5.7 \times 10^8/mm^3$ by 8 mos. of age. Thus, synaptic density is maximal at a time when the visual cortex is developing sophisticated functions. Those synaptic contacts that are utilized, become stabilized and persist; those that are nonspecific regress.[8] By 11 years of age, synaptic density has fallen to adult levels, suggesting that for many years there may be significant plasticity in the cortical visual system. Neuronal density also changes with age and reflects an early overabundance, and with maturity, subsequent elimination. The 25-week fetus has more than a million neurons/mm^3 and the adult only 40,000/mm^3.[7]

Although these studies have been carried out in the neocortex, I believe they allow us to make inferences regarding human spinal cord plasticity. There should be a critical window from birth to perhaps 2 to 3 years of age during which time plasticity permits a child to recover from a spinal cord injury better than an adult.

Mammalian studies on the recovery of spinal cord function after injury suggest that the immature animal has the potential to navigate new or little-used paths within the CNS if damage occurs to the primary, preexisting pathway. The novel trajectory may pass through the CNS at completely different locations or levels, yet ultimately reach the appropriate neuronal targets. Unilateral elimination of a spinal cord tract may result in the remaining tract distributing itself bilaterally, rather than unilaterally. None of these anatomically demonstrated changes has been shown in the adult animal. Let us examine a well studied spinal tract to see if we can support the above hypothesis with data from mammalian experiments. The corticospinal tract is the best studied tract following lesions of the contralateral cortex and lesions of the cord. This "pyramidal" tract has fascinated scientists since Hippocrates (460–377 B.C.) noticed that unilateral head trauma resulted in a contralateral paralysis. Galen (131–200 A.D.) examined transected spinal cord in apes. Mistichelli noted the medullary decussation of the pyramids in 1709, and on into the 20th century the work of Horsley, Sachs, and Penfield, to name only a few, has contributed to our better understanding of the corticospinal tract. In brief, the axons arising in motor cortex (Brodman Area 4) travel through the crus cerebri of the midbrain, the ventral pons, then decussate in the medullary pyramids and segregate into two tracts in the spinal cord, the lateral corticospinal tract and the anterior corticospinal tract (CST). The pyramid refers to the ventral bulge of the CST axons in the medulla. Pyramidotomy (cutting the pyramid) has been employed in rodents to study CST plasticity.[9] In one experiment, the left pyramid (above decussation level) was cut with a fine knife in infant hamsters (day 2–20). Three months later the pyramidal tract was studied using tritiated proline to label axonal projections from the ipsilateral (i.e., left) sensorimotor cortex. The results showed no growth of axons through the cut pyramid, but instead a new growth or sprouting from the severed axons just proximal to their transection. This formed an anomalous and novel pathway not seen in the normal adult hamster; however, the pathway's termination was entirely appropriate in the dorsal column nuclei and cervical spinal cord. The new pathway decussated above the normal level, fanned out in the brain stem, and terminated in the appropriate contralateral sites. The same experiments in adult hamsters resulted in a severe retrograde degeneration of the pyramidal tract back to the midpons. No sprouting was observed. The greatest regrowth occurred if the axons were cut in the first postnatal week. Since the pyramidal decussation is well formed by day 5, labeling of late-arriving (therefore undamaged) axons was not thought to explain the novel pathway. Instead, sprouting or new growth from cut axons was attributed to the greater regenerative capacity of the immature animal. Functionally, these animals had normal gross motor control.

The plasticity of the CST has been extensively studied in the rat, where the CST travels primarily in the ventromedial dorsal funiculus.[10] A minor part of the CST travels in the lateral funiculus. The CST axons terminate unilaterally in dorsal and intermediate gray matter. Rats received a midthoracic cord "over hemisection" (right hemicord and left dorsal funiculus) at birth or at 3 weeks of age (Fig. 3.1). In the newborn rat, the CST axons are not yet at thoracic level so the cord section damages the presumptive

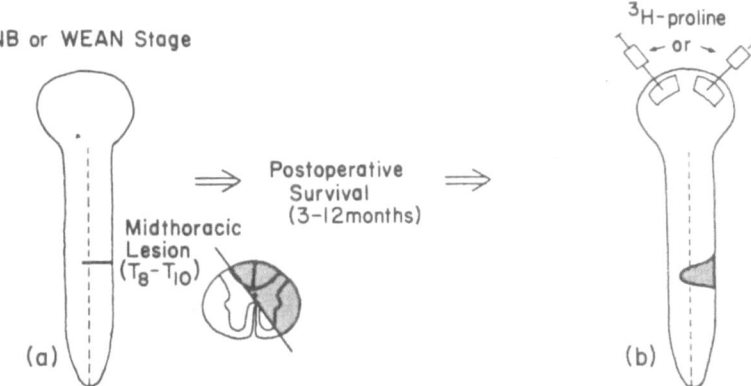

Figure 3.1. Methodologic diagram. Experiment 1. **a**, Neonatal (NB) and weanling (WEAN) stage rat pups received a midthoracic spinal cord overhemisection as illustrated in longitudinal and transverse section. After 3 to 12 months postoperative survival, (**b**) either the right or left CST in each operate group was labeled by unilateral cortical injection of ^{3}H-proline. After delay for label uptake, rats were sacrificed and the CNS tissue histologically prepared for study. (Stippled area indicates the cystic cavity formed in the chronic spinal cord lesion site.) Reprinted with permission of *J Comp Neurol*, from Bernstein DR, Stelzer DJ. Plasticity of the corticospinal tract following midthoracic spinal injury in the postnatal rat. *J Comp Neurol*. 1983;221:382–400.

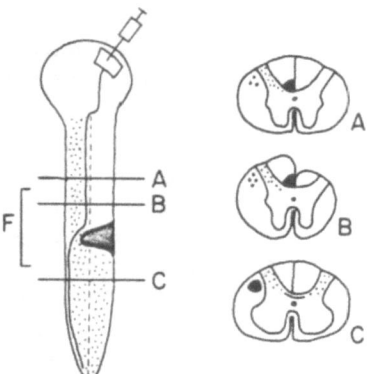

Figure 3.2. Neonatal operate. Rostral to the lesion zone, as shown in upper thoracic cord (A), the CST projection appears normal—most labeled fibers travel in the left dorsal funiculus and terminate unilaterally in the left dorsal and intermediate gray matter. Within 1.5 mm of the lesion site, labeled left CST axons begin to leave the left dorsal funiculus and traverse the left dorsal gray matter to continue their course in the left lateral funiculus. Caudal to the lesion zone, few fibers travel in the appropriate dorsal funiculus but remain in the left lateral funiculus and project to correct CST termination sites bilaterally (C) reaching the right hemicord recrossing the midline in the central gray dorsal to the central canal (C). Reprinted with permission of *J Comp Neurol*, from Bernstein DR, Stelzer DJ. Plasticity of the corticospinal tract following midthoracic spinal injury in the postnatal rat. *J Comp Neurol.* 1983;221:382–400.

cord pathways. In the 3-week-old rat, the injury severs the majority of CST axons.

In the newborn, it was found that the CST axons of the damaged (right) side failed to grow through the lesion but the left CST axons bypassed the left dorsal funiculus lesion by displacement into the lateral funiculus (Fig. 3.2C). The majority of the tract then was rerouted from the dorsal to the lateral funiculus. These axons crossed to terminate contralaterally as well as ipsilaterally in the caudal cord. Three-week operates showed no rerouting, but only minimal sprouting from the few undamaged CST axons. In a second experiment, the right sensorimotor cortex was ablated along with the right cord over hemisection (therefore the left CST input was eliminated along with a right cord section) (Fig. 3.3). In newborns, this resulted in an aberrant pathway for the right-sided CST. This tract grew around the spinal injury into the left lateral funiculus via an abnormally enlarged central gray trajectory, and terminated bilaterally. Two-week-old operates failed to show this rerouted path. The investigators concluded: a) most developing CST axons, were unable to grow through the lesion, but b) the remaining CST axons, ipsilateral or contralateral, could bypass the lesion and terminate bilaterally (i.e., increase their distribution). If any intact

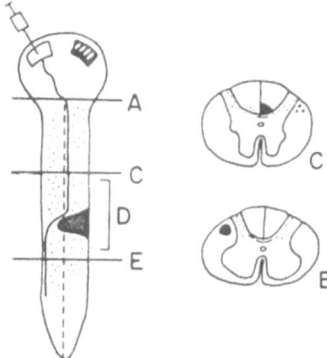

Figure 3.3. Neonatal double lesion operate. Rostral to the injury, right CST axons are located in the right dorsal funiculus and terminate bilaterally (C). At the lesion site, right CST axons pass into the left lateral funiculus where they remain throughout the caudal cord. Reprinted with permission of *J Comp Neurol*, from Bernstein DR, Stelzer DJ. Plasticity of the corticospinal tract following midthoracic spinal injury in the postnatal rat. *J Comp Neurol.* 1983;221:382–400.

spinal cord remained, neonatal CST axons could negotiate a new pathway or shift to an alternative potential pathway. By 2 weeks of age when CST axons were forming synapses, this rerouting was no longer possible.

Barbara Bregman and Michael Goldberger coined the phrase "infant lesion effect"[6,20] to explain the difference in motor function after injury to the neonate versus the adult. They examined locomotion, placing responses of the limb, and contact placing (a postural limb extension reflex elicited by delicate stimuli such as light skin touch or hair displacement). Cord transection in the adult cat results in initial plegia but recovery of gross movement in the fourth to fifth week.[12] Placing responses are poorly executed, require high thresholds to elicit, and provide little weight support. Contact placing is completely abolished in the adult operates. By contrast, if newborn kittens undergo cord transection they recover good placing responses elicited by nearly normal threshold stimuli (Fig. 3.4). Contact placing is also spared. Treadmill-elicited locomotion also recovers to near normal in newborn operates versus adult operates. They attribute this "infant lesion effect" to two factors: a) late-developing CST axons may take an aberrant course around a spinal lesion and redistribute themselves in novel terminations and b) neonatal transection may interfere with the development of normal spinal inhibitory systems, thereby enhancing spinal reflex pathways and autonomous function.[22] (Table 3.2)

Neuroscientists have applied this "adaptability" of immature neural tissue to animal transplantation experiments. Transplants of fetal CNS tissue have shown positive results in neurodegenerative disorders such as Parkin-

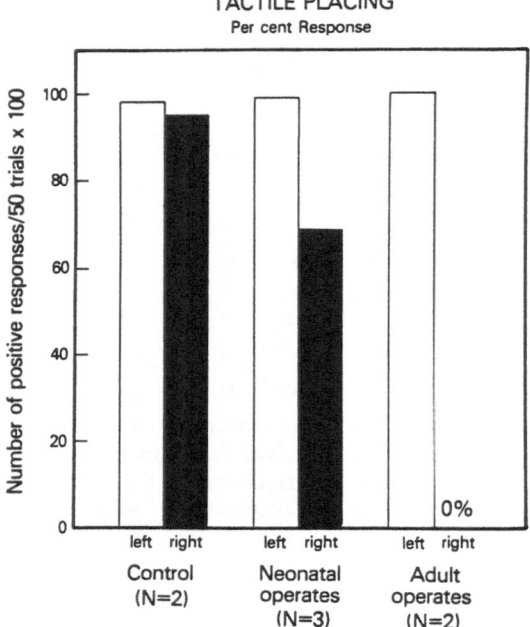

Figure 3.4. Sparing of contact placing after neonatal hemisection is shown by the response frequency of contact placing elicited by a standard stimulus. In normal cats both hindlimbs place in almost all trials. Hemisection in adult operates abolished contact placing permanently in the right hindlimb ipsilateral to the lesion. In neonatal operates, tested as adults, sparing is seen in that the response is not eliminated on the side of the lesion. Reprinted with permission of Humana Press. From Goldberger ME. Mechanisms contributing to sparing of function following neonatal damage to spinal pathways. *Neurochem Pathol.* 1986;5:289–307.

Table 3.2. Mammalian studies.

Injury	Sprouting	Novel path
Pyramidotomy	++	Contralateral
Hemisection		
Rat	+	Contralateral
		Through gray matter
		Bilateral termination
Cat	+	Contralateral
		Through gray matter
Transection		
Cat	+/−	? decreased inhibition

son's disease, in demyelinating disease, and in spinal cord injury. Bernstein and Goldberg report[13] an amelioration of expected limb weakness when a cervical dorsal spinal cord transection is followed by a transplant of fetal spinal cord into the injury site. Even when the host animal is adult, a fetal transplant encourages better recovery from a cord injury. The lesioned animals without transplants had a continued deterioration in motor skills until sacrifice. Lesion plus transplant animals performed consistently better. These results have been attributed to trophic factors secreted by embryonic glia and neurons. However, differences in cellular metabolism or in composition of extracellular matrix substances in fetal versus adult neural tissue may be important. The migratory ability of embryonic versus adult glia is a new area of investigation that may also shed light on the greater "adaptability" of the immature CNS. Molecular neurobiology, as it explores programing differences in the fetal and adult genetic sequence, may help reveal why fetal CNS can tolerate manipulation better than adult CNS. We can look forward to much innovative research in these new areas.

Spinal cord transplantation experiments have been done using neuronal grafts, astroglial grafts, and oligodendroglial grafts. At the Neurological Institute I have been studying oligodendrocyte transplants using a mouse mutant. The shiverer mouse has a gene deletion for the coding sequence of myelin basic protein (MBP), a major CNS myelin component. This protein plays a vital role in formation of the myelin sheath and its compaction. The CNS of these animals shows patchy, noncontinuous myelin that forms irregular loops, is noncompacted, and lacks MBP. The animals manifest a tremor, seizures, and die prematurely. We have taken oligodendrocytes from normal mice (fetal ages to adult) and implanted shiverer mice with these grafts. With no immunosuppression required, the grafts survive, the cells mature and express cell-specific proteins in a correct developmental sequence, and the cells myelinate shiverer axons (Fig. 3.5).[14] It appears the implanted cells migrate out of the graft into the host white matter tracts to myelinate. The new myelin is not random, but is strictly oriented along host commissures. Our technique uses an antibody to MBP so it is strikingly apparent where graft versus host myelin is located. Some of the new MBP-positive myelin is at a distance from the graft, and whether this is due to migration of implanted oligodendrocytes (or their precursors) or cerebrospinal fluid (CSF) dissemination of cells at the time of surgery is unknown. Fetal oligodendrocytes resulted in a much greater degree of myelination than postnatal or adult oligodendrocytes. Currently we are investigating transplants of genetically altered oligodendrocyte precursor cells.

In the fall of 1987 I had the opportunity to work in two European laboratories studying CNS glia. At the Salpetrière in Paris, with Madeleine Gumpel, we transplanted Schwann cells into shiverer spinal cord. The Schwann cells myelinated the cord at their site of implantation, but did

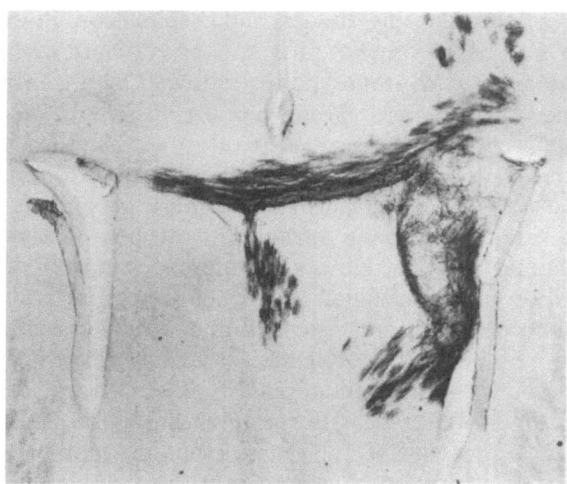

Figure 3.5. Coronal section through shiverer brain (100 μm, Vibratome cut). The transplant is seen in the right lateral ventricle. MBP staining extends from the graft into the deep septal region and crosses to the contralateral hemisphere via the host corpus callosum. MBP reactivity is also seen along the needle tract (×19). Reprinted with permission of *Brain Res*. From Friedman ED, Nilaver G, Carmel P, Perlow M, Spatz L, Latov N. Myelination by transplanted fetal and neonatal oligodendrocytes in a dysmyelinating mutant. *Brain Res*. 1986;378:142–146.

not migrate. Aborted human fetal CNS was also used in transplantation studies and surprisingly, even across major species differences, the human oligodendrocytes formed normal myelin around shiverer axons. In Martin Raff's laboratory in London, cell culture work has revealed an oligodendrocyte–astrocyte precursor cell that can be manipulated to differentiate along either path.[15] These precursor cells are highly mobile and may be the source of myelin distant from our transplants. If we want to enhance remyelination after injury we may have to implant precursor cells rather than differentiated oligodendrocytes, and therefore currently we are isolating and labeling precursor cells.

How can we apply the knowledge gained from research on the fetal nervous system and from animal spinal cord experiments to a better understanding of the pediatric spinal cord? We have learned that the immature animal's spinal tracts are not rigidly delineated but are capable of a) rerouting, b) increasing synaptic terminations, and c) stabilizing neuronal populations that would ordinarily be eliminated. (Table 3.3) We can expect that this is the case in the human neonate also. Until myelination is complete, axon targets can be altered and pathways modified. The human corticospinal tract is myelinated slowly. By 29 weeks the major (anterior) corticospinal tract has partial myelination down to L2-3[16] and by term,

Table 3.3. Why is there sparing of function in neonatal spinal cord injury?

Sprouting
Transfer of function to undamaged neurons
Failure of retraction of "exuberant" projections
Interference with normal development of supraspinal inhibition

there is partial myelination of the corticospinal tract into the sacral level. Since the human spinal cord has not completed myelination until age 2 to 3 years, there is a greater chance for remodeling if the cord is injured within the first 3 years of life. This means that there is the potential for plasticity.

Is there any human evidence of pediatric cord plasticity? Unfortunately there is little documented evidence, although plenty of clinical examples that children recover from spinal cord tumors or injury with remarkably no deficit. A brief review of the literature on outcome after spinal cord injury in children does not support our hypothesis, but for different reasons. The newborn child has such ligamentous elasticity and the spine and discs are so mobile, that they are able to sustain severe traction and torsional forces without bony and ligamentous disruption. However, in the process the cord has been stretched to its limit. This is why the syndrome of *SCIWORA* exists: *Spinal Cord Injury Without Radiographic Abnormality*.[17] What few autopsy studies have been done in children show gliosis (reactive astrocytes in increased number) and scarring (increased glial fibrillary protein and increased fibrosis) at the level of the lesion.[21,7a] These children do not recover. Pang reviewed 25 children that had cord injury, comparing their age to the severity of injury (Fig. 3.6). In general, the younger the child, the more severe the cord injury. The ligaments and bones were so

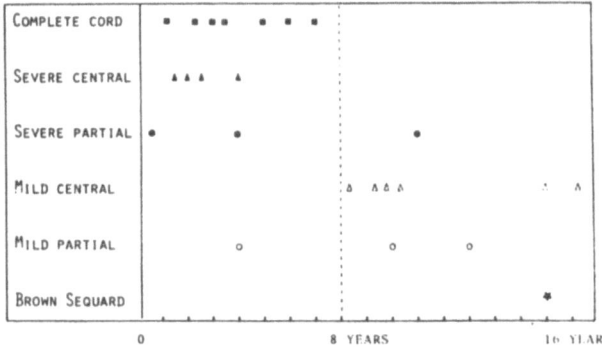

Figure 3.6. Correlation between patients' age and neurological syndromes. Reprinted with permission of *J Neurosurg*. From Pang D, Wilberger Jr, JE. Spinal cord injury without radiologic abnormalities in children. *J Neurosurg*. 1982;57:114–129.

elastic that they had tremendous cord damage, whereas the older children with less flexible spinal columns were less damaged. The strength and rigidity of the older spine protected the cord from torsional and stretching injury. An autopsy study on newborns[18] documented that the spinal column in a newborn can stretch 2 inches but the spinal cord cannot, so there is a discrepancy between spinal column and spinal cord stretch. This is why the infant cord can be functionally transected with an apparently nondisrupted spinal column. Reports of hyperextension birth injuries to the cord also confirm the severe cord trauma with minimal spine disruption.[19]

Unfortunately then, no literature exists to support directly the greater resiliency of the human pediatric versus adult spinal cord. Perhaps new technological developments in neuroimaging or in electrophysiology will confirm recovery of the pediatric spinal cord after trauma or injury due to tumor compression. In the interim, we can be encouraged by the results of animal studies on spinal cord recovery mechanisms, and be cautiously optimistic when faced with a cord injury in a child.

References

1. Kennard MA. Cortical reorganization of motor function. *Arch Neurol Psychiatry*. 1942;48:227–240.
2. Merzenich MM, Nelson RJ, Stryker MP, Cynader MS, Schoppmann, Zook JM. Somatosensory cortical map changes following digit amputation in adult monkeys. *J Comp Neurol*. 1984;224:591–605.
3. Bjorklund A, Stenevi V, eds. *Neural Grafting In the Mammalian CNS*. Amsterdam: Elsevier, 1980.
3a. Schneider GE. Is it really better to have your brain lesion early? A revision of the "Kennard principle." *Neuropsychologia*. 1979;17:557–583.
4. Lenn NJ. Plasticity and responses of the immature nervous system to injury. *Semin Perinatol*. 1987;11(2):117–131.
5. Hamburger V, Oppenheim RW. Naturally ocurring neuronal death in vertebrates. *Neurosci Comment*. 1982;1:39–55.
6. Innocenti GM. Growth and reshaping of axons in the establishment of visual callosal connections. *Science*. 1981;212:824–827.
7. Huttenlocher PR. Synaptic density in human frontal cortex—developmental changes and effects of aging. *Brain Res*. 1979;163:195–205.
7a. Burke DC. Spinal cord trauma in children. *Paraplegia*. 1971;9:1.
8. Huttenlocher PR, De Courten C. The development of synapses in striate cortex of man. *Hum Neurobiol*. 1987;6(1):1–11.
9. Kalil K, Reh T. Regrowth of severed axons in the neonatal central nervous system: establishment of normal connections. *Science*. 1979;205:1158–1160.
10. Bernstein DR, Stelzner DJ. Plasticity of the corticospinal tract following midthoracic spinal injury in the postnatal rat. *J Comp Neurol*. 1983;221:382–400.
11. Bregman BS, Goldberger ME. Infant lesion effect: III. Anatomical correlates of sparing and recovery of function after spinal cord damage in newborn and adult cats. *Dev Brain Res*. 1983;9:137–154.
12. Goldberg S, Frank B. Do young axons regenerate better than old axons? *Exp Neurol*. 1981;74:245–259.
13. Bernstein JJ, Goldberg WJ. Fetal spinal cord homografts ameliorate the severity of lesion-induced hind limb behavioral deficits. *Exp Neurol*. 1987;98:633–644.
14. Friedman E, Nilaver G, Carmel P, Perlow M, Spatz L, Latov N. Myelination by transplanted fetal and neonatal oligodendrocytes in a dysmyelinating mutant. *Brain Res*. 1986;378:142–146.
15. Raff MC, Miller RH, Noble M. A glial progenitor cell that develops in vitro into an astrocyte or an oligodendrocyte depending on the culture medium. *Nature*. 1983;303:390–396.
16. Kappers, Ariens CU, Huber GC, Crosby EC. *Comparative Anatomy of the Nervous System of Vertebrates, Including Man*. New York: Hafner Publishing Co; 1960.
17. Pang D, Wilberger Jr, JE. Spinal cord injury without radiographic abnormalities in children. *J Neurosurg*. 1982;57:114–129.
18. Leventhal HR. Birth injuries of the spinal cord. *J Pediatr*. 1960;56:444–453.
19. Abrams IF, Bresnan MJ, Zuckerman JE, Fischer EG, Strand R. Cervical cord

injuries secondary to hyperextension of the head in breech presentations. *Obstet Gynecol*. 1973;41:369–378.

20. Robinson GA, Goldberger ME. The development and recovery of motor function in spinal cats. 1. The infant lesion effect. *Exp Brain Res*. 1986;62:373–386.
21. Ahmann PA, Smith SA, Schwartz JF, Clarke DB. Spinal cord infarction due to minor trauma in children. *Neurology*. 1975;25:301–307.
22. Goldberger ME. Mechanisms contributing to sparing of function following neonatal damage to spinal pathways. *Neurochem Pathol*. 1986;5:289–307.

Discussion

Factors Surrounding Remyelination

Dr. Kliot raised two questions: The first concerns the implantation of embryonic tissue. What evidence is there that remyelination is not secondary to the release of trophic factors or is it strictly due to the cells being implanted. Have you labeled those cells and shown that they are the ones bringing about remyelination?

Dr. Friedman responded that we are still looking for good labels for transplantable cells and that is why I mentioned the BUDR and that's the interest in retrovirus. Molecular biologists have developed viruses that can package genetic information to give an artificial label to a cell that the cell will not lose because it is incorporated into their genome. The problem with identifying a transplanted oligodendrocyte and its connection to a myelin sheath is that your normal oligodendrocyte will myelinate 30 to 40 axons in the CNS and to get a cut, an electron microscopic cut through its trajectory in continuity with the cell body is nearly impossible. A few people have done it in their lifetime, but it is nearly impossible.

The evidence therefore is indirect that it is not trophic factors. If one uses cultured oligodendrocytes and removes them from their natural environment you still will get myelination and also if you take this shivera optic nerve and put it in a culture dish with normal oligodendrocytes I suppose you cannot rule out completely that trophic factors are involved. I do not know if anyone has taken the medium that the oligodendrocytes were sitting in and then put it in optic nerve shivera cultures to see if they myelinate. I do not think that has been done. The fact now is that there is a genetic marker for the shivera mouse that is due to a gene deletion and that replacing that gene, the myelin basic protein gene, corrects the shivera defect. I think that weighs against trophic factors.

Dr. Kliot's second question concerned Schwann cell implants. Dr. Friedman responded that when we used Schwann cell implants in the spinal cord there was local remyelination, but they were not able to migrate within the central nervous system terrain. They stayed locally especially around the pial surface. This contrasted with the oligodendrocyte transplants, which migrated 1 to 2 cm.

Dr. Kliot asked if these were young Schwann cells. Dr. Friedman answered that they were taken from the sciatic nerve of the young rat pup.

Dr. Holtzman asked if anyone had considered using peripheral nerve to bridge a gap in the spinal cord. Would the Schwann cell help to create the tube or would oligodendrocytes and astrocytes create the tube. Dr. Friedman responded: that's the problem with Schwann cells, even though they can encourage axonal growth outside the CNS when they get into the CNS there is some barrier to their ability to remyelinate and to migrate. In fact, we are hoping that the oligodendrocyte precursors have a greater ability to migrate. These precursor cells may be the ones migrating in the CNS rather than oligodendrocytes themselves. There is some experimental evidence in optic nerves that the migratory cells are the precursors and not the mature oligodendrocytes. Oligodendrocytes that mature and no longer undergo cell division may have a mature function to perform, making it no longer biologically advantageous for them to maintain migratory capabilities.

Unmasking

Dr. Marin-Padilla emphasized that when we are talking about the formation of new pathways, as was the case in the discussion on regeneration, the question of unmasking of existing pathways cannot be excluded. In development multiple alternative pathways may be formed, of which only a few are utilized. It is conceivable that what we term regeneration may in part or wholly be a reflection of an unmasking phenomenon.

Dr. Friedman responded: I believe that the statement that exuberant projections along with an overabundance of pathways initially in many systems may occur early in development and persist unrecognized into adulthood, has validity and if a major pathway is lesioned and then alternative pathways can be used.

Dr. Marin-Padilla added that the existing systems may hypertrophy rather than regenerate in the face of an insult if unmasking is the mechanism.

Dr. Friedman agreed and indicated that in Cunard's work in the 1930s in monkeys she found that you lesion the motor cortex, and the monkeys regain motor function. When these animals matured their motor function was not perfect, showing that it was not the dominant pathway; rather, alternate pathways that were able to take over and be effective but with imperfect functioning. We pay a price for our plasticity. The recovery of function is not absolute and the neonatally lesioned cat that still retains contact placing, the contact placing that is seen in normal animals, is much more exquisitely sensitive and deformable by lesser force than was seen in the transected animals. They had it, but qualitatively the function was not as good.

Immunological Considerations

Dr. MeCormick asked if some comments could be made on the immunologic ramifications of xenographic transplantation to mammalian central nervous system. Dr. Friedman replied that it can be looked at from an afferent or an efferent point of view. From an afferent viewpoint what the peripheral immune system sees in regard to the nervous system is limited and that is because there are virtually no lymphatics in the brain and so foreign antigens are not transported out of the brain to the peripheral immune system to thymus or spleen or anywhere that white blood cells are made. Therefore, we do not develop antibodies to foreign substances that are put into the brain. Also antibodies cannot get in because of the brain barrier. You can suggest that when a transplant is performed the blood–brain barrier is destroyed but that is probably reestablished relatively soon, and whatever blood–brain barrier is destroyed is relatively small so that our peripheral immune system does not detect it. This may be one of the reasons why ventricular shunts do not excite a huge reaction.

Despite the fact that antibodies and white blood cells do not get into the CNS to stimulate our immune system, there is evidence that astrocytes and macrophages that are in the CNS can recognize foreign antigen and be stimulated to turn on white blood cells. Just exactly how this is accomplished is unknown, but it appears as though astrocytes can be activated and endothelial cells may also play some role in activating the peripheral immune system. This is becoming a very exciting area in the wake of transplantation.

To respond to Dr. Holtzman's question about why the gray matter is on the inside rather than the outside of the spinal cord, if you think that neurons in the cortex spread out over the entire surface of the cortex and there are a multitude of association pathways permissible because of this huge mass of gray matter it may enable us to free associate . . . it may enable us to have higher thinking function. On the other hand, we would not want our spinal cord to be an independent thinking mechanism. We would not want free association to be occurring in our lumbar spinal cord such that it might be firing off in every which direction. Therefore, perhaps by containing the pool of motor neurons with a column of white matter this might restrict and confine it, thereby honing its responses from above. There is some evidence that once myelin is laid down it may inhibit neuron outgrowth.

Regeneration Versus Reorganization

Dr. Lazorthes spoke about the three processes that were discussed during this morning's talks concerning recovery of function after a lesion in the central nervous system namely, regeneration, unmasking of preexisting pathways, and reorganization. It was his strong feeling that in reality reorganization is the mechanism most often used by the nervous system in recovery of function.

Dr. Friedman responded by saying in a sense regeneration means reorganization. There does not appear to be evidence that the mature animal has the ability for reorganization of neural pathways and that is part of the problem we are dealing with, namely, whether we can restore the fetal environment with trophic factors or fetal cells. We are optimistic that the fetal potential for growth will be understood during our lifetime.

Dr. Stein offered the opinion that he felt it was just the other way around. The young animal has the potential for regeneration and there may be reorganization of the regenerating pathways, but there is regeneration. The older animal, up to a point, has the ability to reorganize pathways and circuitry. That can be the only explanation for the fact that patients can recover from horrendous lesions of the central nervous system if given time. This must be reorganization. I cannot believe that it represents regeneration.

Dr. Marin-Padilla added that it could also represent unmasking. Dr. Stein responded that what they have shown with the transplantation of fetal cells is that there is actually regeneration occurring. Dr. Marin-Padilla added that when lesions are produced it is possible that unmasking may occur and despite the appearances of regeneration, that may be the mechanism of functional recovery.

Dr. Kliot added any time you do these kinds of experiments on a developing pathway it is important to note development first and then compare regeneration, because a lot of examples of what people thought was regeneration was just a failure to retract. I agree with Dr. Lazorthes that the terminology we use is very important and that reorganization occurs more frequently than we expect. I would like to hope that the approach we took in which we actually tried to demonstrate that fibers from the dorsal root ganglia were growing back into the spinal cord after they had been cut or crushed were true examples of regeneration, because there was nothing to reorganize. We cut them and they regrew. In addition, perhaps reorganization is also occurring in the spinal cord as well. That is why I made the point that all the animals get better. That is probably, to a certain extent, reorganization. The part that got worse when we recut that root I would attribute to regeneration.

Neurogenic Ischemia

Dr. Antunes thought that we should also be reminded that in the clinical settings lesions are not pure lesions. In other words, even when you implant something, something else is happening. Of course, you cannot forget that there is edema around the lesion and there are probably some cells that become nonfunctional because of "neurogenic ishemia." It is not regeneration or reorganization that is involved in the recovery of activity of these neurons. I must say that is the clinical setting I have always been very puzzled why after removing a herniated disc at the L4–5 level the L5 nerve root rapidly recovers motor function and full power is restored to the foot. This is not an uncommon observation. What is the mechanism in that instance is something other than reorganization or regeneration and it is quite puzzling.

CHAPTER 4

Vascularization and Vascular Pathophysiology of the Spinal Cord

Guy Lazorthes

Three events between 1957 and 1967 shed new light on spinal cord pathology. Research into the vascularization and circulation of the neuraxis carried out in the 1950s and 1960s not only called attention to the older, and frequently ignored, developments of Adamkiewicz,[1] Kadyi,[2] and Tanon,[3] but also brought new findings from Lazorthes.[4-6]

More systematic anatomic and clinical studies of spinal cord pathology have also led to some very interesting observations by Ullmann and Alajouanine,[7] Garcin, et al.[8] Jellinger,[9] Neumayer,[10] and Fazio.[11]

New exploratory techniques by Houdart et al.[12] and di Chiro,[13] in particular, arteriography of the spinal cord arteries by selective injection, placed the anatomical findings to be applied directly to a clinical and surgical context.

Spinal cord pathology was for many years dominated by myelitis. However, it is now thought that many syndromes that were given that name are in fact vascular myelopathies. Moreover, disturbances of spinal cord circulation can be found in conjunction with many neurological or vascular diseases.

A final analysis clearly shows that associated with the complexity, the fragility of the neuraxis (brain, brain stem, and spinal cord), and the sensitivity of the neurone to ischemia and anoxia is, fortunately, a vascularization and circulation that differs from those of the other viscera. Indeed, the neuraxis has:

1. safety systems in the arterial vascularization that can become replacement channels; these systems can be compared with no others found anywhere else in the organism
2. multiple drainage channels in the venous vascularization
3. protection from regulatory mechanisms.

We studied the role played by the different arteries in the vascularization by microangiographically injecting colloidal barium sulphate into each one, and by the diaphanication technic. However, the functional value of anatomical compensation can only be estimated with in vivo observation, that is, by experiments on animals or thanks to fortuitous clinical observations. In the monkey, dog, cat, and rabbit we obtained information on the functional territories of the arteries by injection of biological fluorescent compounds.

Arterial Vascularization and Compensatory Channels

In the spinal cord, as in the whole neuraxis, safety systems of anastomoses are found distributed at several levels going from the aortic trunk to the spinal cord. They come into play in the event of physiological or pathological circulatory failure and can constitute efficient compensatory vessels.

One system, which is extraspinal, links the arterial supply vessels. Two systems that are intraspinal can be called periaxial and intraaxial, according to their location.

We shall consider the supplying vessels, the perimedullary arteries, and the intramedullary arteries.

Arterial Supplying Vessels

The arterial supplying vessels of the spinal cord are more numerous and spread out than those of the brain. Their possible substitution was less well known than those of the brain and the brain stem.

The division of the spinal cord into three parts distinguished by their differing vascularization, which we proposed in 1957[4] and which was adopted by all authors, must be maintained for the study of the circulation. Each of the three parts, that is, each of the three vascular territories, represents not only an anatomic unit but also a functional unit; this division therefore is not only morphological, but to an even greater extent is physiological (Fig. 4.1).

Supperior or Cervicothoracic Territory

Upper Cervical Cord. The first four cervical segments (C-1 to C-4) generally have no or little radicular supply. They are vascularized by the anterior spinal artery. This artery originates from the convergence of two affluents of the vertebral arteries. The compensatory system is composed of the "suboccipital anastomotic confluent" formed by the anastomosis of the vertebral, the occipital, and the ascending and deep cervical arteries.[14] It is capable of supplying the terminal segment of the vertebral artery and hence of protecting the circulation of the brain stem and the brain, but especially that of the upper cervical cord, which depends on it. In thrombosis of the vertebral artery, its distal segment can be supplied by the occipital, deep cervical, ascending cervical arteries.

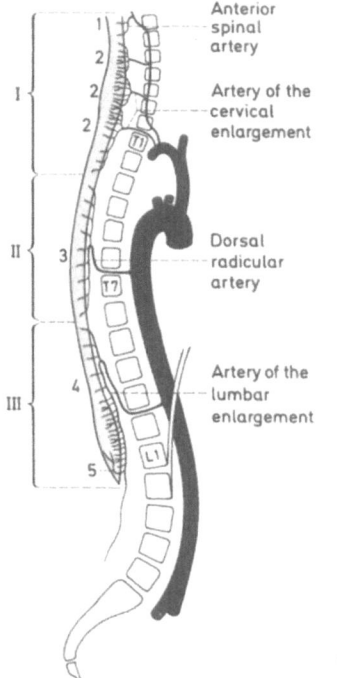

Anterior
spinal
artery

Artery of the
cervical
enlargement

Dorsal
radicular
artery

Artery of the
lumbar
enlargement

Figure 4.1. The three vascular territories. (G. Lazorthes, 1957.)

The Cervical Enlargement. The last four cervical segments and the first two thoracic (C-5 to D-2) constitute the functional unit of the upper limb and their vascularization is autonomous. They are, in fact, vascularized by two to four large radiculomedullary arteries that arise from the vertebral arteries and from the deep and ascending cervical arteries; the lowest artery, arriving with the seventh or eighth cervical radical, is the largest and we call it the cervical enlargement artery[15] (Fig. 4.2).

We were able to demonstrate that the subclavian and external carotid systems are capable of assuring vascularization of the cervical cord after ligation of the two vertebral arteries.

The anastomotic collaterals of the external carotid irrigate the upper two thirds of the cervical cord; the subclavian arteries irrigate the cervical enlargement. Finally, if one vertebral artery is ligated the whole cervical cord is supplied by the other[14] (Fig. 4.3).

The second thoracic medullary segment represents a line of division located between the upper territory, vascularized by collaterals of the subclavian artery, and the intermediate and lower territories, whose vascularization arises directly from the thoracolumbar aorta. Naturally, this line of

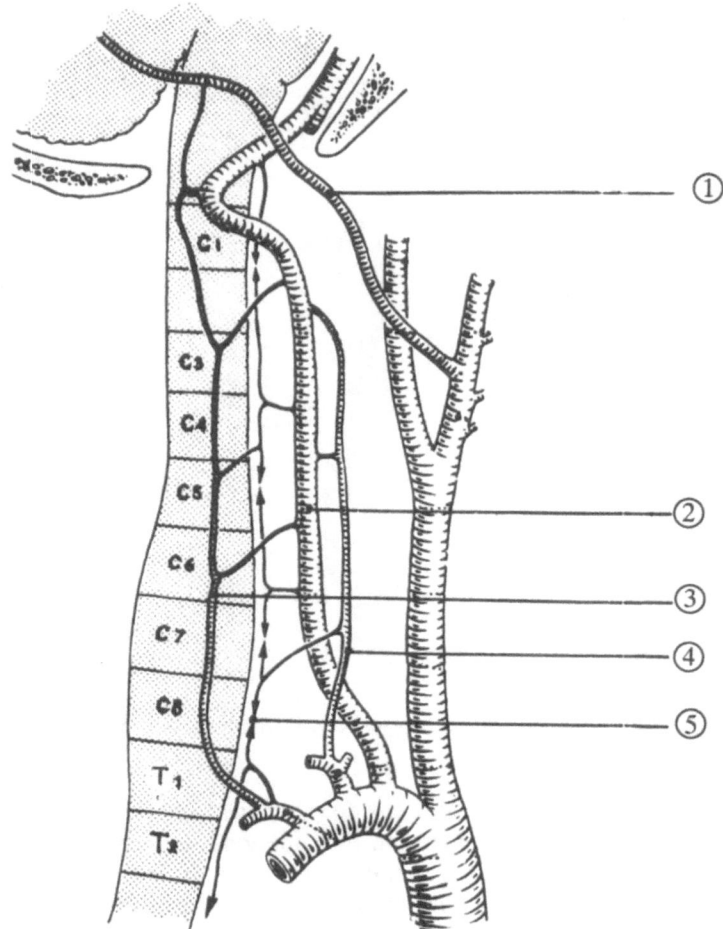

Figure 4.2. Vascularization of the cervical spinal cord. 1, Occipital artery; 2, vertebral artery; 3, deep cervical artery; 4, ascending cervical artery; 5, anterior spinal artery.

separation is subjected to large individual variations that lead to it being raised or, more frequently, lowered to D-3. The zone deprived of arterial afference generally corresponds to the second and third thoracic segments.

Intermediate or Middle Thoracic Territory

The third, fourth, fifth, sixth, seventh, and eighth thoracic segments usually receive a single artery that penetrates with the fifth, sixth, or seventh thoracic ñerves.

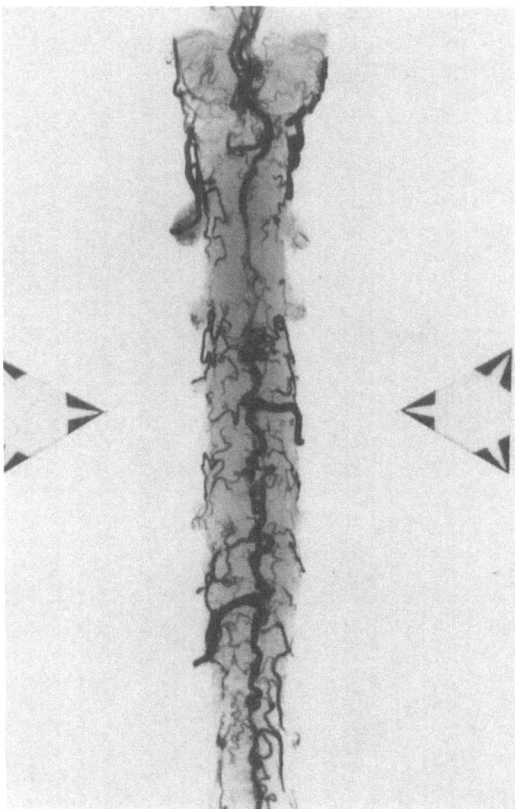

Figure 4.3. Cervical spinal cord is vascularized by two or four large radiculomedullary arteries. The lowest artery is the largest.

It should be noted, however, that when one of the dorsospinal arteries is injected at the point where it leaves the aorta, after having ligated the actual intercostal artery, the bulk of the injection soon finds its way to the opposite side and to the levels above and below. The dorsospinal arteries are in effect linked by their various collaterals in the vertebral, intravertebral, and retrovertebral planes. Selective aorta angiographs demonstrate their existence. However, insofar as the spinal cord is concerned, there are few alternative channels at this middle dorsal level. It remains particularly vulnerable and is a favored site for ischemic lesions. We tried to evaluate it with the following experiment.

The thoracic aorta was ligated below the origin of the subclavian artery, which gives rise to the cervicointercostal artery (itself giving the last radiculomedullary artery that vascularizes the upper or cervicothoracic region) and above the intercostal or lumbar artery where the lumbar enlargement

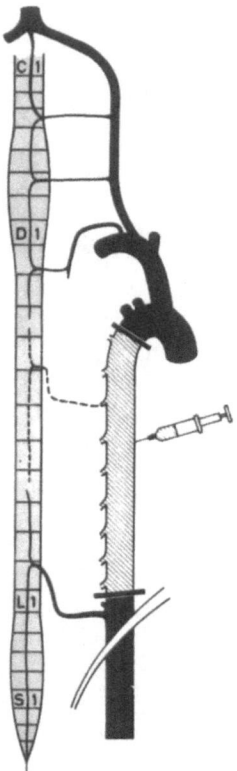

Figure 4.4. Experiment to show the vascularization of the intermediate cord territory.

artery arises (this irrigates the lower territory) (Fig. 4.4). An injection of the segment of aorta isolated showed the small supply from the aorta to the middle thoracic cord, the slight alternative supply possible, and the precariousness of the vascularization of the intermediate cord territory.

Lower or Thoracolombosacral Territory

The rich vascularization of the lower thoracic, lumbar, and sacral medullary segments most often essentially depends on one artery called the "great radicular anterior artery" by Adamkievicz and for which we proposed the name "lumbar enlargement artery" (because it is not only anterior)[4] (Fig. 4.5). It is most often the only arterial supply to this territory, which represents approximately the lower third of the cord (Fig. 4.6). When its origin is high up and it arrives with the seventh, eighth, ninth, and tenth

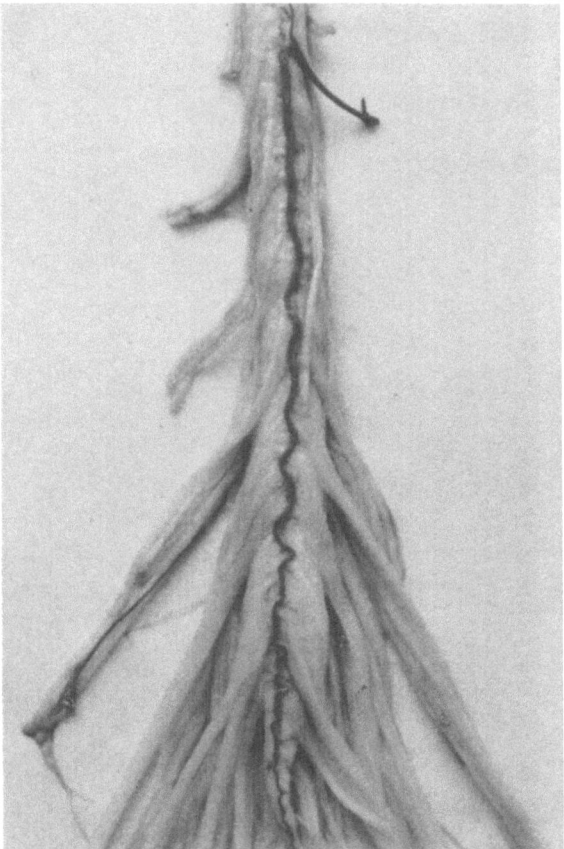

Figure 4.5. Lumbar enlargement artery.

thoracic nerves, a second anterior radiculomedullary artery can occur lower down. The posterior radiculomedullary arteries are more numerous.

The lower or thoracolombosacral territory constitutes the functional unit of the lower limbs. This unit is also one of arterial vascularization since a single artery generally ensures the supply.

The compensatory systems mainly comprised "lower radicular supply vessels" that we described in 1962.[15] On each root of the cauda equina, above the lumbar enlargement artery, there are one or several arteries that, although they are fine, do exist and terminate at the anterior spinal chain for the anterior arteries and the posterior spinal chain for the posterior arteries. We have shown in animals (monkey and dog), by means of in vivo injection of neurotrophic fluorescent tracers,[14] that these radicular

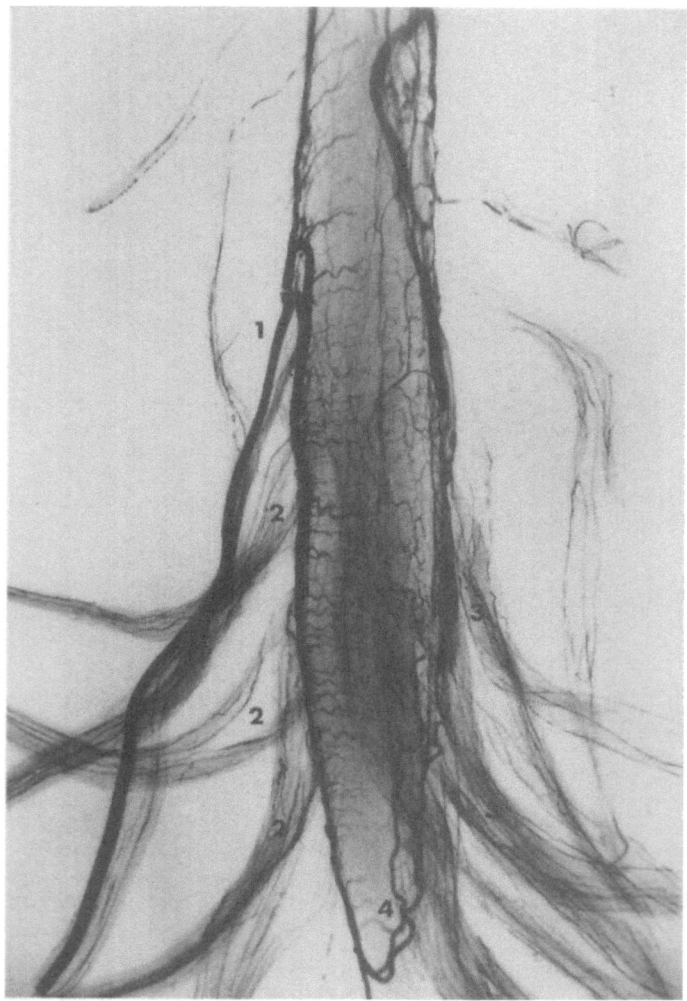

Figure 4.6. Lumbosacral territory. 1, Lumbar enlargement artery; 2, lumbar and sacral arteries on the cauda equina roots; 4, anastomotic conus ansa. (G. Lazorthes, 1957.)

vessels can play an important role in the event of failure of the main supply and that they may assure the vascularization of the lumbar enlargement (Fig. 4.7).

In man, if a solution of colloidal barium sulphate is injected into the abdominal aorta, below the origin of the lumbar artery, which gives rise to the lumbar enlargement artery, the contrast medium is found throughout the lumbar enlargement. It doubtless arrives there by the arteries associ-

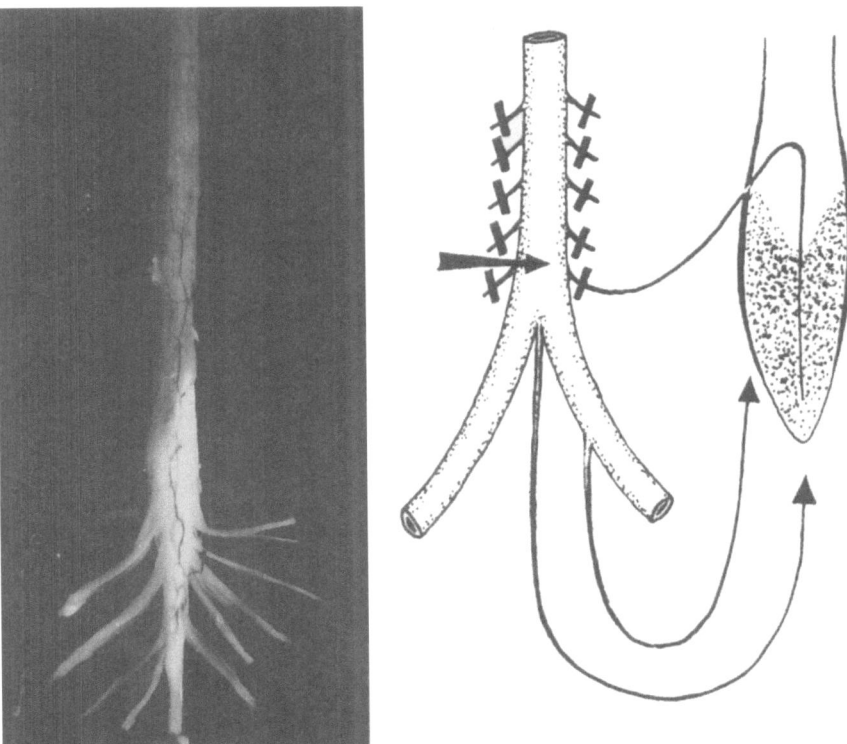

Figure 4.7. Demonstration in vivo by inspection of neurotrophic fluorescent tracers of the role of the sacral radicular vessels to assure the vascularization of the inferior extremity of the spinal cord.

ated with the cauda equina roots arising from the lumbar, iliolumbar, and median and lateral sacral arteries and then by the anastomotic conus ansa.[4]

Perimedullary Arterial System

In the brain, two levels can be distinguished along the periaxial arterial plane: first, the anastomotic circle of the base (polygon of Willis), which represents a theoretically ideal security system and which is unique in the body, and second, the cortical network, which is made up of the three cerebral arteries and their anastomoses (Fig. 4.8).

In the spinal cord there is nothing comparable: the periaxial network is made up of a widespread anterior and median longitudinal channel that is a continuation of the vertebrobasilar trunk onto the spinal cord and of other longitudinal channels of lesser importance and finally of the transverse anastomoses that link them.

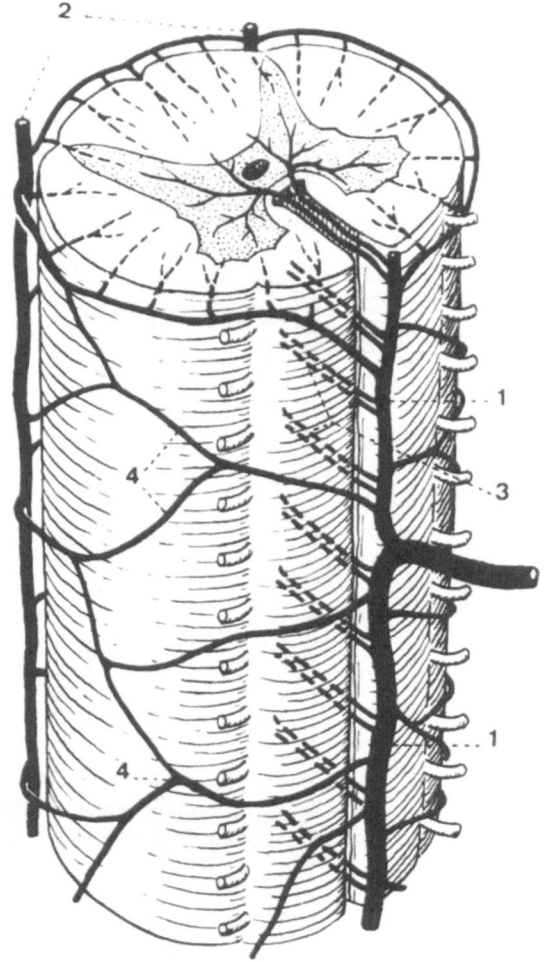

Figure 4.8. The perimedullary network. 1, Anterior spinal artery; 2, posterior spinal arteries; 3, central arteries; 4, perimedullary arteries.

The Longitudinal Spinal Pathway

Two questions arise: the continuity of these longitudinal channels and the direction of flow in the anterior spinal channel.

What is known of the anterior spinal pathway? Suh and Alexander[16] observed that if an injection is made into the arteries of the first cervical segments, the radioopaque substance does not go farther than the cervical cord and that if it is made into the arteries of the lumbar region it rises into the lower and medium thoracic segments (Figure 4.9). This observation prompted the authors to hypothesize that the flow in the anterior arterial

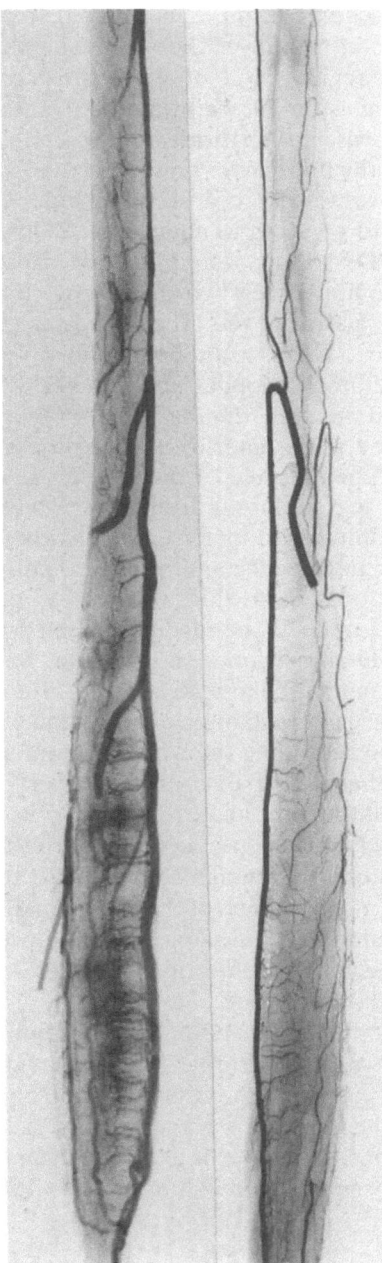

Figure 4.9. The longitudinal anterior spinal way. We can see poor vascularization of the dorsal spinal cord and on the contrary rich vascularization of the lumbosacral spinal cord.

channel is reversed: descending in the upper part (cervical) and rising in the lower part (lombosacral and lower thoracic). The perimedullary arteries of the upper thoracic region, point of convergence of the two flows, is thought to represent an anastomotic pathway that is totally insufficient to link the upper and lower vascular territories.

Zulch[17,18] accepts that the flow moves upward in the ascending branch of a radicular artery and downward in its descending branch. For the cervical cord the flow is thought to go down to about D-4. Below, on the thoracic cord, it would rise from D9-10 to D-4 and go downward until the start of the lumbar cord. For the lumbosacral cord, the flow goes upward over a short distance above the arrival of the great radicular artery (about L-2) and goes downward below. There would be a vulnerable point at D-4 between the cervical and thoracic supplies and another at L-1 between the lower thoracic supply and the upper lumbar (Fig. 4.4).

In order to study the flow in the anterior spinal pathway, we carried out a certain number of experiments[5]; one of them seems particularly demonstrative. We ligated the two vertebral arteries of a fetus after the point where they cross the occipital dura mater. By injection under pressure of the basilar trunk, we then injected the anterior spinal pathway from the top to the bottom. The radioopaque medium was seen to go no farther than the cervical enlargement; none of the medium injected was visible in the thoracic perimedullary arterial network. The medium, however, was found much lower down in the lumbar enlargement artery. It did not find its way there via the perimedullary network but by leaving the spine by one of the cervical radicular arteries and filling the whole arterial system, the aorta, and the artery leaving the lumbar enlargement artery (Fig. 4.10). This experiment proves that in the fetus and even more so in the adult, neither the anterior spinal pathway nor the perimedullary arterial network constitutes a longitudinal anastomotic channel able to fulfill the role of supplement in the event of obstruction of one of the supply paths. It seems logical to assume that, in the adult, the functioning of this pathway can be counted on even less. This impossibility of injection beyond C-4 or C-5 was also reported by Corbin[19] and by Taylor.[20]

In a second set of experiments, in 1962, we first confirmed the fact that injection into one of the vertebral arteries in its intracranial section rarely allows the medium to be pushed farther than C-4[15]; in one case it did reach D-6 but the pressure of the injection was rather high, exceeding that found in physiological conditions. Then we injected the lumbar intumescence artery four times and observed the medium fill the whole anterior spinal

───▷

Figure 4.10. An injection of radioopaque medium in the basilar trunk after ligature of the two vertebral arteries do not go farther than the cervical enlargement. It leaves the spine, fills the whole arterial system, and appears on the spinal cord by the lumbar enlargement artery.

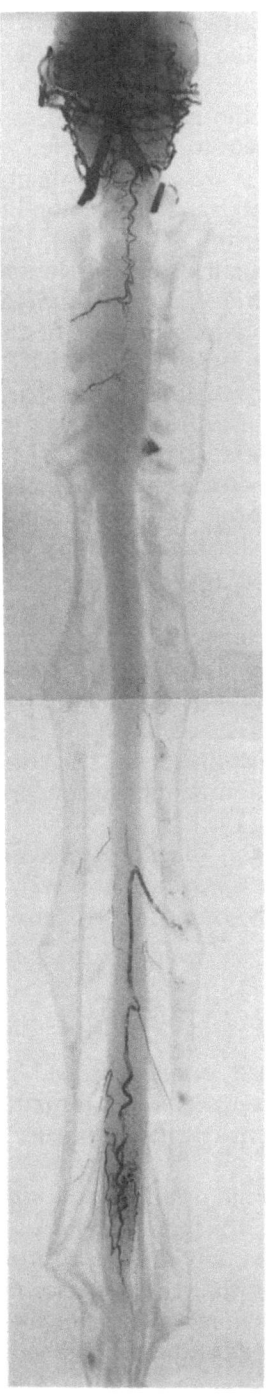

pathway from the bottom to the top. It can be noted that this injection only acted at the surface since, from the middle thoracic region, it never reached full depth.

In conclusion, the continuity of the anterior, and especially the posterior, spinal pathways does not appear to be complete.

Concerning the direction of flow in the anterior spinal pathway, we can grant that, at the level of the first cervical segments the blood flows craniocaudally, that on the lumbosacral cord it also flows downward, below the arrival of the lumbar enlargement artery (great radicular artery of Adamkiewicz), and that in the intermediate region the flow is not in one direction only but in opposing directions in each of the branches. The downward flow seems, in general, to be preponderant.

The perimedullary network has a debatable role. Charpy[21] and Testut[22] suggest that it represents a sort of blood reservoir that receives the blood of the radicular arteries and redistributes it all along the cord: its physiological homogeneity counteracting the inequality of the original segmentary distribution, making uniform the flow through the cord. This vision is certainly too optimistic: the perimedullary network is not an irreproachable anastomotic back-up system and does not protect the whole organ.

The small diameter of the vessel suggests that the compensation arising from the perimedullary network cannot go farther than the neighboring medullary segments and only protects the peripheral or superficial compartment (i.e. just the white matter).

It is not justifiable to make a distinction between an anterior arterial plan and a posterior arterial plan in the perimedullary network as proposed by certain authors.[23]

Schematization of this order appears to us to be excessive. The separation of two perimedullary planes is not clear. It is even more difficult to accept elective disease of one or the other and the possibility of distinct syndromes appearing.

Intramedullary Arteries

Inside the whole neuraxis, spinal cord, brain stem, and brain two vascular systems exist that, according to whether reference is made to their location or their territory, can be called anterior or central system and posterior or peripheral system.

In the spinal cord, unlike in the brain or brain stem, the two systems are hardly separated at the surface (Fig. 4.11). Although it can be seen that the anterior radiculomedullary arteries supply the anterior spinal channel and go essentially to the central territory while the posterior radiculomedullary arteries go to the posterior spinal channels and mainly become distributed through the peripheral territory, in fact, the perimedullary network links them closely (Fig. 4.12).

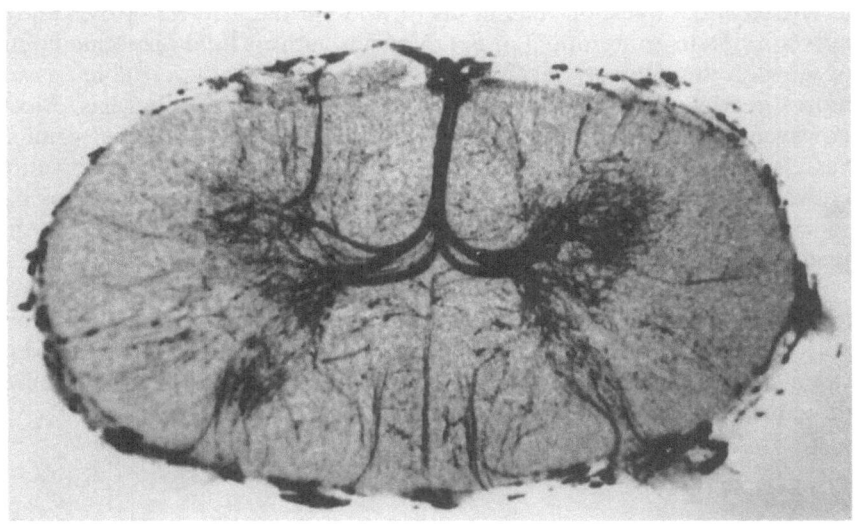

Figure 4.11. Intramedullary vascularization of the cervical spinal cord C-6.

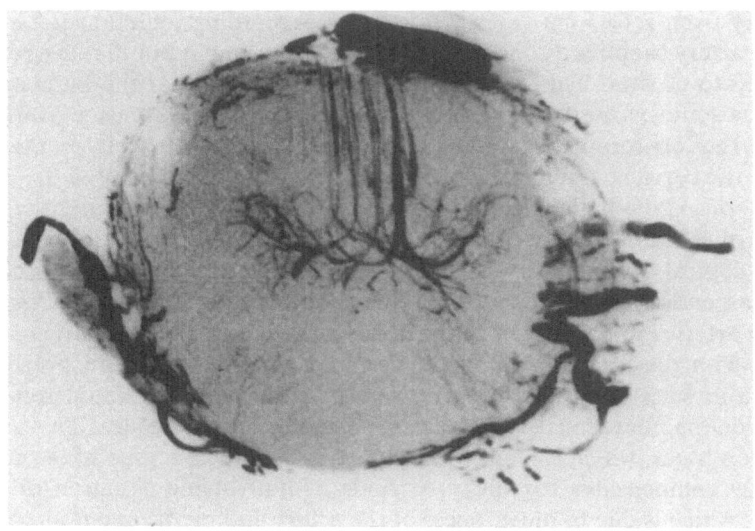

Figure 4.12. Intramedullary vascularization of the sacral spinal cord S-2.

The essential question remains as to whether the arteries of the central nervous system are terminal or not. Various authors hold diverging points of view on this subject. Several support the existence of veritable anastomoses between the different vascular territories of the neuraxis. Most, however, uphold the view that the intraaxial arteries act like terminal vessels, as defined by Conheim,[24] that is, that the only communication between them is a network of capillaries 7 to 13 μm across which is not functional. This microscopic anastomotic network is not crossed by injections of colored or radioopaque substances.

This seems to be the case in the brain where central and peripheral territories are separate, independent, and with no possible system of compensation. A central artery or a peripheral artery only assures sufficient vascularization of the territory around its terminal capillary network. Does the same hold for the spinal cord?

The Peripheral Arteries

The peripheral arteries are linked by a network of such small diameter that it cannot be functional. The anastomoses, if indeed they exist, seem to be small and have no functional role.

The Central Arteries

The central arteries, on the other hand, are anastomosed. One should first picture that each of them spreads its terminal branches over a height that can vary from 2 to 3 cm (Figs. 4.13, 4.14). According to Jellinger,[9] each central artery supplies a zone from 15 to 20 mm in height but that can reach up to 50 to 60 mm. This is implies, since it is known that the number of central arteries varies from 1 to 8 per cm,[4] that there is extensive overlapping of the territories irrigated by the central arteries especially in the region of the cervical and lumbar enlargements where the density of the central arteries is the highest (Fig. 4.15). Each central artery supplies several groups of cells and each group of cells is irrigated by several arteries.

The central arteries are also anastomosed: a) a first anastomosis comprises ascending and descending branches that come off the trunk of the central arteries in the region of the commisura grisea and that are anastomosed with the branches of the corresponding underlying and overlying arteries in such a way as to form a paramedian vascular canal running alongside the neurocanal, as already reported by Adamkiewicz. This anastomotic system, which is mainly developed in the dorsal region of the cord, partially compensates for the precarious hemodynamic situation of this region, which is due to meagreness of the artery and the frequent interruptions of the anterior spinal artery and to the paucity of central vessels, and b) transverse anastomoses are reported to exist between the central

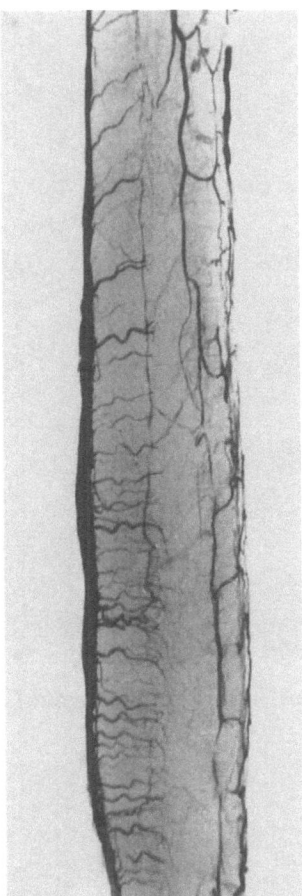

Figure 4.13. Central arteries by angiographic technique (sagittal section).

arteries of a given level and to link the arteries from one side to those on the other side either by passing in front of or behind the neurocanal.[25]

The central arteries and the peripheral arteries communicate only by the capillary network. The intramedullary arteries can be considered to be terminal, as defined by Conheim.[24]

The area encompassed by the central and peripheral territories varies from one region to another. The peripheral territory is greater in the cervical and thoracic regions than in the lumbosacral region. The central territory covers a greater area in the cervical and lumbar intumescences. These differences correspond to the relative size of the white and gray matter.

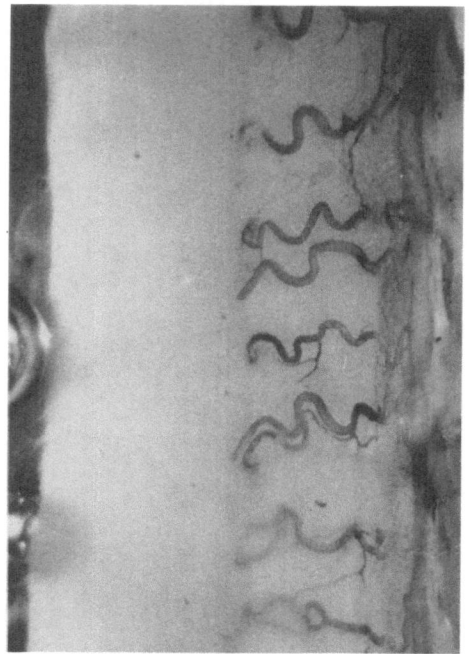

Figure 4.14. Central arteries by angiographic technique (sagittal section).

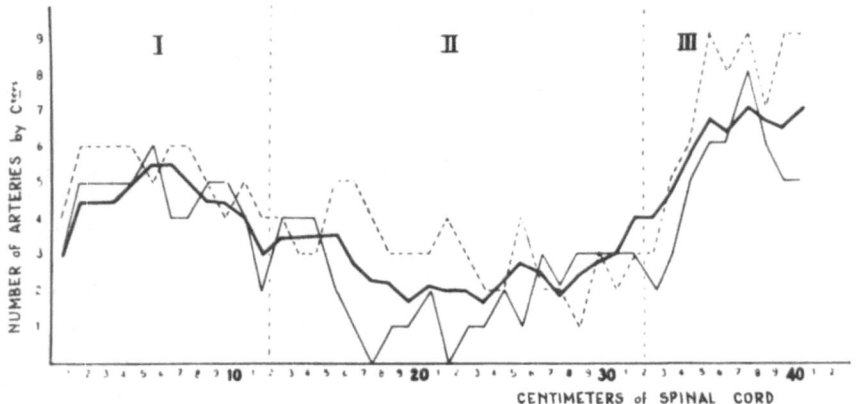

Figure 4.15. Variations of the number of central arteries. (G. Lazorthes, 1957.)

Can it be concluded that disease of the anterior spinal way is more serious in the cervical and lumbosacral regions than in the thoracic region?

Is there a clear-cut boundary zone between the central and peripheral territories? Some think there is and have proposed detailed limits. Others, however, have described an overlap of the territories. Turnbull and colleagues[26] in particular defined the areas of overlap where the two territories meet. This zone would therefore not be vulnerable, as it had been suggested, but, to the contrary, favored by the double origin of its vascularization.

Conclusions

Compensatory pathways for arterial blood flow exist at all levels but they do not all have equivalent capacities and their functional ability is limited. For the supply channels, especially in the region of the intumescences, afferent paths are numerous; compensation for a flow deficit is possible through collateral afflux. The perimedullary network is only anastomotic within certain limits. The intramedullary anastomoses between the central and peripheral arteries also play only a functional role in a narrow boundary zone.

Vascular Pathophysiology of the Spinal Cord

All these studies have led neurologists and neurosurgeons to think of the possible involvement of a vascular factor in a certain number of poorly understood medullary syndromes.

Circulatory failure of the spinal cord can result from narrowing or obstruction of one of the arterial paths, from general circulatory failure, or, often, from a combination of both anatomic and hemodynamic failure.

The Cellular Factor

A decrease in arterial blood supply to a given territory necessarily means that the quantity of blood arriving is not sufficient or adequate for the metabolic requirements. In the neuraxis, this quantity is probably directly proportional to the number of neurones and to the density of the synaptic endings; this means that it must be greater in the cervical and lumbar intumescences.

The General or Hemodynamic Factor

With normal arteries a drop in blood pressure will only cause disturbances or medullary ischemic lesions if it reaches the very low figure of 40 to 50 mm Hg. In the brain, the lower threshold level is about that of a blood flow of under 70 mm Hg. Association with arteriosclerosis raises the safety threshold since medullary blood flow decreases earlier.

The rate at which a drop in blood pressure occurs is extremely rapid. In sudden hypotension from cardiovascular collapse during myocardiac infarction or traumatic shock, ischemia is less well compensated than when it is progressive, since the back-up systems are slow to fulfill their function.

The territories most at risk are those distant from the nutrient trunks: those situated in the boundary zones and those where vascularization is least rich. This is true for the medullary circulation as well as for the cerebral circulation.

Vertically, the least well vascularized region is the middle thoracic cord. Consultation of neurological works and anatomical accounts in observations published concerning myelopathies have confirmed this. The authors report, without particularly calling attention to it, that the lesions brought about by medullary arteriosclerosis, neuroanemic syndromes, Foix and Alajouanine's necrotic myelitis, periarteritis nodosa, and myelopathy brought about by radiotherapy and radiumtherapy, are most serious around the central thoracic medullary segments. This preferential location probably also explains that, in their study of the spinal cord in the elderly, Graux et al.[27] bring forward the notion of discrete neurological disease of the upper limbs and top half of the trunk, which is more disease in the lower limbs and bottom half of the trunk.

Transversely, in each segment there is a boundary zone at the borders of the central and peripheral arterial streams. The two streams are quite independent and hardly anastomosed. Many authors describe them as being juxtaposed, which suggests that the circular limiting zone which is at the edge of the two territories should be the first affected by ischemia. On the other hand, Turnbull et al.[28] acknowledge the existence of a circular zone common to both territories where the central and peripheral arteries superimpose their endings; this would, on the contrary, create a particularly protected zone.

The Local Vascular Factor

Location and Syndromes

As for disturbances of cerebral circulation, it has been discovered during the last few years that the circulatory failure responsible is not solely located in the periaxial or intraaxial ramifications but often it is quite remote—in the original large trunks.

Lesion of the Arterial Supply Paths. When there is a problem with a vertebral artery, the other artery easily compensates the arterial supply of the cervical cord but less easily for the brain stem. If the other artery is of smaller diameter, compensation can also come from the collaterals of the subclavian arteries (i.e., the cervical arteries). The distal segment of the vertebral artery can also be supplied by the occipital arteries.

One of the intercostal arteries or lumbar arteries that arise from the aorta bears one of the important radiculomedullary arteries. The danger comes at two points in particular: between D-5 and D-7, which is the origin of the artery that vascularizes the middle thoracic segment, and between D-11 and L-2, which is the origin of the lumbar enlargement artery on which the vascularization of the lower part of the cord depends. These two arteries most often arise on the left.

Total transverse medullary syndrome or Charcot's medullary ictus is characterized by paraplegia that can be sudden, preceded by intermittent claudication, or become progresssively more serious.

Lesion of the Juxtamedullary and Intramedullary Arteries. As soon as the radiculomedullary arteries reach the cord, they divide into an ascending and a descending branch; the ischemic territory will therefore generally spread above and below. It covers a greater area in the central territory, where compensatory channels are less frequent, than in the peripheral territory where the perimedullary network is supplied by several radicular arteries.

Obstruction of the radiculomedullary artery of the lumbar enlargement (great anterior radicular artery of Adamkiewicz) causes flaccid paraplegia with sensory disturbances that spread upward to a varying degree depending on the location of the artery (Cossa's syndrome) of the lumbar enlargement artery. Stenosis or spasm of this artery gives rise to an intermittent medullary claudication syndrome. Obstruction of the median dorsal radiculomedullary artery can bring about flaccid paraplegia unless the anterior spinal channel compensates. Obstruction of the anterior spinal channel generally causes a central, plurisegmental softening covering a variable area. The consequence of this is either a total anterior syndrome or a partial anterior syndrome affecting the anterior horns, or a central syndrome by central myelomalacia or Zulch's softening "en crayon."[17]

Obstruction of a single central artery (sulcocommissural artery) in theory should cause a unilateral central segmental softening. In fact, however, if we first accept the overlapping of the territory of the superimposed central arteries whose terminal ramifications interpenetrate, and second, the existence of vertical periepandymal anastomoses, several neighboring central arteries would have to be blocked to create an ischemic center.

Obstruction of the peripheral network, rarely complete and circular, in theory gives rise to softening of the white matter and of the head of the posterior horn. This obstruction, which is limited to the posterior spinal channels and the posterior arterial plane, would give rise to what Perier et al.[29] called a posterior spinal syndrome.

Causes

Causes of different kinds, intrinsic or extrinsic, spontaneous or induced, can, at any given point, interrupt the corticomedullary way of the nutrient arteries of the cord.

Arterial Compression. On spinal trauma with widespread skeletal damage, vascular compressions are often ignored in the overall clinical picture. On spinal trauma without skeletal lesion, however, circulatory disturbances can play the main role; sudden cervical hyperextension movements can cause medullary compression and vascular compression, and it is difficult to define the respective responsibilities.

Cervical, dorsal, and lumbar discopathies are rarely at the origin of medullary softening. Medial cervical or dorsal hernias compress the cord as well as the anterior spinal artery. Paramedial hernias compress half the cord and give rise to Brown-Séquard syndrome. Lateral hernias can compress the roots and sometimes a radiculomedullary artery.

Primitive or secondary, spinal or intraspinal, tumors can cause ischemia and necrosis by compression of the root or meningeal neoplastic infiltration. This should be borne in mind when paraplegia occurs suddenly or evolves rapidly. We reported from statistics obtained personally the particular susceptibility of the middle dorsal segment of the cord.

Degenerative conditions of the spine can also become complicated by medullary circulation disturbances and lesions. With vertebral diseases, it is the radicular arteries, the anterior spinal artery, or the anterior spinal artery that are compressed. With cervical diseases it is sometimes the vertebral artery. With kyphoscoliotic deformation it can be the perimedullary arteries.

In conclusion, it is difficult to evaluate the respective responsibility of direct compression and vascular compression in the appearance of medullary disturbances: a shift in the level between the site of the causal lesion and the medullary symptom should be reason for reflection.

Arterial Obstruction. Obstructive atherosclerosis of the aorta or the intercostal arteries can cause acute, subacute, or chronic ischemia of the cord. Dissecting aneurysm is responsible for massive necrosis of the cord. Thrombosis of the subclavian artery or vertebral artery is seldom responsible for medullary ischemia since compensation is provided by the opposite vertebral artery and by the ascending and deep cervical arteries.

Periarteritis nodosa can be detected by inaugural myelomalacic accident or by medullary disturbances occurring as part of a general picture of neurological signs.

Emboli of the medullary arteries are rare whereas they are frequent in cerebral pathology. This difference is in accordance with the laws of hemodynamics; the embolus generally takes the large diameter and most direct arterial path, that is, the carotid system rather than the vertebrovascular system. The arteries of the cord are of average diameter and come off the aorta at right angles. The embolus can be cruoric (blood clot) (from valvular cardiopathies) or noncruoric; bacterial, parasitic, or gaseous (after accidents of rapid decompression).

Stenosis of the aortic isthmus seldom causes medullary complications since the development of sufficient collateral circulation compensates the disturbances caused by the coarctation. Ischemic vascular complications through hypovascularization downstream of the malformation are rare. Those resulting from hypervascularization occurring upstream of the stenosis arise from the compression of the cord by the dilated arterial vessels. These complications occur on the lower cervical and upper dorsal cord.

Interruption of Arterial Flow by Surgery. As early as the 17th century, Swammerdam[30] and Stenonis[31] discovered that prolonged occlusion of the aorta in animals was followed by paralysis. Cardiovascular and thoracic surgery has stimulated new interest.

Curative treatment of congenital or acquired diseases of the large arteries requiring prolonged clamping and even the sacrifice of compensatory arterial channels can cause a risk of medullary complications. An excellent study was carried out by Adams and Van Geertruyden[32]. The question is dominated by the reestablishment of collateral circulation, which is itself dependent on functional and anatomic factors: the functional value of the anterior spinal channel, the number of radiculomedullary arteries, and the

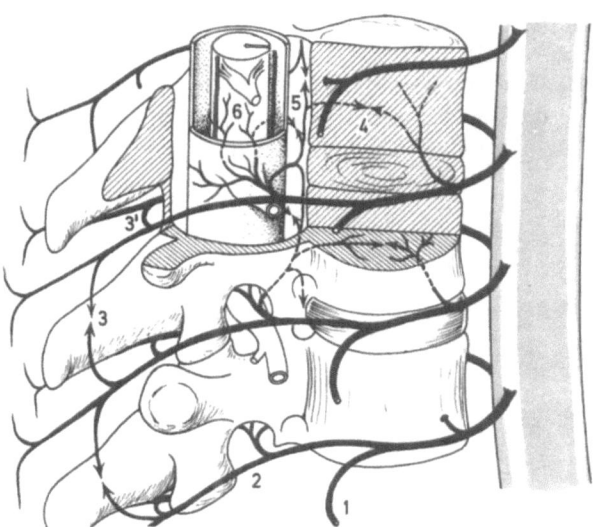

Figure 4.16. 1, Intercostal artery; 2, dorsospinal artery; 3, retrovertebral; 4, vertebral; 5, intravertebral planes; 6, intradural vessels.

level at which the lumbar enlargement artery arises. The danger of ischemia and medullary necrosis increases when the occlusion of the aorta is associated with that of the last intercostal arteries, especially on the left; it increases if there is no efficient compensatory way and if the general condition of the patient's arteries is poor.

Thoracoabdominal operations [thoracolumbar sympathectomy for arterial hypertension (Smithwick type), pneumonectomy, thoracoplasty, requiring ligation of one or several intercostal or lumbar (D-8 to L-2) arteries especially on the left] can result in paraplegia (Fig. 4.16). It is recommended to ligate the intercostal or lumbar arteries far from the aorta, that is, after the dorsospinal artery comes off.

Abdominal aortography can cause medullary necrosis with vascular and toxic pathology. The first observation was reported by Antoni and Lingren in 1949[33]; since then, numerous cases have been published. All the factors that contribute to a concentration of contrast medium favor the occurrence of cord necrosis. Djindjian reported the danger of aortography carried out at high pressure.

Conclusions

1. In circulatory failure of the spinal cord, both hemodynamic circulatory disturbances and narrowing of the vascular lumen of the cord arteries are partially responsible.
2. Possibilities of compensation, when an artery is affected, are greater if the obstruction is distant from the cord. There are arteries, however, where compensation cannot occur (e.g., arteries of the central segments of the dorsal cord).
3. The more rapidly the failure of the medullary circulation occurs the less the chance the compensatory systems have of acting efficiently since it does not have a sufficient adaptation time.

References

1. Adamkiewicz A. Die Blutgefässe der menschlichen Rückenmarkoberfläche. *Verh Kon Akad Wissensch Wien Math Nat Kl.* 1882;85:101.
2. Kadyi H. *Über die Blutgefässe des menschlichen Rückenmarkes.* Lemberg: Gubrinovicz und Schmidt; 1889.
3. Tanon 1910.
4. Lazorthes G, Poulhes J, Bastide G, Roulleau J, Chancholle A. Researches on arterial vascularization of the medulla spinalis. Applications in medullar pathology. *Bull Acad Nat Med.* 1957;41:464.
5. Lazorthes G, Poulhes J, Bastide G, Roulleau J, Chancholle A. Arterial vascularization of the medulla spinalis. Anatomical researches and application in medullar pathology and aortal pathology. *Neurochirurgia.* 1958;4:3–19.
6. Lazorthes G, Gonaze A, Djindjian R. Vascularization et circulation de la moelle efiriese. Anotomie. Physiologie. Pathologie. Angiographie. 286 pages 211 figures Masson edit 1973.
7. Ullmann and Alajouanine 1938.
8. Garcin, Godlewski, and Rondot 1963.
9. Jellinger 1966.
10. Neumayer, 1967.
11. Fazio 1970.
12. Houdart, Djindjian, Hurth 1965.
13. di Chiro 1967.
14. Lazorthes and Gouaze 1968.
15. Lazorthes 1962.
16. Suh and Alexander 1939.
17. Zulch KL. Mangeldurchblutung an der Grenzzone zweier Gefäbgebiste als Ursache bisher ungeklärter Rückenmarksschädigungen. *Dtsch Zschr Nervenhk.* 1954;172:31–101.
18. Zulch 1962.
19. Corbin 1961.
20. Taylor 1964.
21. Charpy 1921.
22. Testut 1928.
23. Lhermitte and Corbin 1961.
24. Conheim 1872.
25. Pitzorno.
26. Turnbull IM, Brieg A, Hassler O. Blood supply of cervicäl spinal cord in man. A microangiographic cadaver study. *J Neurosurg.* 1966;XXIV(6):951–965.
27. Graux et al 1962.
28. Turnbull et al 1962.
29. Perrier et al 1960.
30. Swammerdam 1667.
31. Stenonis 1669.
32. Adams and Van Geertruyden.
33. Antoni and Lindgren 1949.

II-B. RADIOLOGY AND NEUROIMAGING

CHAPTER 5

The Role of Neuroimaging in Regeneration and Recovery of the Spinal Cord

Jacqueline A. Bello

Neuroimaging plays a crucial role in establishing a perspective on the potential for spinal cord recovery and/or regeneration in various clinical settings. Within the field of neuroimaging, it is essential to select the proper modality for the information needed, realizing that conventional ("plain film") radiography is still the state of the art in addressing certain clinical problems, and, at the opposite extreme of the technological spectrum, magnetic resonance (MR) imaging, MR contrast agents, MR angiography, MR spectroscopy and positron emission tomography (PET) scanning have their unique applications as well. In addressing the questions related to spinal cord recovery and/or regeneration, neuroimaging actually plays several different roles: (a) diagnostic initially, (b) therapeutic occasionally, with interventional procedures, and (c) prognostic, through radiographic monitoring of the clinical course.

From a "preventive perspective," accurate diagnoses in terms of lesion characterization and extent will minimize the *need* for recovery and/or regeneration of the spinal cord. In certain instances, neuroimaging facilitates less invasive closed rather than open biopsy procedures, and allows appropriate treatment formulation to maximize sparing of vital neural tissue. Correct lesion characterization in various clinical settings is modality dependent. Accurately defining the extent of a lesion is dependent on visualizing its anatomic margins, adequately assessing the immediate adjacent tissues, appropriately investigating potential avenues of spread, and considering associated lesions.

Congenital malformations, with the exception of exclusively bony anomalies, are most efficiently examined by magnetic resonance imaging (MRI). Careful analysis of T2- and T1-weighted images defines the extent of cord tethering, and differentiates among fat, soft tissue, and fluid signal intensity for the detection of lipomas, and "celes" of various descriptions (i.e., meningoceles, myelomeningoceles, and lipomyelomeningoceles) (Fig. 5.1). If preliminary AP and lateral L-S spine radiographs are obtained, dysraphism will not be missed, and patients with pronounced scoliosis may be spared a nondiagnostic MR exam and undergo computed

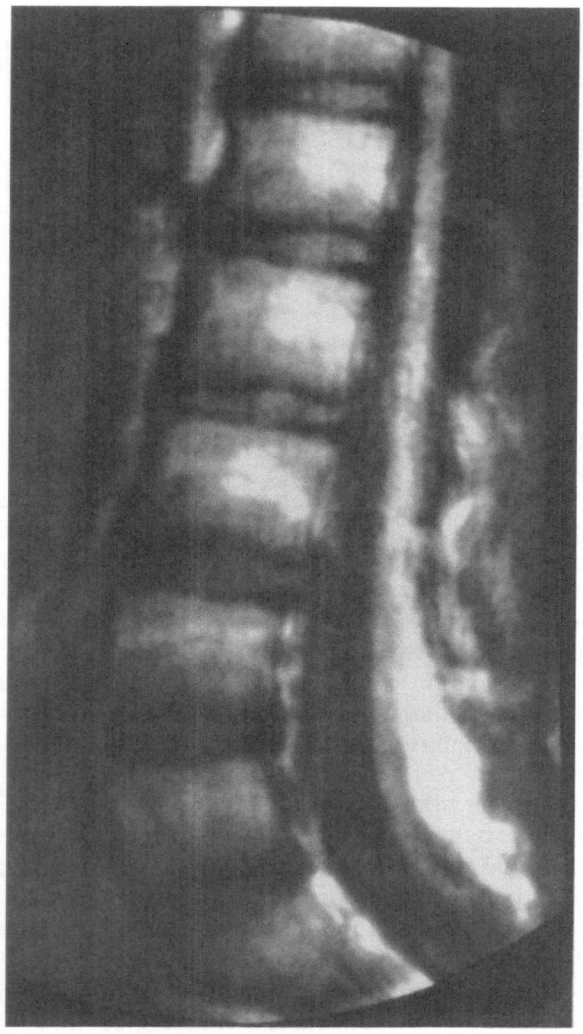

Figure 5.1. A: Sagittal T1 MRI demonstrates high signal due to fat (lipoma) posterior to a tethered cord. CSF anterior to the cord is *hypo*intense on T1.

tomography (CT) myelography instead. CT is capable of differentiating fat, soft tissue, and fluid by density (and therefore x-ray attenuation coefficient), and detects calcification with greater sensitivity and specificity than MRI. In posttreatment follow-up examinations, MRI noninvasively defines the extent of "untethering" and effective surgical treatment of "celes" (Fig. 5.2).

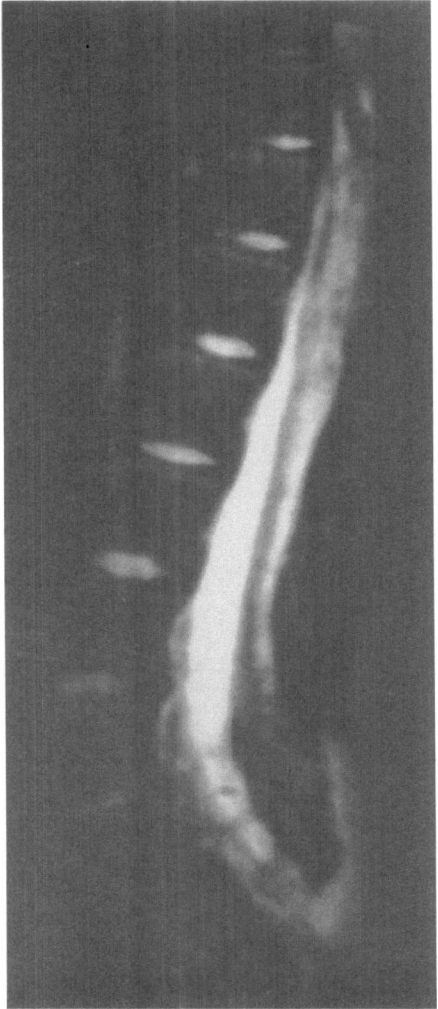

Figure 5.1. B: Sagittal T2 MRI demonstrates *hyper*intense signal due to CSF anterior to the cord and lower signal intensity posteriorly in the lipoma.

Acute spinal trauma is most practically evaluated using conventional radiography and CT for the evaluation of stability of the spinal canal and CT myelography for consequent neuraxial impingement (Fig. 5.3). Although sagittal MRI is capable of doing this, it requires a stable, cooperative patient (Fig. 5.4). MRI is perhaps the modality most capable of specifically diagnosing and dating hemorrhage, due to the characteristic

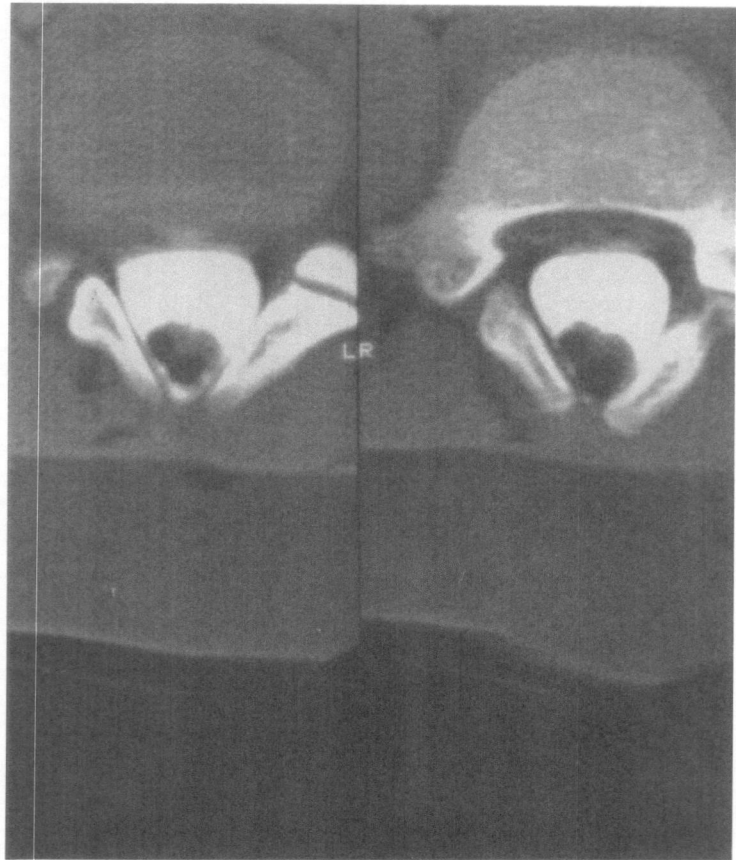

Figure 5.1. C: Axial postmyelography CT images demonstrate contrast within the thecal sac anterior to the soft tissue density of the cord as well as lucency in the posterior lipoma. Spinal dysraphism is noted.

appearance of blood acutely, and of blood degradation products subacutely and chronically on T1- and T2-weighted images (Fig. 5.5). Nerve root avulsions are optimally evaluated by myelography (with option for post-myelography CT) (Fig. 5.6) and acute injury to vascular structures by subtraction arteriography (Fig. 5.7). In evaluating (chronic) posttraumatic sequelae, MRI, unequaled by other modalities, obviates the need for delayed postmyelography CT scanning for the detection of syrinx/cysts (Fig. 5.8). However, spinal cord cavities, which either result from expansion of the central canal (classical hydromyelia) or replace cord substance (syringomyelia) may be mimicked on both T1- and T2-weighted images by pro-

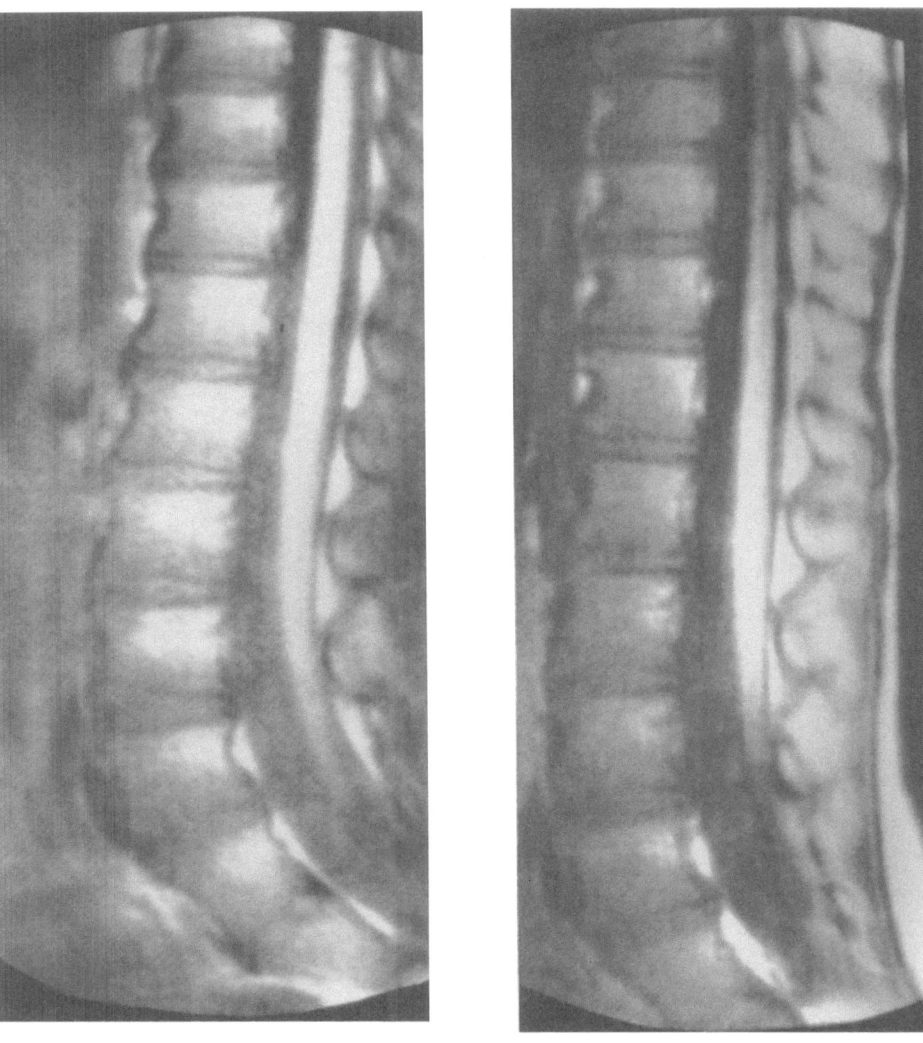

a

b

Figure 5.2. A: Sagittal T1 MRI of a tethered cord terminating at L5-S1. **B:** Post-operative sagittal T1 image demonstrates the cord terminating at L4-5.

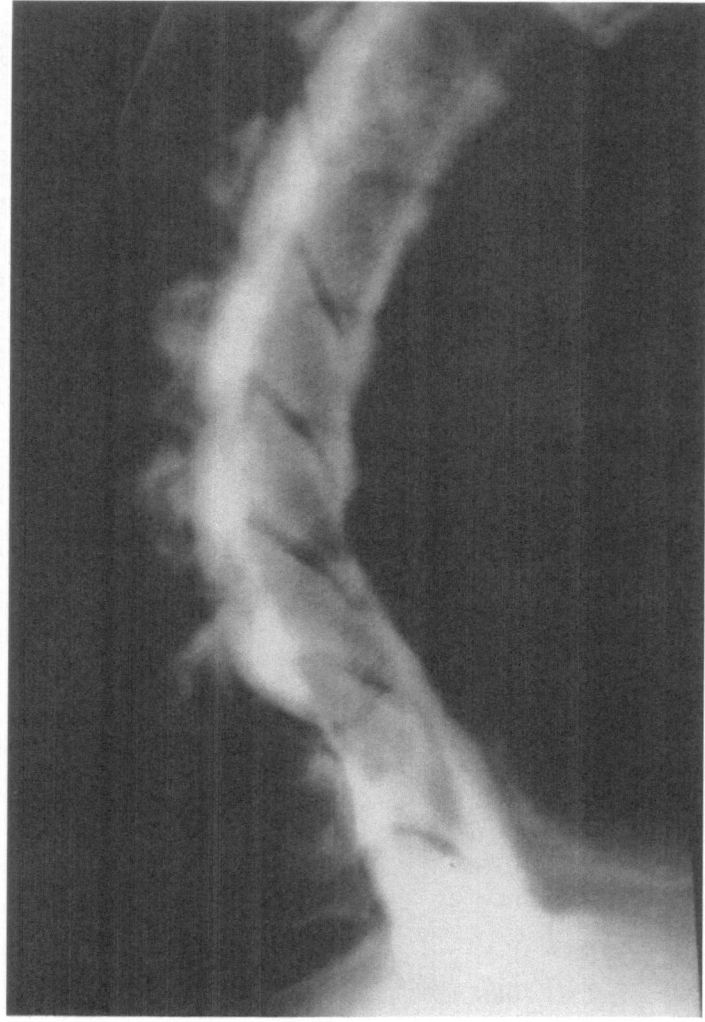

Figure 5.3. A: Myelography, in the lateral projection demonstrates traumatic cervical subluxation at C6-7.

nounced cord edema, myelomalacia, and by "syrinx-like" artifacts also known as truncation artifacts (Fig. 5.9). "Balanced" (proton density) imaging may help distinguish the former two entities from true cavities. Once the diagnosis of a spinal cord cavity is made, cine MR is useful in the detection of pulsatility within these cord cysts. Pulsatility has been shown to correlate with clinical deterioration in patients, and the elimination of

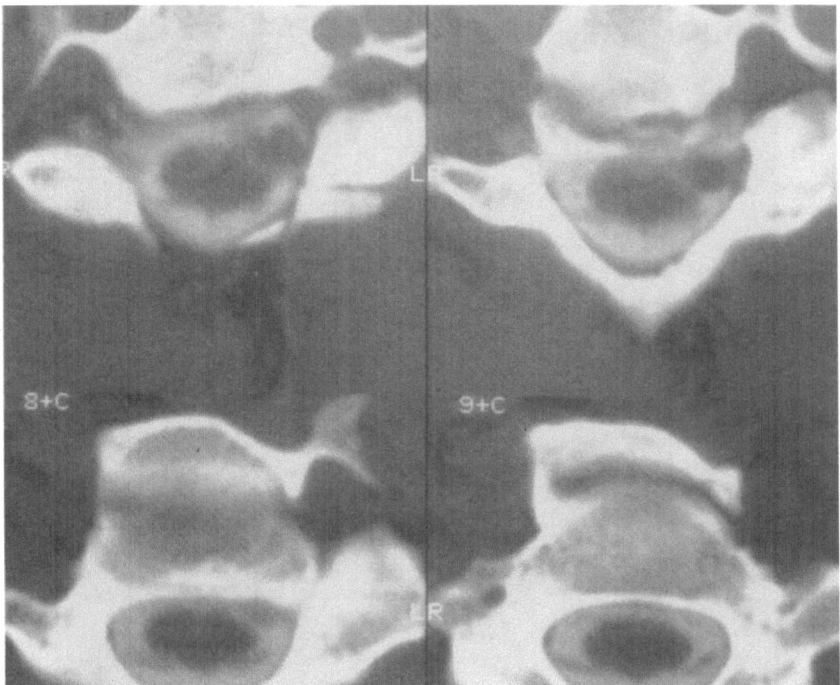

Figure 5.3. B: Axial postmyelography CT further demonstrates cord impingement due to the subluxation as well as root avulsions.

pulsatility within cysts by shunt procedures has been shown to correlate with clinical improvement. Cine MRI also depicts the lack of normal CSF flow within the spinal subarachnoid space surrounding these pulsatile posttraumatic spinal cord cysts, and documents the return of normal CSF pulsations within the spinal subarachnoid space after these cysts are shunted. This is perhaps one of the most exciting frontiers in neuroimaging in terms of its prognostic potential for cord recovery. In the long-term evaluation of trauma patients status post–open reduction and internal fixation of mechanical spinal injury, the presence of hardware may preclude diagnostic CT/MR scanning, thus elevating conventional tomography (in conjunction with myelography) to "state-of-the-art" status.

Truly cystic intramedullary cavities also exist outside the clinical setting of trauma, in association with congenital malformations (such as syrinx with Chiari malformations) (Fig. 5.10), arachnoiditis, and neoplasms. In the latter case, using intravenous paramagnetic contrast agents (e.g., gadolinium) with T1-weighted pulse sequences may best distinguish cord tumor

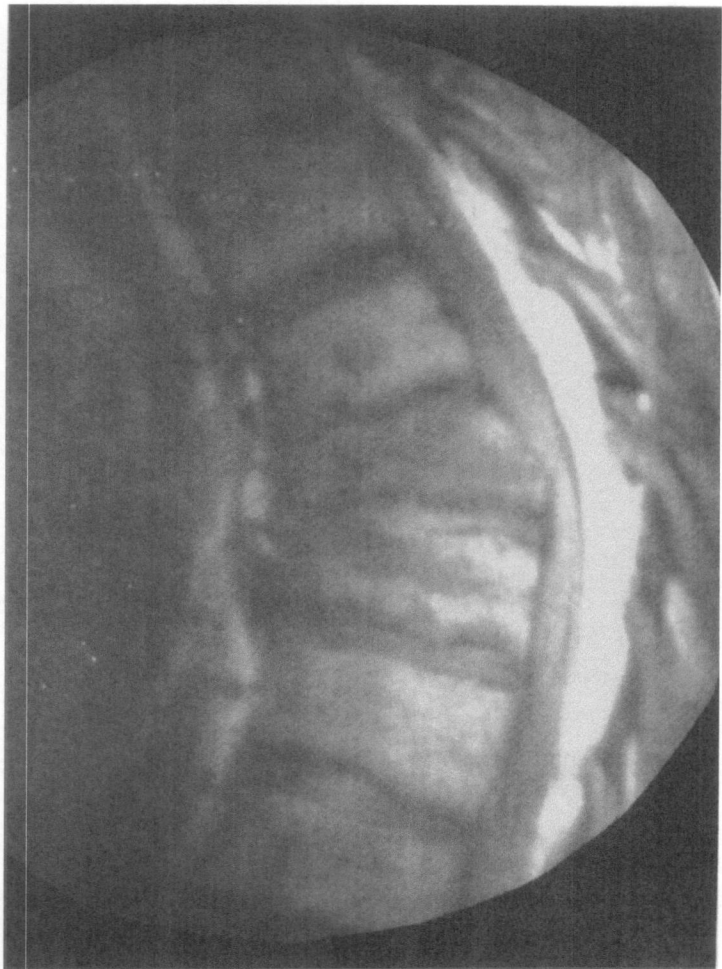

Figure 5.4. Sagittal T1 MRI demonstrates a traumatic thoracic vertebral compression with cord impingement.

Figure 5.5. **A:** Axial postmyelography CT demonstrates extradural soft tissue in the canal posteriorly on the right, deforming the sac and compressing the cord. **B,C:** Axial T1 MRI (with a short "flip angle" for a T2 /myelogram effect) and sagittal T1 demonstrate the extradural lesion posterior to the sac. Signal hyperintensity within the lesion on both pulse sequences is characteristic of subacute hematoma.

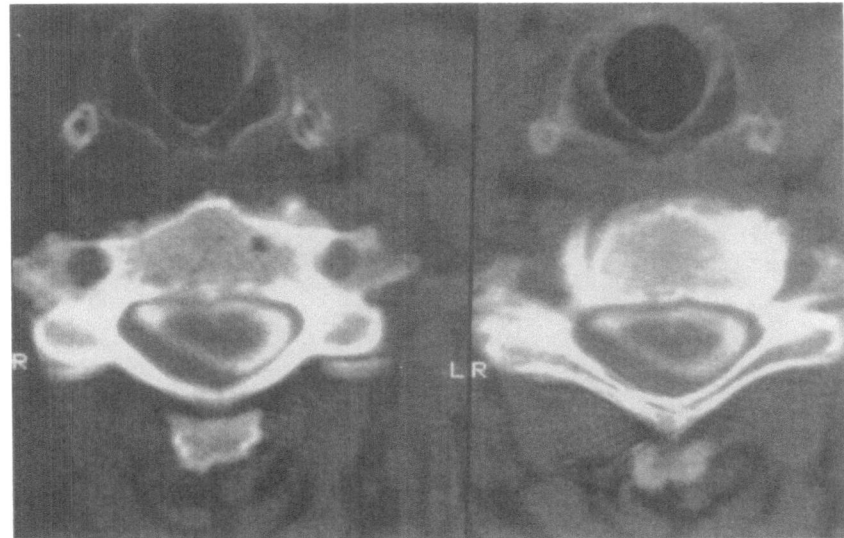

A

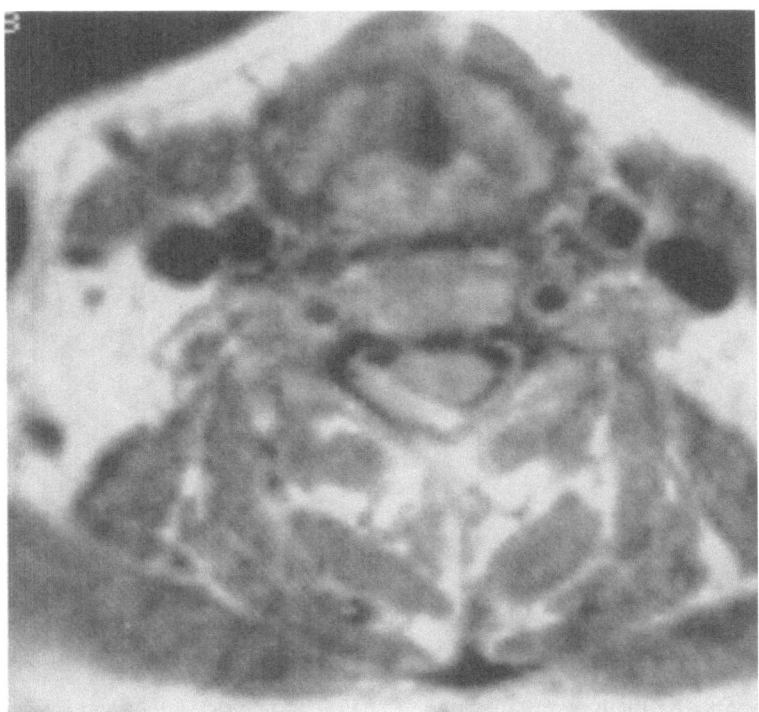

B

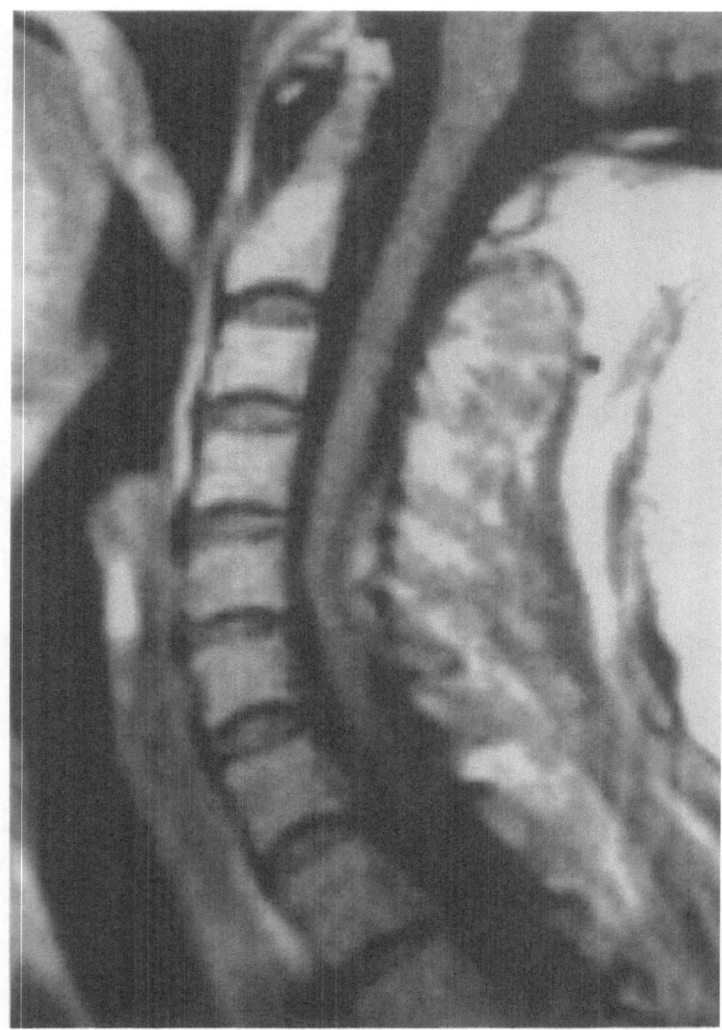

Figure 5.5. C

Figure 5.6. A: Pantopaque myelogram, AP view demonstrates right C8 and T1 root avulsions. **B:** Axial postmyelography CT in a different patient (same patient as Figure 3) demonstrates left-sided cervical root avulsions.

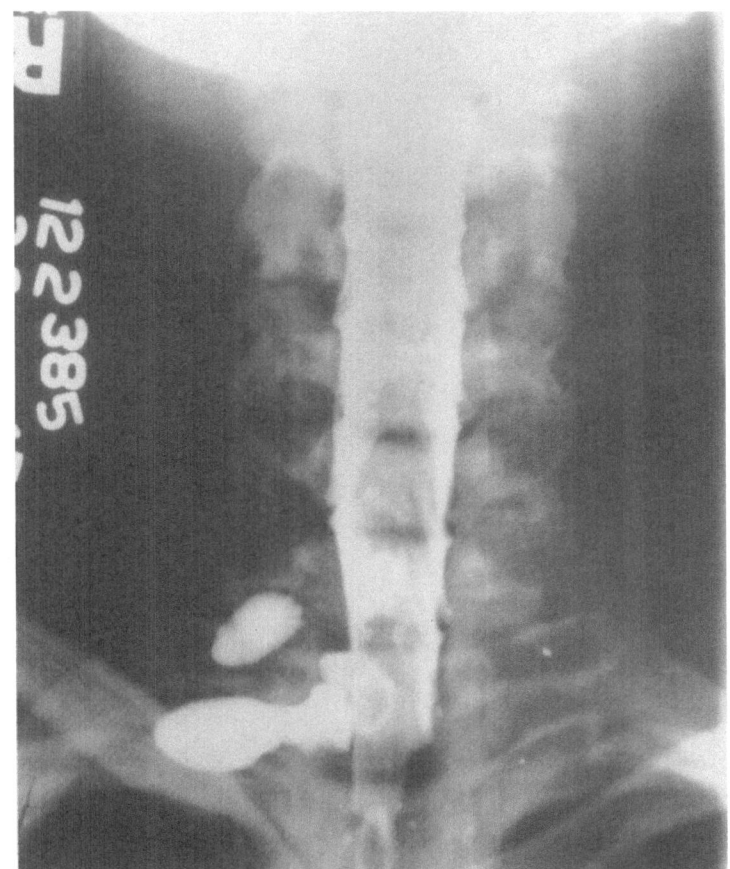

A

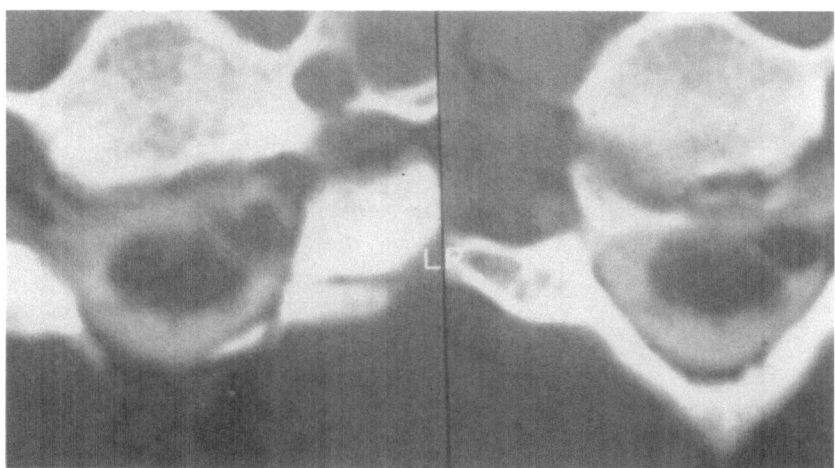

B

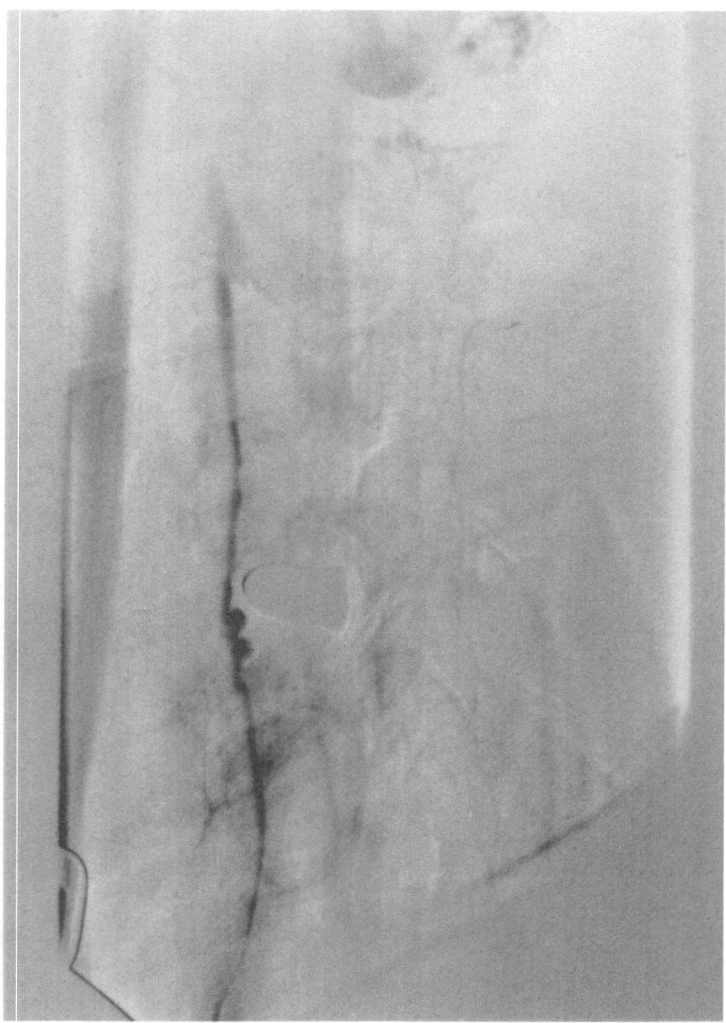

Figure 5.7. Lateral view, vertebral angiogram (subtraction film) demonstrates a bilobed traumatic pseudoaneurysm of the vertebral artery at the level of the bullet (seen posteriorly).

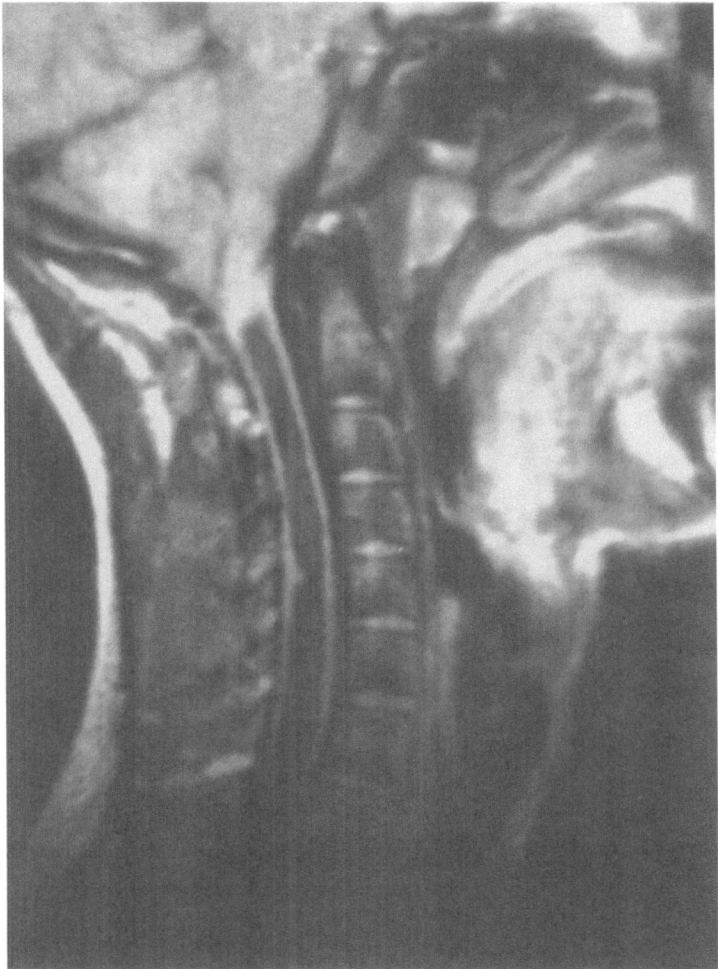

Figure 5.8. Sagittal T1 MRI demonstrates low (CSF) signal intensity within a large posttraumatic cervical syrinx.

from associated cyst by its enhancement (Fig. 5.11). *Extra*medullary, extradural cysts may occur as congenital diverticulae of the thecal sac, which may or may not contain nerve roots. These are easily diagnosed by MR if both T1 and T2 imaging is performed. Extradural spinal meningeal cysts may also occur posteriorly in the spinal subarachnoid space where they may result in neuroaxial compression/"block." These are best examined by CT myelography following sequential cyst and sac punctures for contrast instillation, which are separated in time (Fig. 5.12).

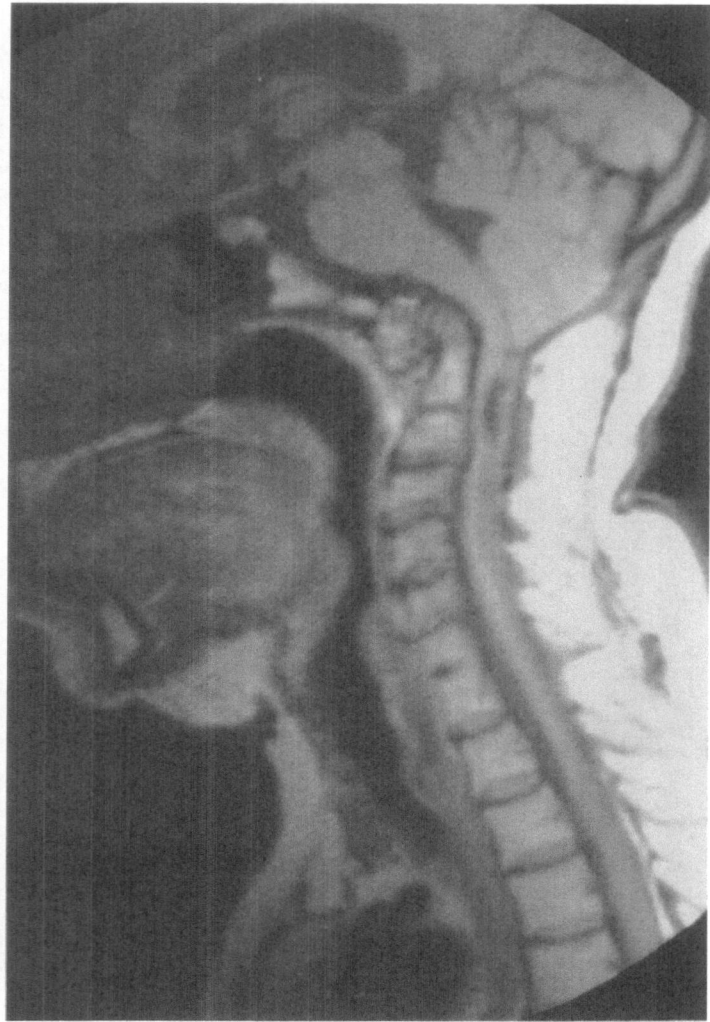

Figure 5.9. Sagittal T1 MRI demonstrates intramedullary low signal intensity due to myelomalacia in a patient with congenital C1-2 anomaly that resulted in chronic cord impingement.

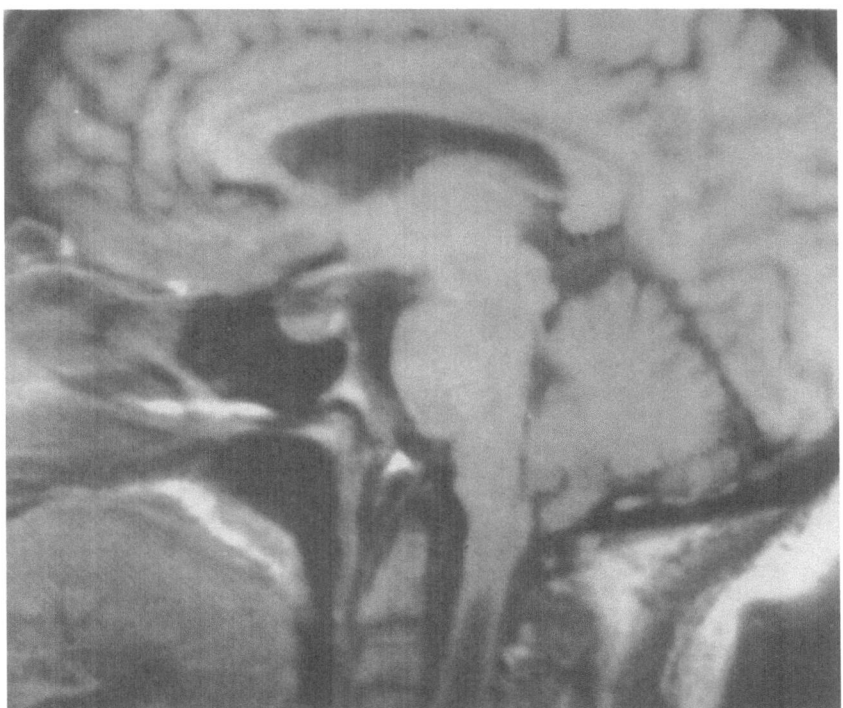

Figure 5.10. Sagittal T1 weighted MRI shows hypointense signal due to CSF within a syrinx in a patient with a Chiari I malformation.

Spinal vascular malformations, which include Arteriovenous Malformations AVMs (fistulous communications between arteries and veins) (Fig. 5.13) and cavernous hemangiomas (dilated sinusoids lacking normal intervening neural tissue) are easily detected by MRI due to the characteristic signal void of flowing blood and the easily recognized MR characteristics of hemorrhage. Thus, AVMs are typically diagnosed by their serpiginous signal void—with attention to potential confusion with artifact due to CSF flow phenomena. CSF pulsations around exiting nerve roots and the septum posticum are especially prominent in the thoracic region. This altered flow results in oval/curvilinear "pockets" of altered signal intensity within the spinal subarachnoid space, which demonstrate intermediate signal intensity on T1-pulse sequences and appear hypointense on T2 imaging—hence the confusion with serpiginous signal void due to flow in AVMs (Fig. 5.14). With true AVMs, concomitant cord edema due to venous congestion may occur and is readily apparent by MR imaging. Cavernous malformations have the pathognomonic appearance of a

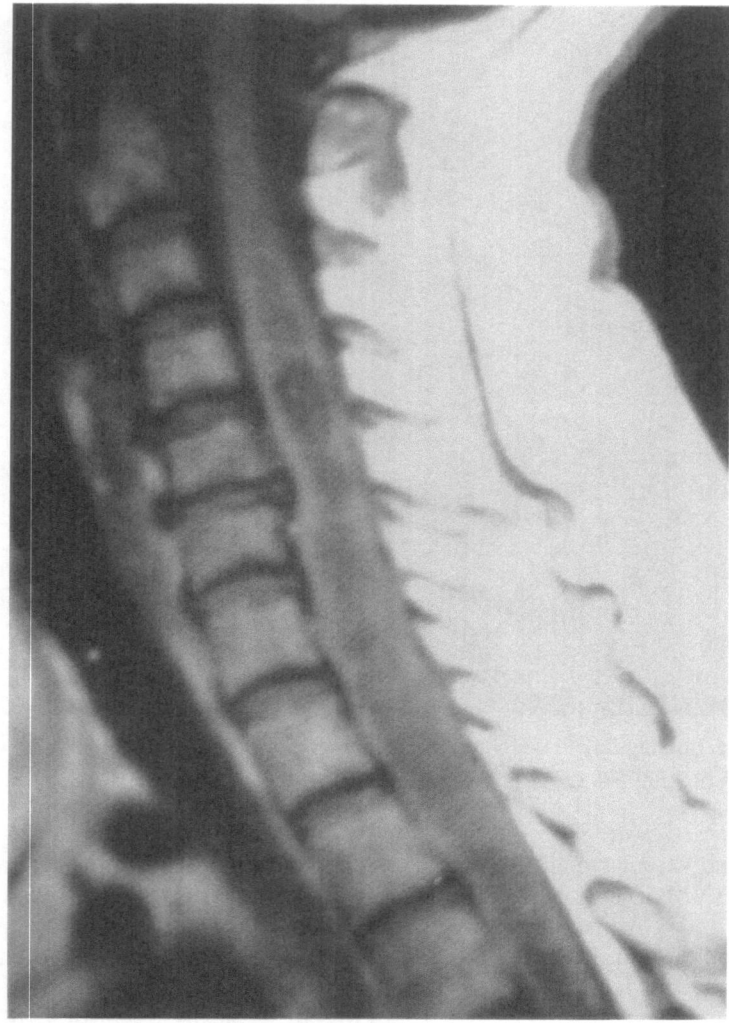

Figure 5.11. A: Sagittal T1 MRI demonstrates intramedullary low signal due to cyst and tumor.

peripheral ring of hypointensity surrounding a focus/foci of hyperintensity—characteristic of different blood breakdown products (Fig. 5.15). From a more interventional perspective, neuroimaging is an important adjunct to certain therapeutic procedures, in particular, the embolization of spinal vascular malformations performed preoperatively in some cases, and as an alternative to surgery in others.

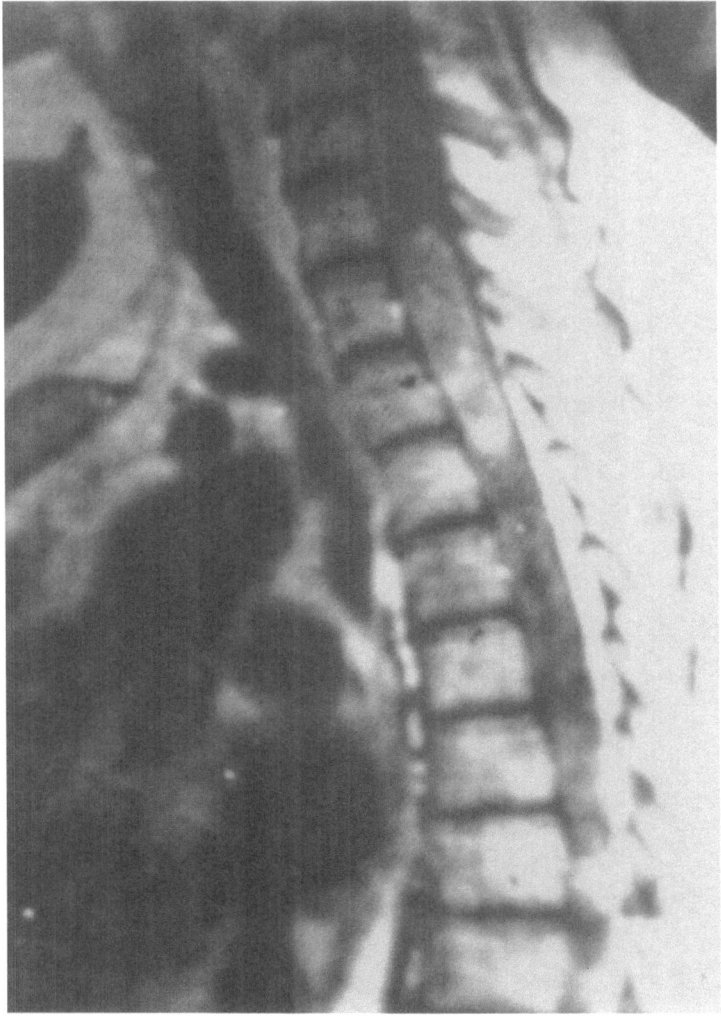

Figure 5.11. B: Repeat T1 MRI with gadolinium contrast demonstrates tumor enhancement distinct from the cyst above the lesion (ependymoma).

As applied to tumors of the spine, neuroimaging's classic role has been to define their anatomic relationship to the neural axis as intramedullary, intradural extramedullary, or extradural. Until the advent of MRI, lesion identification was on the basis of morphology and anatomic compartmentalization according to the above scheme by myelography combined with CT. MRI has two distinct advantages over these modalities—one is the capabil-

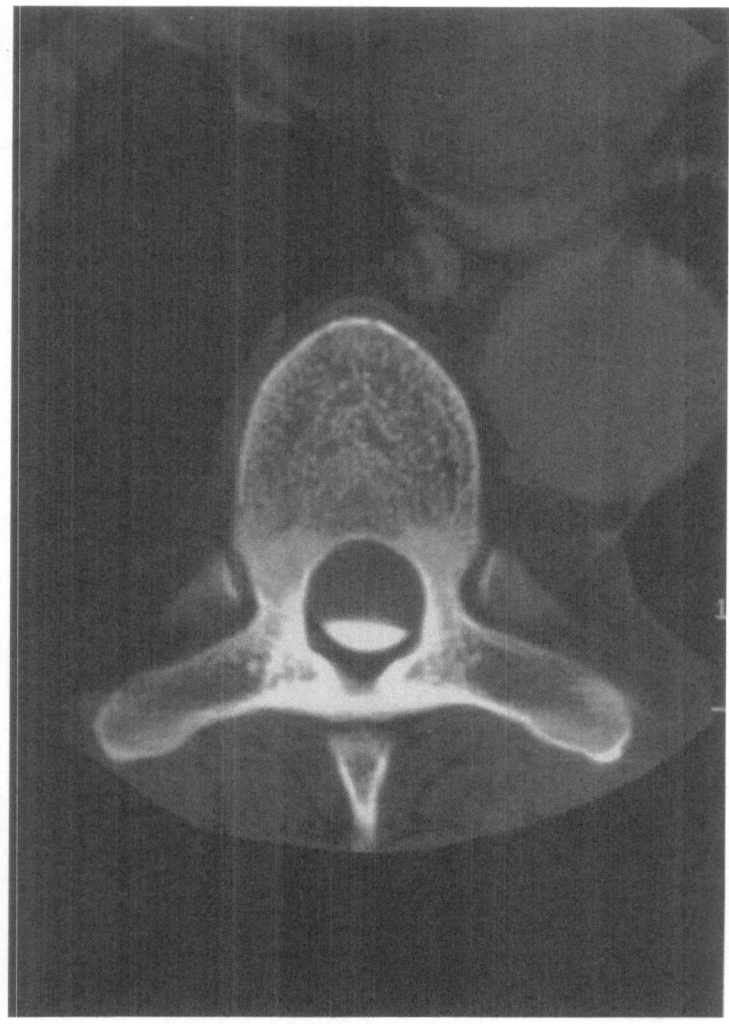

Figure 5.12. A: Axial CT, midthoracic level following instillation of water-soluble iodinated contrast by lumbar puncture. Filling of a posteriorly situated arachnoid cyst is demonstrated.

ity for *direct multiplanar* imaging, obviating the need for CT reconstructions from axial to sagittal, coronal and/or oblique planes; the second is lesion characterization, especially *within* the cord (Fig. 5.16). The appropriate combination of pulse sequences and utilization of intravenous paramagnetic contrast agents (gadolinium) has improved the detection of tumor extent and its differentiation from associated cyst/edema (Fig. 5.17).

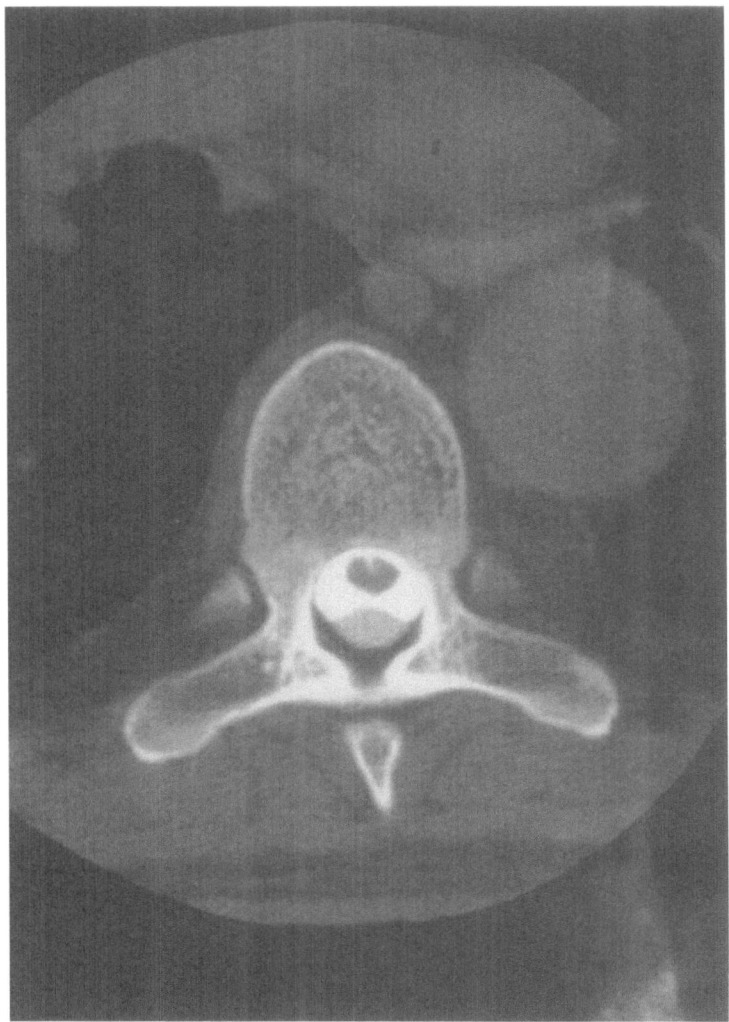

Figure 5.12. B: Axial CT at the same thoracic level following instillation of contrast by C1-2 puncture the following day. Note dense contrast within the subarachnoid space surrounding the thoracic cord and residual contrast appearing relatively less dense within the posteriorly situated cyst.

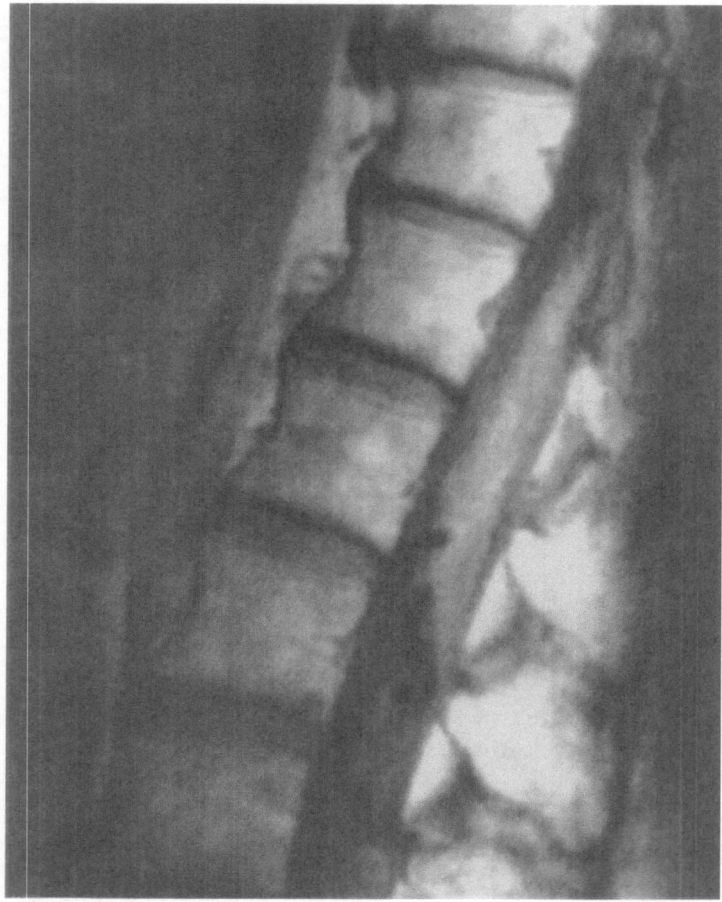

Figure 5.13. A: Sagittal T1 MRI demonstrates serpiginous signal void (due to flow) within prominent vessels surrounding the conus.

Hemorrhage into neoplasms can also be detected. Whereas the myelography-CT appearance of astrocytoma, ependymoma, and hemangioblastoma may be similar, their more *unique* features are better characterized with MRI. Contrast enhanced T1 MRI has higher sensitivity than any modality for intramedullary metastases and approaches myelography CT in detecting intradural tumor spread (Fig. 5.18). Extradural primary and secondary neoplasms can be characterized using MRI with the added advantage of directly visualizing neuroaxial impingement (Fig. 5.19). Complete block can be detected with T2 imaging, comparing pulse sequences with and without "flow compensation."

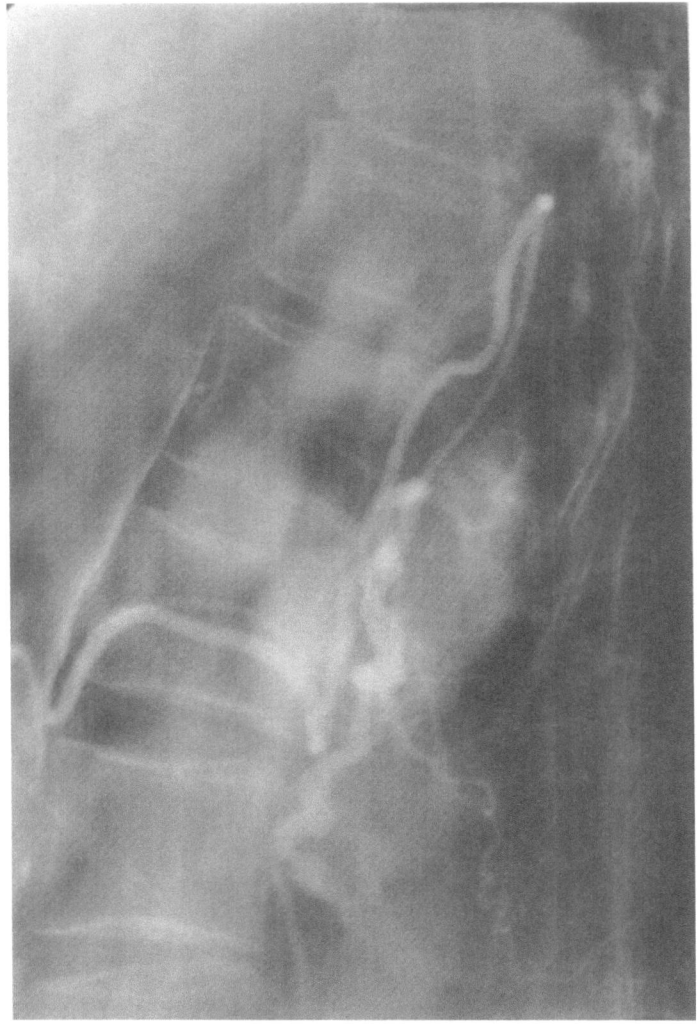

Figure 5.13. B: Spinal angiography in the lateral projection demonstrates the AVM, providing excellent correlation with the signal void structures seen on MRI.

Degenerative disease of the spine and its sequelae in the neural axis is perhaps the largest single etiologic component to spinal neurologic functional impairment. The anatomy, and to some extent the pathophysiology of this process, are exquisitely demonstrated by neuroimaging with myelography CT and MRI. Since the basis for standard MRI is proton imaging, the decrease in disc water content with disc degeneration is readi-

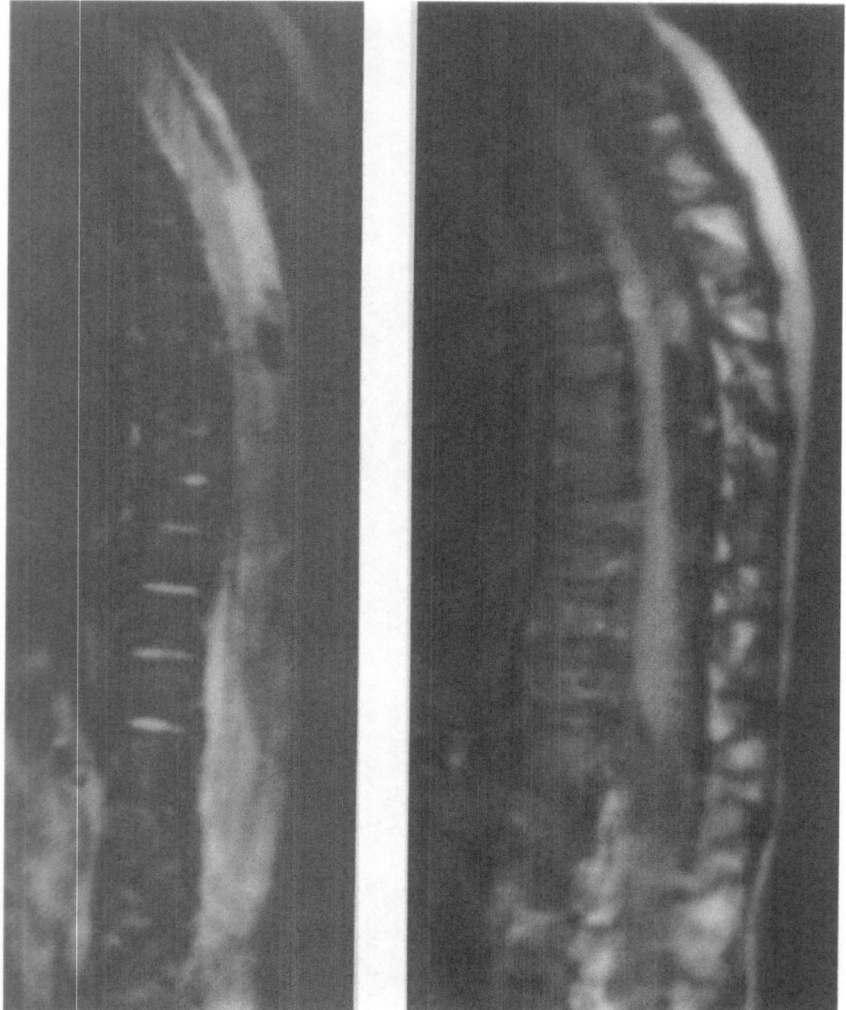

A   B

Figure 5.14. A: Sagittal T2 MRI demonstrates *apparent* signal void dorsal to the cord, within the hyperintense CSF. **B:** Corresponding T1 MRI demonstrates intermediate signal dorsal to the cord within the hypointense CSF.

ly apparent. Disc herniation, including free fragments can be diagnosed noninvasively by MRI using the correct combination of imaging planes and pulse sequences (Fig. 5.20). With MRI, bony degenerative changes are manifested by altered signal intensity within the marrow of involved vertebrae. The central and peripheral components to spinal stenosis (both congenital and acquired) can be assessed by combined axial and sagittal

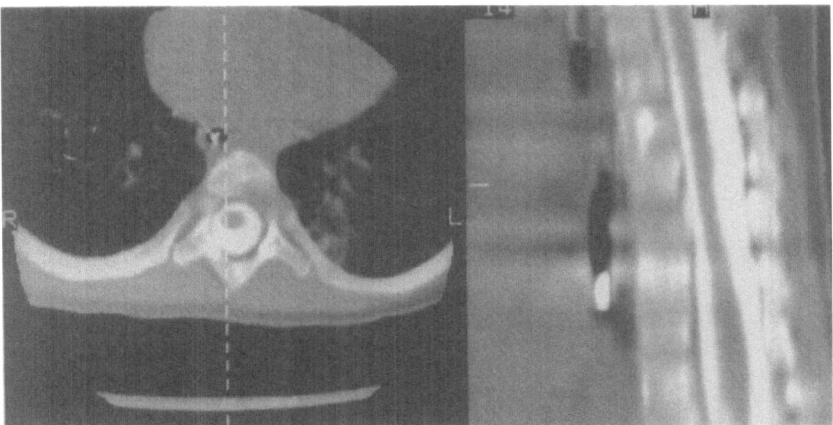

Figure 5.14. C: Axial postmyelography CT through the same thoracic level as well as a sagittal reconstruction demonstrate *only* CSF dorsal to the cord. This CSF flow phenomenon was accentuated by vertebral anomalies in this child with mild scoliosis. (Hence the apparent thinning of the cord, which is actually slightly out of plane of section).

MR imaging. Cord and/or root impingement by any of the above mechanical factors can also be detected, as well as underlying cord edema, myelomalacia, or frank cavitation (Fig. 5.21).

In the realm of primary neurodegenerative disease processes MRI is sensitive to demyelination, which is manifest by signal hyperintensity on T2 pulse sequences. This, however, is more easily achieved in cerebral than spinal imaging, due to the need for spine surface coils and cardiac gating, among other technical factors. These requirements are more easily met in cervical than thoracic imaging due to the prominent thoracic CSF pulsations described above. As the resolution of *axial* imaging improves, correlation of different patterns of cord atrophy can be made with primary and secondary degenerative disorders as has been done with CT myelography, and follow-up of treatment can be achieved noninvasively.

Postoperatively, MRI is valuable in defining fluid collections and in excluding hematoma. In addressing the postoperative question of disc versus scar, preliminary experience suggests that early imaging (i.e., within 15 minutes) post–gadolinium injection may show enhancement of epidural fibrosis, whereas herniated disc enhancement is reported to occur later (30 minutes postinjection).

In inflammatory conditions, conventional radiography and CT lag behind radionuclide imaging in the detection of disc space infection and osteomyelitis. MRI approaches the *early* sensitivity of the nuclear medicine techniques and exceeds that imaging modality in anatomically defining

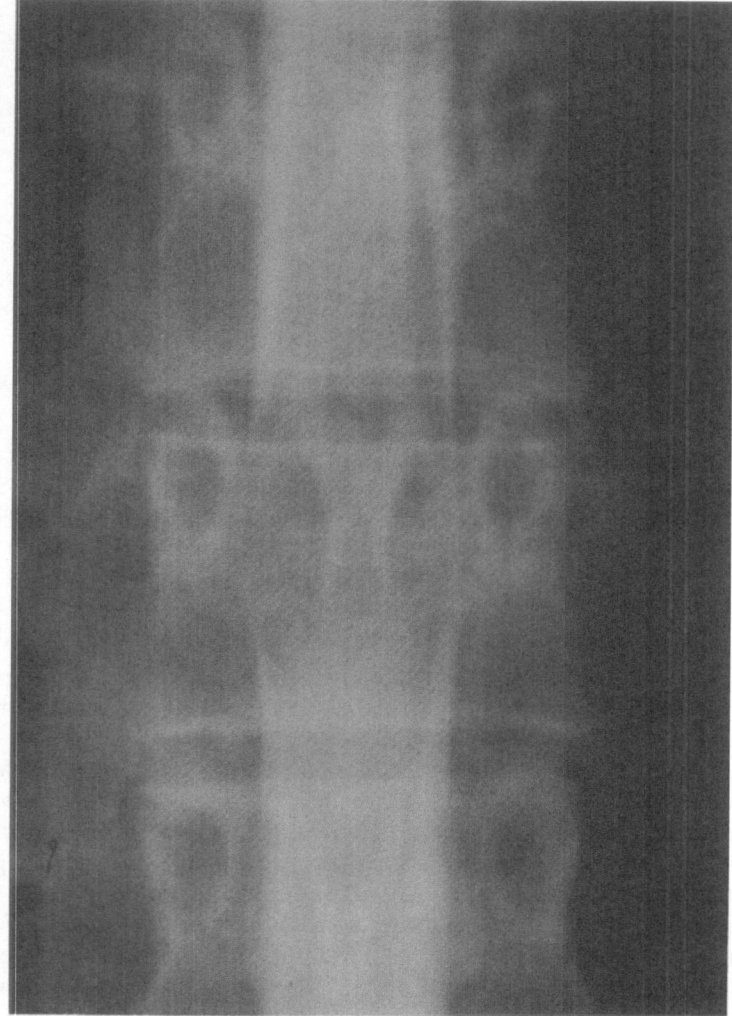

Figure 5.15. A: AP myelogram demonstrates focal intramedullary lesion in the thoracic cord.

epidural and paraspinal components of infection. MRI differentiates osteomyelitis from degenerative and neoplastic bony changes better than conventional radiography or radionuclide studies. With respect to intradural inflammation, the very modality, myelography, which has been regarded as the "gold standard" for diagnosing arachnoiditis may, depending on technique and circumstances, be among the contributing etiologic fac-

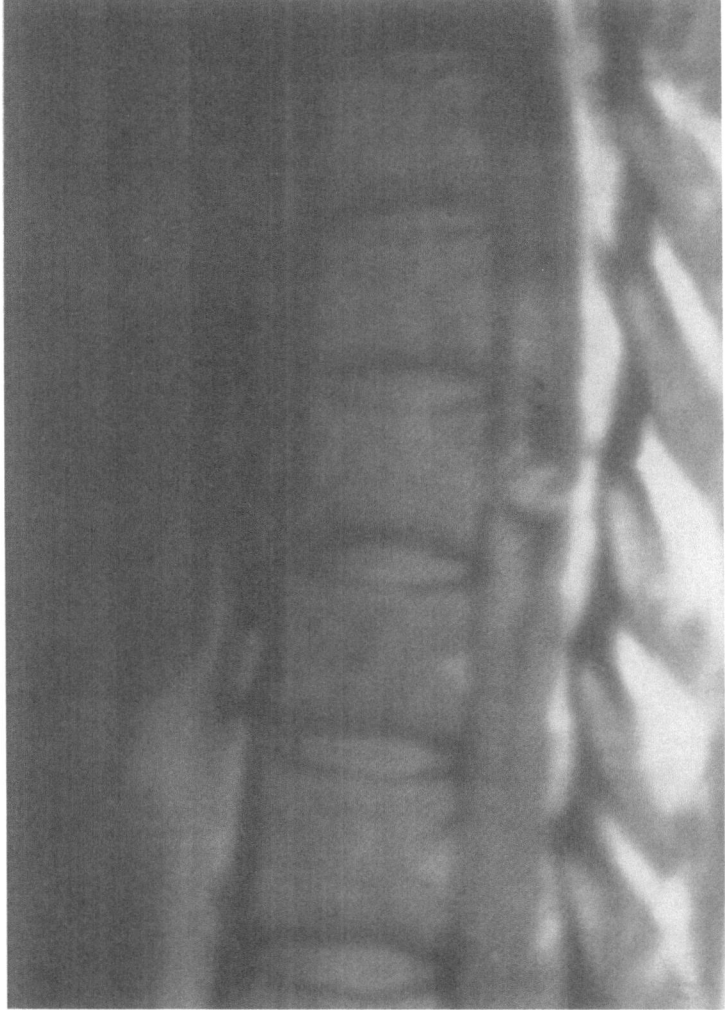

Figure 5.15. B: Sagittal T1 MRI characterized the lesion as a cavernous malformation by the pathognomonic mixed signal intensity due to hemorrhage in various stages.

tors. Therefore, the capability of MRI to make the diagnosis is an important issue. Clumping of nerve roots can be seen on high resolution sagittal and axial images, especially at the lower lumbar levels where normal variation is less confusing than at L2 and L3. Intradural neoplastic seeding may be more difficult to exclude, even with the use of paramagnetic contrast.

With the advent of high field MRI, neuroimaging "has arrived" at its

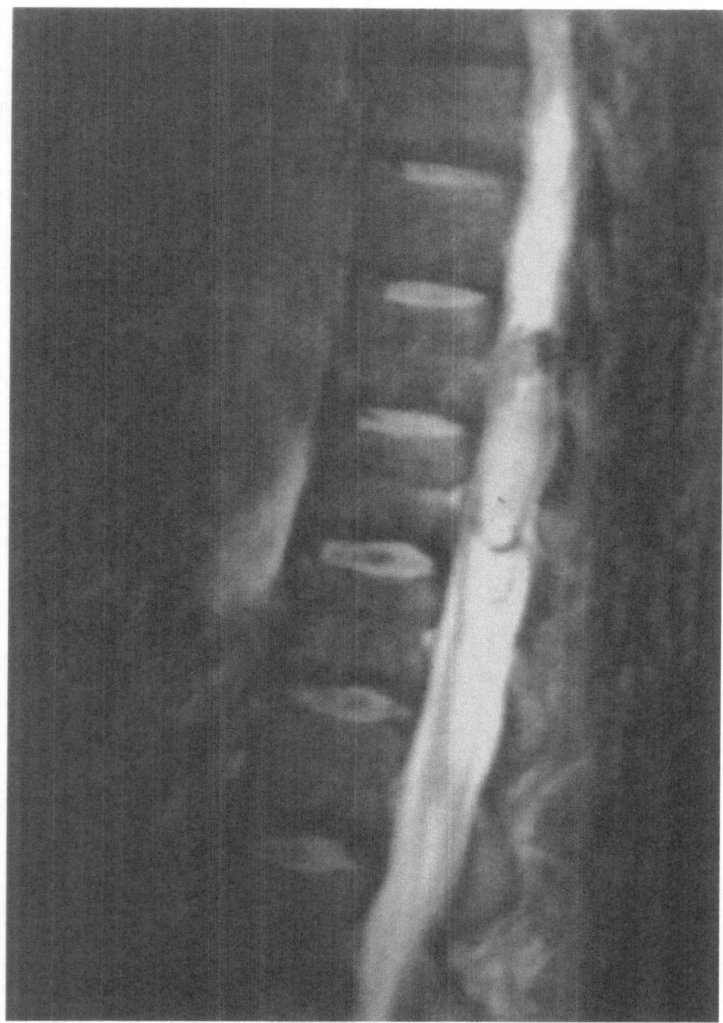

Figure 5.16. A: Sagittal T2 MRI shows a well-encapsulated lesion with edema above and below.

role of defining neuroanatomy and pathology. With advanced MR technology and new modalities on the horizon, neuroimaging can address functional anatomy with MR angiography; MR spectroscopy, in addition to PET and single positron emission computed tomography (SPECT) imaging have potential applications in studying neurophysiology. Understanding the functional anatomy and neurophysiology is crucial to establishing the potential for cord regeneration and recovery.

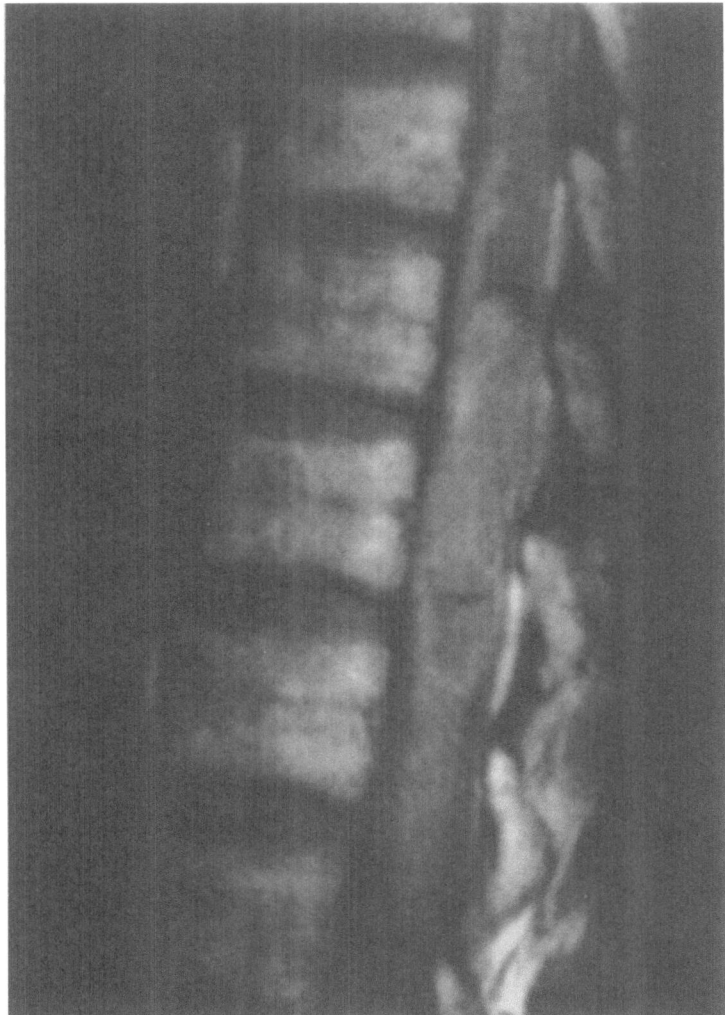

Figure 5.16. B: Sagittal T1 MRI demonstrates high signal within the lesion (a pigmented schwannoma) due to the paramagnetic effect of melanin.

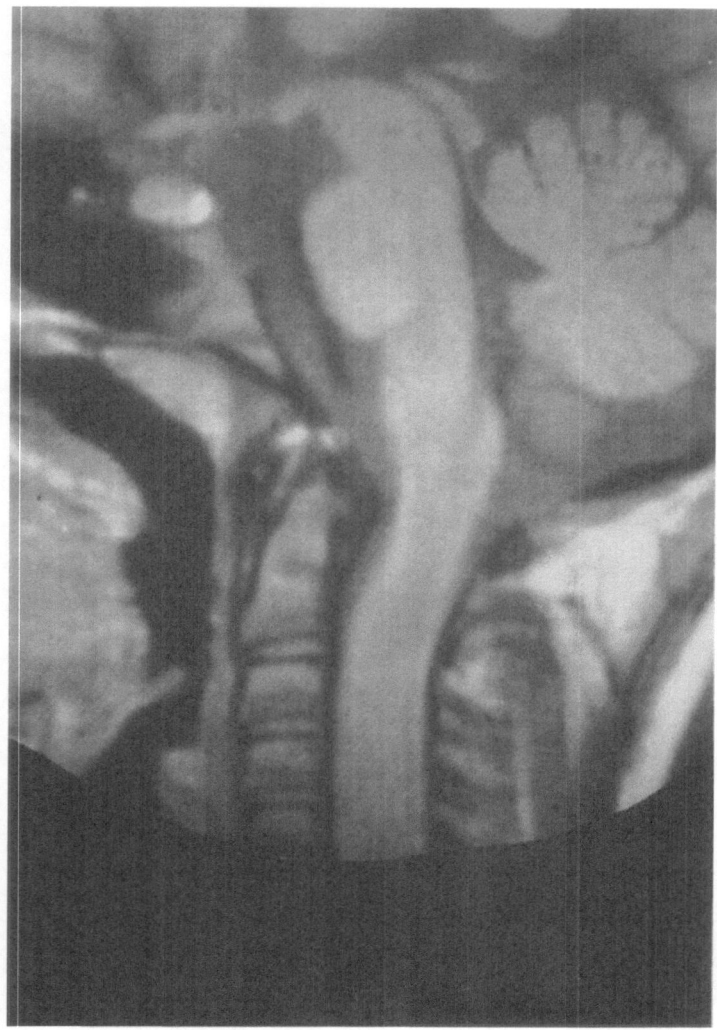

Figure 5.17. A: Precontrast sagittal T1 MRI shows enlargement of the upper cervical cord from C2 through C5.

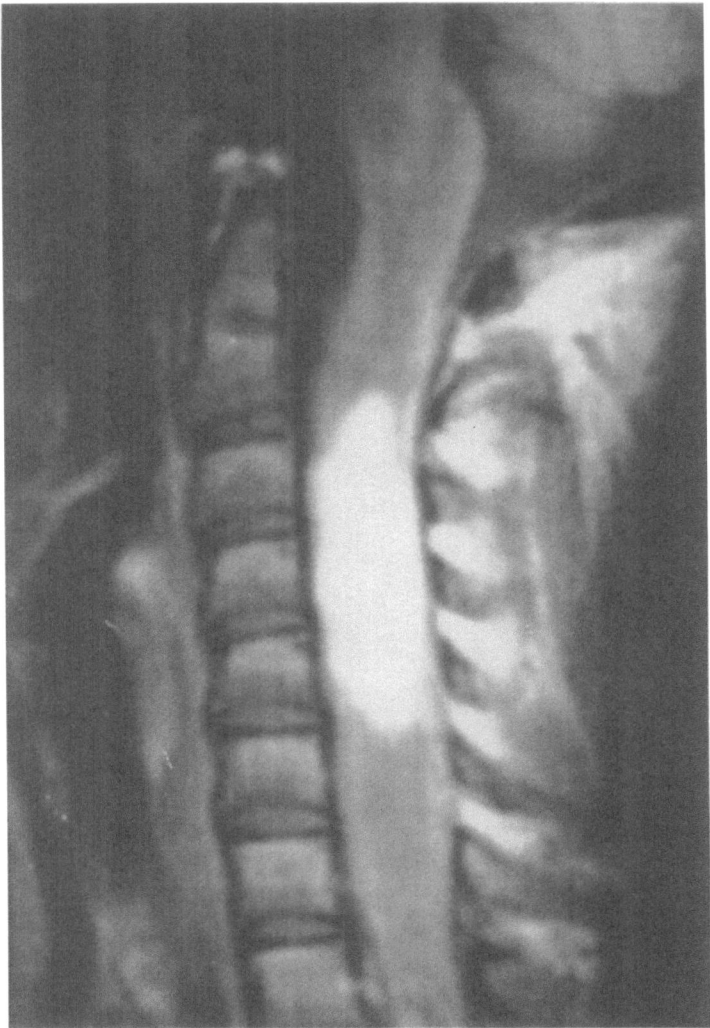

Figure 5.17. B: Sagittal T1 MRI postcontrast (gadolinium) defines the intramedullary neoplasm (a primitive neuroectodermal tumor) within the cord, which is diffusely widened due to edema above and below the lesion.

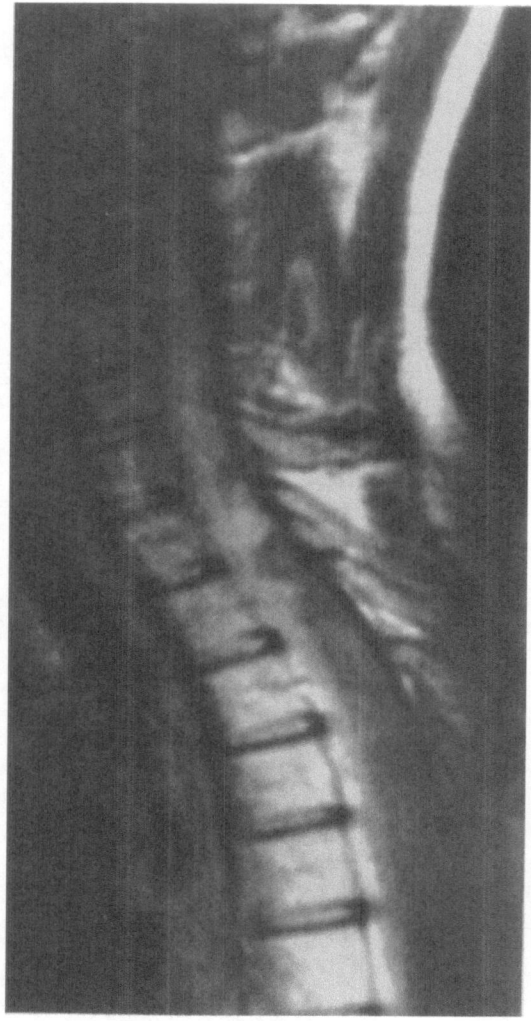

Figure 5.18. A: Precontrast sagittal T1 MRI demonstrates faint nodular soft tissue signal along the dorsal aspect of the cord.

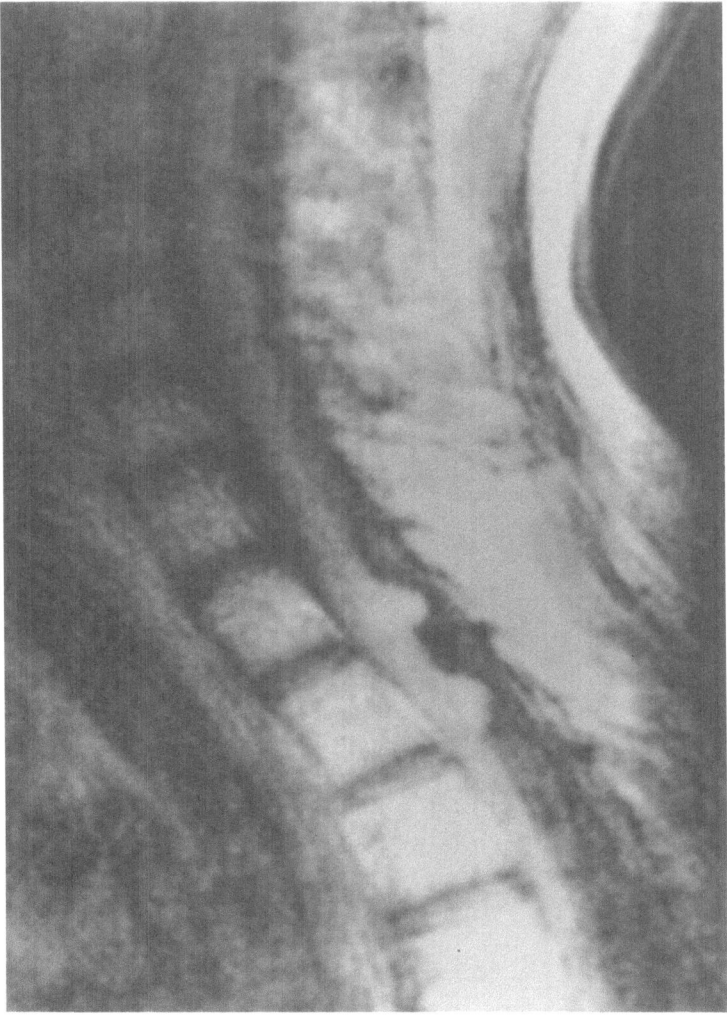

Figure 5.18. B: Gadolinium administration enhances the conspicuity of the intradural metastases on T1 imaging in this patient with ependymoma seeding.

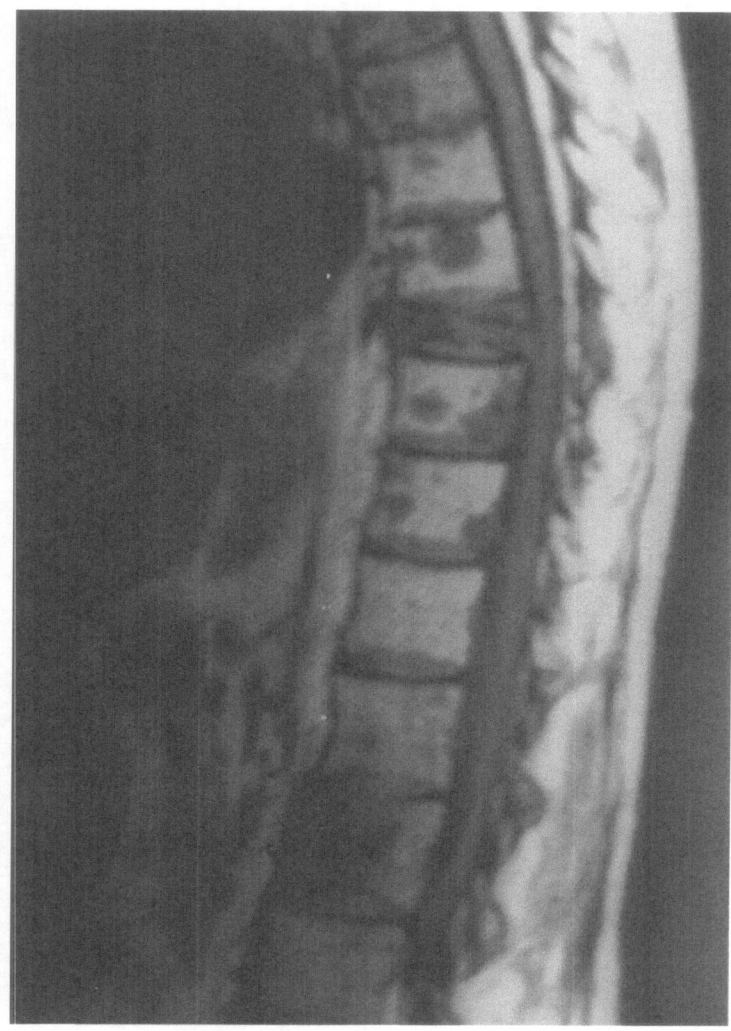

Figure 5.19. Sagittal T1 MRI shows extensive vertebral body metastases as nodular soft tissue signal replacing the normally hyperintense signal due to marrow fat. Note *complete* marrow replacement in the collapsed vertebra and cord compression.

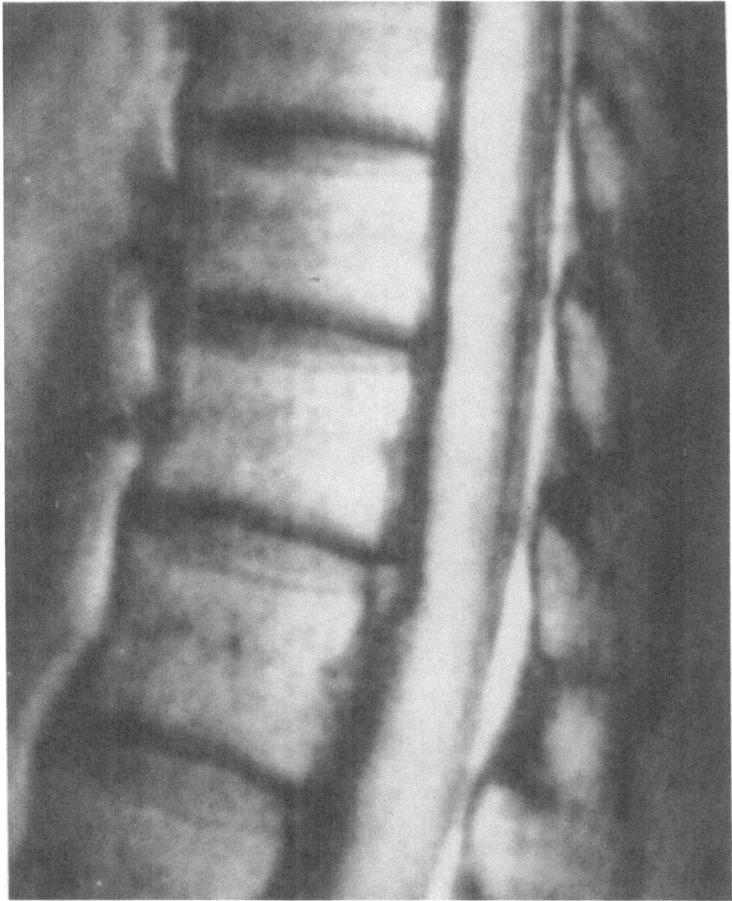

Figure 5.20. Sagittal T1 MRI demonstrates herniated thoracic disc with cord impingement by disc fragment.

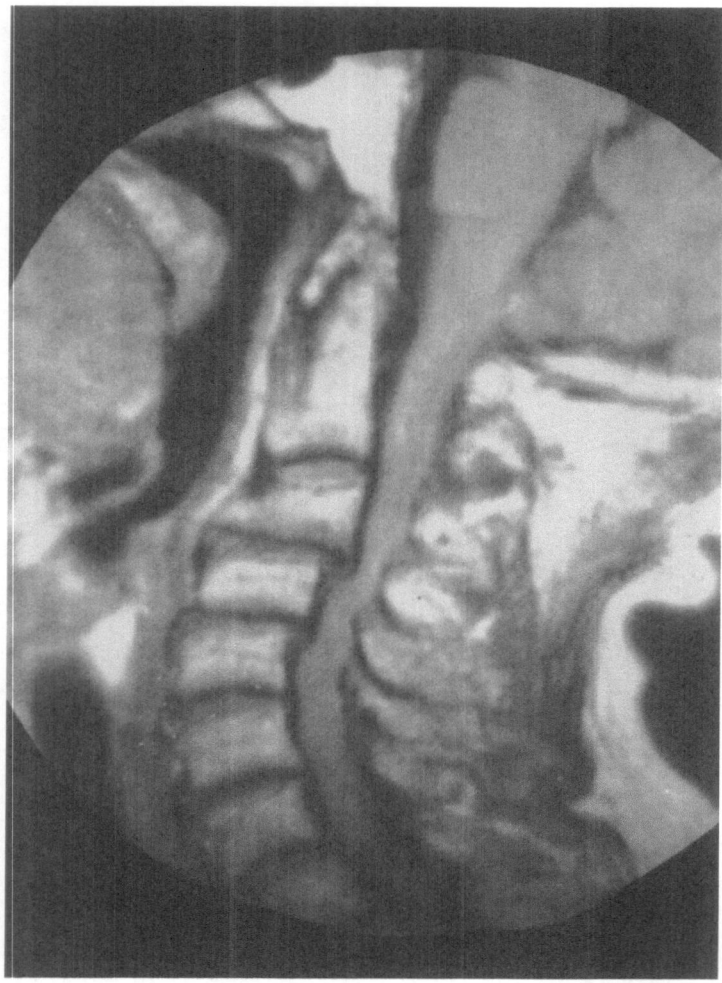

Figure 5.21. A: Sagittal T1 MRI shows mechanical cord impingement with acquired segmental stenosis due to severe cervical spondylosis.

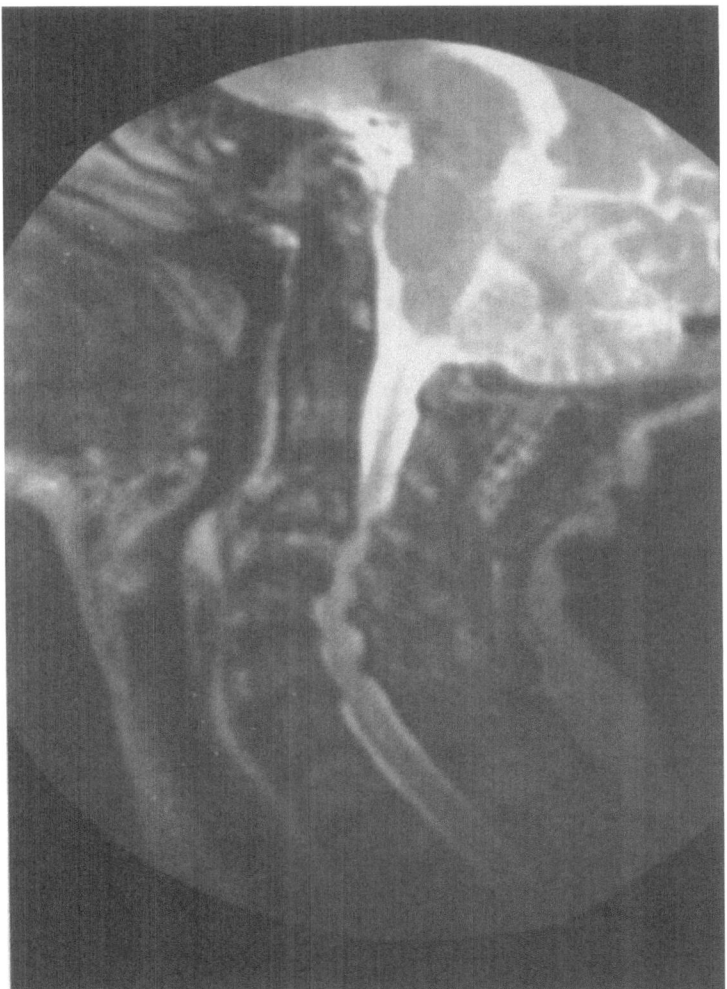

Figure 5.21. B: Sagittal T2 MRI (note "myelogram effect" due to hyperintense CSF signal surrounding the cord) demonstrates obliteration of the CSF signal ventral and dorsal to the cord with impingement at multiple cervical levels.

Bibliography

1. Bronskill MJ, McVeigh ER, Kucharczyk W, Henkelman RM. Syrinx-like artifacts on MR images of the spinal cord. *Radiology*. 1988;166:486–488.
2. Enzmann DR, O'Donohue J, Rubin JB, et al. CSF pulsations within nonneoplastic spinal cord cysts. *AJR*. 1987;149:149–157.
3. Fontaine S, Melansun D, Cosgrove R, et al. Cavernous hemangiomas of the spinal cord: MR imaging. *Radiology*. 1988;166:839–841.
4. Hueftle M, Modic MT, Ross JS, et al. Lumbar spine: post-operative imaging with GD-DTPA. *Radiology*. 1988;167:817–824.
5. Haughton VM. MR imaging of the spine. Radiology. 1988;166:297–301.
6. Hyman RA, Gorey MT. Imaging strategies for MR of the spine. *Radiol Clin North Am*. 1988;26(3):505–533.
7. Levy LM, DiChiro G, Brooks RA, et al. Spinal cord artifacts from truncation errors during MR imaging. *Radiology*. 1988;166:479–483.
8. Modic MT, Masaryk T, Paushter D. Magnetic resonance imaging of the spine. *Radiol Clin North Am*. 1986;24(2):229–245.
9. Modic MT, Masaryk TJ, Ross JS, eds. *Magnetic resonance imaging of the spine*. Chicago: Year Book Medical Publishers, 1988.
10. Mawad ME, Hilal SK, Fetell MR, et al. Patterns of spinal cord atrophy by metriazamide CT. *AJNR*. 1983;4:611.
11. Rubin JB, Enzmann DR. Imaging of spinal CSF pulsation by 2DFT MR: significance during clinical imaging. *AJNR* 1987;8:297–306.
12. Sze G. Gadolinium-DTPA in spinal disease. *Radiol Clin North Am*. 1988;26(5):1009–1023.
13. Sze G, Krol G, Zimmerman RD, Deck MDF. Intramedullary disease of the spine: diagnosis using Gadolinium-DTPA-enhanced MR imaging. *AJNR*. 1988;9:847–858.

Discussion

Dr. Hecht-Nielsen said that he had considerable experience with magnetic resonance when it was used to determine polymer structure. It had nothing to do with medicine at that time. All we used it for was spectroscopy and it's unbelievable, too. You can actually see how the molecules are put together. When do you believe that that technique will be exploited in medicine and what do you see as the early impact it will have?

Dr. Bello responded that it is already being done in terms of sodium scanning and the distribution of sodium and its role in cerebral edema. The spectroscopy that we use in terms of imaging actually generates an MR scan. The resolution of that scan is not nearly as anatomically clear as what you've seen presented here. The signal is coming from sodium atoms rather than the hydrogen of water.

Dr. Hecht-Nielsen asked, So is that the big thing? The proton signals are so much stronger than the signals from any of the other atoms that you lose spatial resolution. You have to sacrifice a great deal of that to get chemical resolution.

Dr. Bello: Yes. I've not seen beautiful resolution (in sodium scanning), but that's not really the information that's being looked for. It is the distribution of these elements and the significance of them in that distribution that is being searched for.

Dr. Hecht-Nielsen continued, because from a chemical engineering standpoint there is in principle no reason why you couldn't pick a particular molecule like choline and literally build a cross-sectional map of choline density or for that matter any other molecule. So it would seem that the future is very bright, but it may take magnetic fields, which would be rather daunting, to achieve that.

Signal Voids in Cysts

Dr. Friedman asked, Do you think that the presence of a signal void in a cyst within the spinal cord would give you the same information that this cine MR would? Is the signal void going to tell you that there is abnormal flow and movement within the syrinx such that it will have the ability to predict that a given syrinx will progressively enlarge and lead to clinical disturbances.

Dr. Bello responded, No, the people who are trying to derive this same information from static images are doing it in the following way. They do an image that is flow-compensated, which constitutes most of the images that you see. These images look very nice and the anatomic resolution is great and there is a cyst on that image and the flow-compensation takes care of flow that would degrade the image. Then they do a non–flow-compensated image and it is a poorer quality image, but you can at least still see where the cyst is. If there is flow in that cyst, its configuration and its signal should degrade, just like the rest of the scan where you have flow in the vessels and flow in the CSF, and if it remains very sharp then they try to infer that the flow is significant everywhere else on the scan and not in the cyst. It's slightly inferior to the method where you actually have the cine, but the people who are trying to do it from static images are doing a flow-suppressed or flow-compensated scan and a non–flow-compensated scan and comparing them. So you can get information from plain images, not quite as well, but two sets of images, not just by looking at a signal void on one image.

The Question of Toxicity of Large Magnetic Fields

Dr. Holtzman asked if there is any known toxicity from exposure to large magnetic fields.

Dr. Bello responded that heat is what most people have been concerned about, not in amounts that have been biologically or physiologically significant in any known setting.

Dr. Hecht-Nielsen added that several of his friends have spent years working in and around magnetic fields that are much greater, from 8 to 20 tesla, without any known physiological changes or symptomatology.

Dr. Leeds noted that is true but those magnets are not the magnitude that are being used clinically today. You don't need the protection because of the gauss. You are discussing two different tools. The main factor is the heat. The current factor is 4 watts per kilogram, which is about 2 tesla.

Disadvantages of MRI

Dr. Leeds mentioned that the point concerning MR microscopy, which we have not yet developed, and MR spectroscopy is that it will require magnetic fields of 8 or 12 tesla and we are using 2 tesla. Therefore we are handicapped even with sodium and phosphorus and there is no way that one can image in depth, and that is the great disadvantage of the present system. We can obtain a gross image, but it is impossible to obtain 1-mm-, 3-mm-, or even 5-mm-thick slices and identify focal structures at this time.

CHAPTER 6

Neuroradiologic Features of Spinal Cord Pathology

Norman E. Leeds

The first point I would like to make is that one would like to avoid technical errors that tend to mislead and point in the wrong direction. The first pitfall to be avoided is that which results in an apparent normal image when, in fact, a lesion exists. In one of the patients to be presented by Dr. Holtzman subsequently, the magnetic resonance image (MRI) appeared normal, but the computed tomography (CT) revealed cord atrophy. The reason for this was that averaging of information occurred because of patient motion, resulting in a normal-appearing spinal cord on MR. The neurologist did not accept this information since he was convinced that the patient had a cord abnormality. This was subsequently substantiated. Persistence of examination is important even with misleading information. Thus, MR may not reveal appropriate information in some instances.

Partial volume phenomena occur because of slice thickness variations and lack of precision in contiguous slices. Thus, one may observe in some cases a pseudosyringomyelia. This results from a superimposition of cerebrospinal fluid (CSF) appearing to be within the cord (Fig. 6.1). This false appearance may be confirmed by using an axial slice, which reveals the true location of the "cavity" in questionable cases. The appearance of the central black line on sagittal T_1 MRI images may also be due to truncation artifact.

In a patient with cervical spine trauma, the objective is to identify the pathology, and with this noninvasive examination one may exclude the presence of a surgical lesion. I believe the important key, and it is a big key, that was alluded to in this morning's presentation, is the presence of cord edema. Edema may be focal or diffuse. Diffuse edema is difficult to visualize. An extruded disk may be observed after trauma. In addition, because of increased intensity on T_1, balanced imaging, and T_2 weighted images, hematomas may also be recognized.

Another patient presented to the neurologist with a story that was bizarre, but suggestive of spinal multiple sclerosis. On the proton density image, a focal density was observed overlying the spinal cord. The neurologist substantiated his clinical diagnosis based on this hyperintense signal

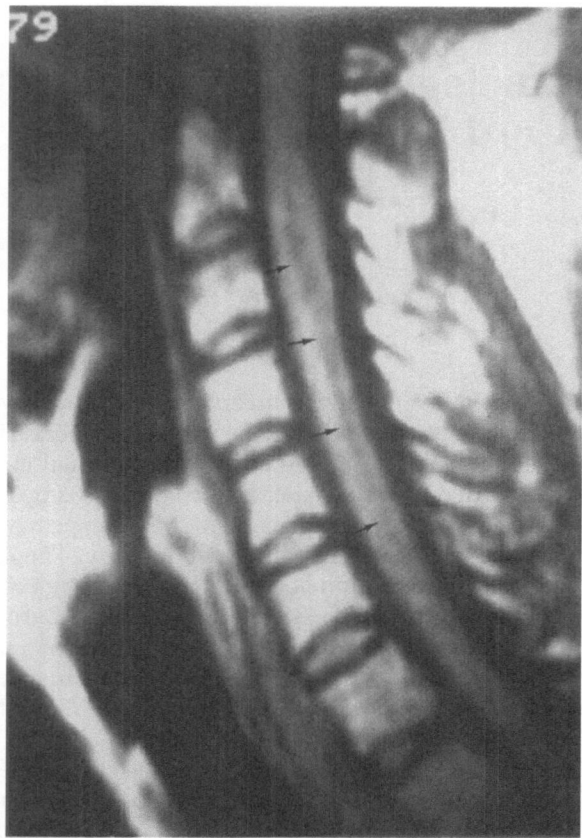

Figure 6.1. Spurious central cavity (*arrows*) as a result of a truncation artifact.

within the spinal cord (Fig. 6.2). Note that it extends beyond the confines of the cord and is not an intrinsic image, but represents an artifact.

In the next example, a Gradient Recall Acquisition in Steady State (GRASS) density image or field echo is used. Gradient or field echoes are used with angles less than 90° and are acquired with shorter acquisition times. The advantage of this technique is to visualize vascular structures. The next patient had bizarre symptoms related to the spinal cord. In this case, the patient had an arteriovenous malformation demonstrated by the flow void that reveals abnormal vessels on this MR gradient echo image (Fig. 6.3). On the myelogram, the presence of a vascular malformation may be recognized by noting the abnormal vascular pattern (Fig. 6.3). In this case, the advantage of the noninvasive MR is observed.

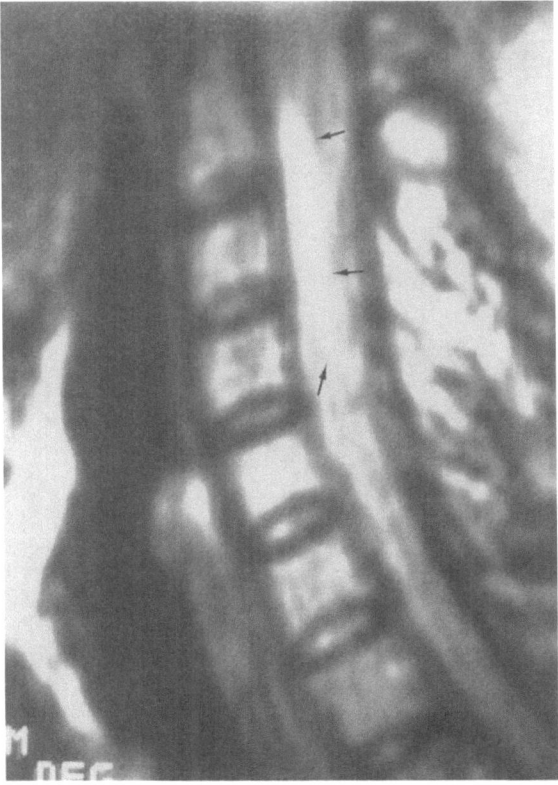

Figure 6.2. Hyperintense signal (*arrows*) representing an artifact extending beyond confines of spinal cord.

MR is often now the first study being done in the investigation of spinal lesions since it can solve many problems. It will help in revealing spinal cord changes that demonstrate the potential for spinal cord recovery (Table 6.1). I believe, just as pneumoencephalography disappeared, myelography will continue to diminish and eventually may disappear with the continued improvement in MRI.

The next is a spectacular case. This is a young woman with bizarre cerebral and spinal symptomatology. Imaging studies revealed a cystic collection in the posterior fossa in the inferior vermis, compressing the medulla (Fig. 6.4A,B). In this case the answer is on the films. A prominent posterior inferior cerebellar artery demonstrated by the presence of a flow void was observed on another image.

The presence of this abnormal vessel, plus the cyst, allows one to make a

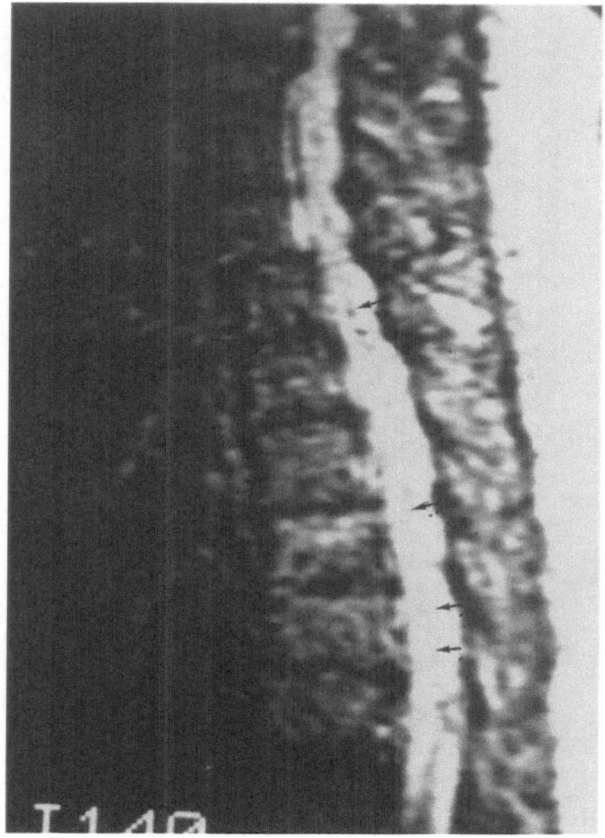

Figure 6.3A. GRASS density image of thoracic region reveals dilated tortuous vessels "signal void" of spinal AVM (*arrows*).

Table 6.1. Potential for recovery following spinal cord compromise.

Vascular insult	Demyelinating lesions
Ischemia	Inflammatory lesions
Infarction	Congenital lesions
Compressive lesion	Diastematomyelia
Degenerative disease of spine (spondylosis)	Tethered cord
Disk herniation	Neoplasms
Trauma	Tonsillar ectopia
Hematoma	
Contusion	
Bone compression	
Neoplasm	

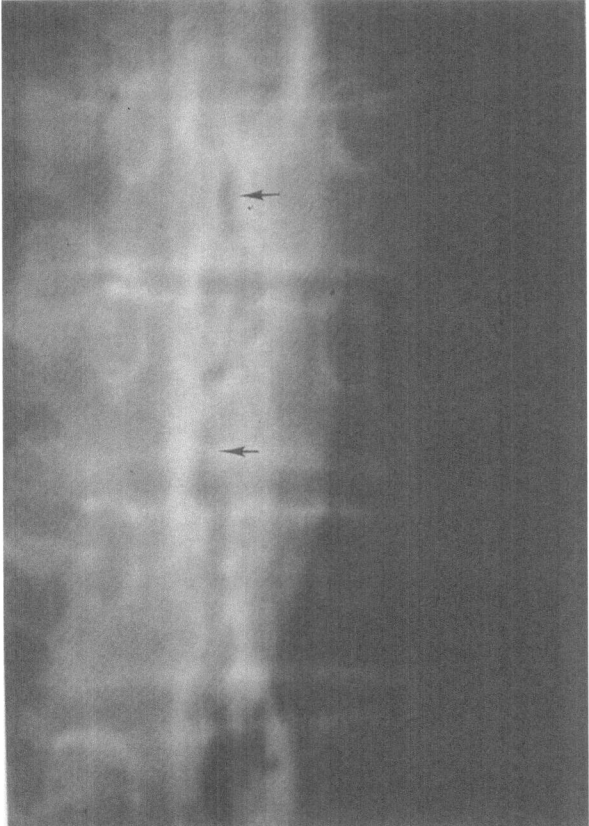

Figure 6.3B. Thoracic myelogram confirms presence of dilated vessels (*arrows*).

diagnosis of a hemangioblastoma. This case is complex as you will soon see. In addition to this cyst, which was part of the hemangioblastoma, there is a syrinx or hydromyelia. Using various planes (Fig. 6.4C,D), the extent of the cyst and its location can be appreciated.

The patient appears to have a hemangioblastoma and a syrinx. In addition to the expanded cord from the syringohydromyelia, hyperdensity from a nodule in the cervical region can be recognized as well as the extent of the cavity in the dorsal area. Prominent vessels with variations in intensity because of the alterations in flow pattern also may be recognized. The cavity extends all the way down to the caudal portion of the thecal sac (Fig. 6.4D). In fact, this patient has cystic cavities related to hemangioblastomatosis. In addition, multiple nodules are recognized throughout (Fig. 6.4D)

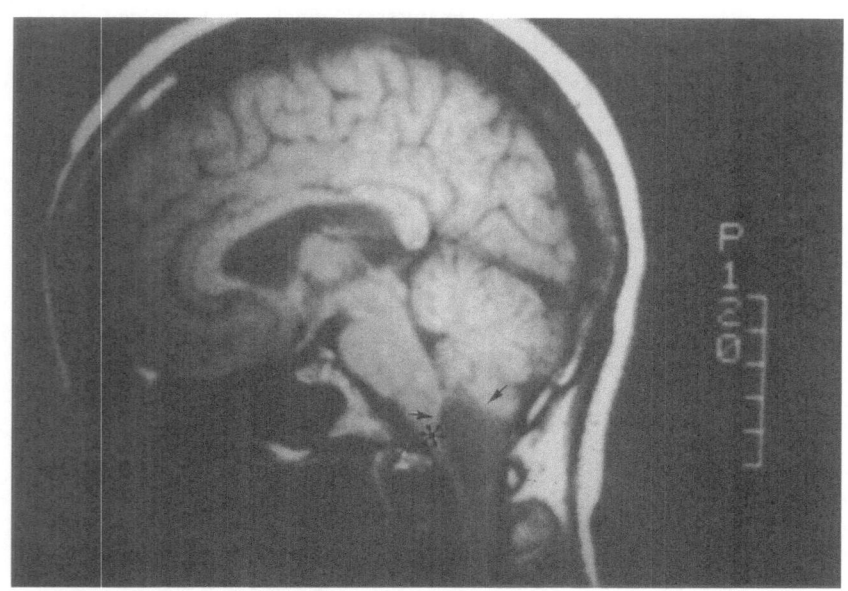

A

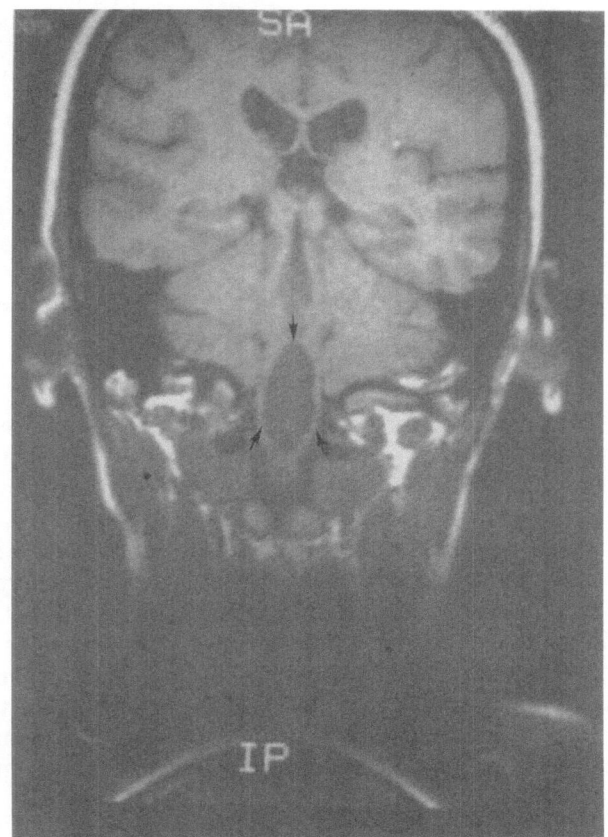

B

142

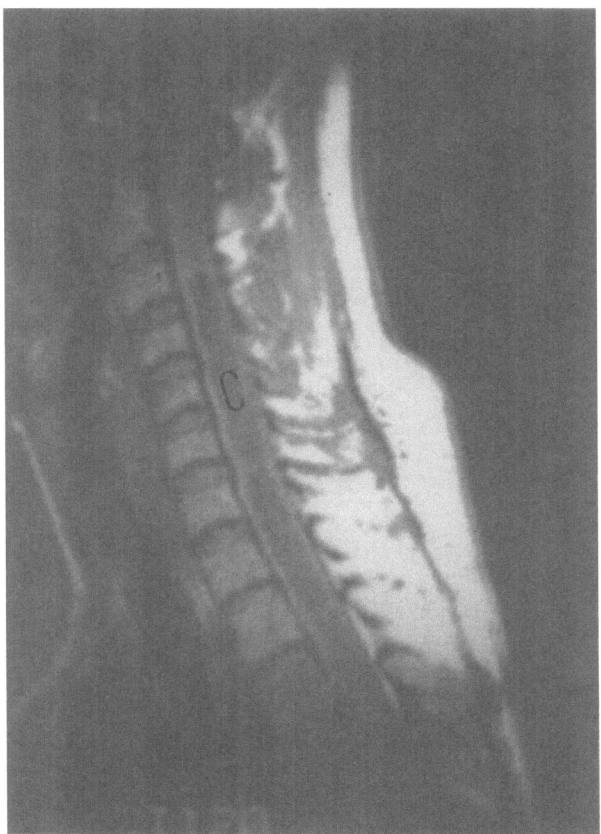

Figure 6.4C. Sagittal T_1 image of cervical spinal canal reveals a dilated spinal cord with a large central cavity (C).

and are substantiated by contrast CT in the dorsal region, which resulted in opacification of these nodules (Fig. 6.4E).

Thoracic spinal arteriogram further confirms the identification of the abnormal vessels (Fig. 6.4F) and establishes the diagnosis of hemangioblastomatosis within the spinal cord, as well as in the posterior fossa (Fig. 6.4G). I have come to the conclusion that portions of multiple hemangioblastomas may be hamartomas, because on follow-up studies some lesions

◁―――――――――――――――――――――――――――――――――――――――

Figure 6.4A. A midline sagittal T_1 image of the brain demonstrates a cystic lesion in the inferior vermis (*arrows*) compressing the medulla (*).
Figure 6.4B. Coronal T_1 shows also the cystic lesion (*arrows*).

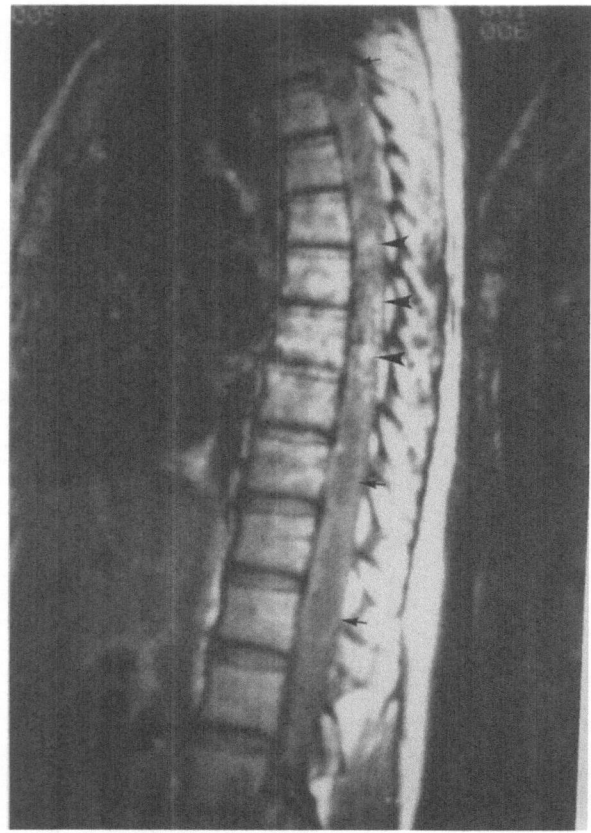

Figure 6.4D. Sagittal T_1 image of thoracic spinal canal reveals a discontinuous cavitary lesion (*arrows*) as well as nodular zones of hyperdensity (*arrowheads*).

may spontaneously disappear. Dr. Yang artistically diagrammed the nodules visualized during posterior fossa angiography (Fig. 6.4).

This patient had hemangioblastomatosis and the syrinx cavity was a secondary phenomenon due to involvement and expansion of the central canal. Therefore, this is a fascinating case in which MRI performed its imaging task well, demonstrating the nodules, cystic cavity, and abnormal blood vessels as well as compressed medulla and spinal cord.

The next case illustrates the significant value of MR in trauma. This was a patient who was seen acutely with rending back pain and progressive paraplegia. Instead of having a myelogram acutely, the patient was taken to the MR suite, and from the MR suite directly to the operating room. Now, this morning we heard about regeneration of the spinal cord (see

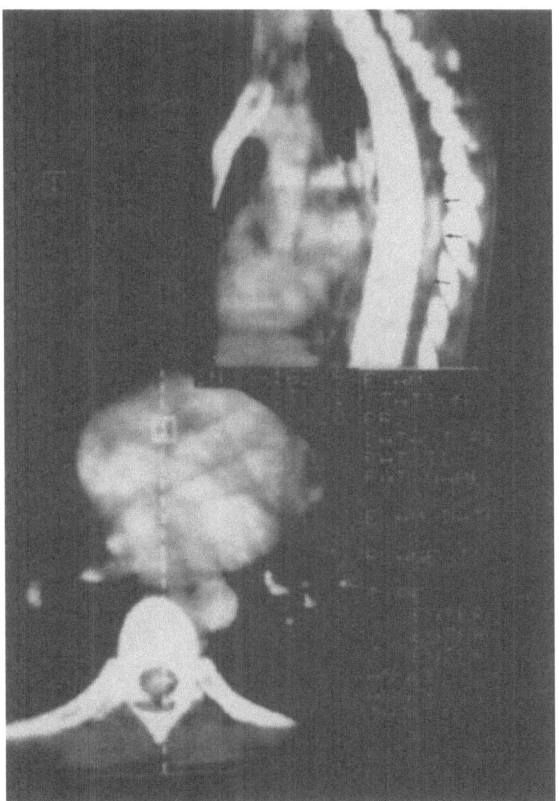

Figure 6.4E. Sagittal reformatted CT image of thoracic spine after intravenous contrast shows hyperdense lesion (*arrows*).

Table 6.1). The spinal cord is markedly compressed by spinal epidural hematoma (Fig. 6.5A,B). This patient was operated on immediately, made an uneventful recovery, and regained strength in his lower extremities. I believe the fact that he was taken immediately to the MR, at which time accurate localization and diagnosis was made, and then directly to the operating room, resulted in the excellent result.

In patients with spinal trauma, the evaluation with MR is obviously advantageous because of the outstanding visualization of spinal cord and overlying structures. In this next case, the spinal cord is compromised due to forward displacement of C-1 on C-2. One may appreciate the constriction of the spinal cord due to the osseous displacement (Fig. 6.6).

In another case, one may observe the bony configuration at the level of the foramen magnum and the compression at the level of the medulla, as

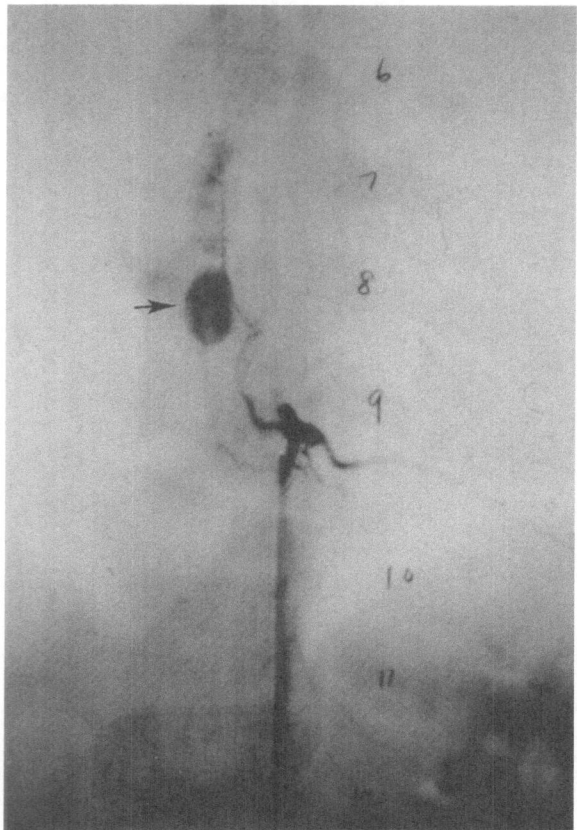

Figure 6.4F. Enhancing nodule (*arrow*) visualized during spinal arteriography.

well as the superior placement of the odontoid (Fig. 6.7). Basilar invagination is present, and the tonsil is slightly below the foramen magnum—tonsillar ectopia—Chiari 1 malformation; the constriction in this instance is the result of the basilar invagination and the medullary compression.

Next, a child with Trisomy 21 and instability of C1-2. One may appreciate on the plain roentgenogram the forward displacement of C-1 (Fig. 6.8A); the marked constriction of the spinal cord is seen on MR at the level of the odontoid (Fig. 6.8B). In this case the tonsils are well above the foramen magnum. The anatomy is therefore well demonstrated using MR in these patients with abnormalities at the foramen magnum. In the axial plane at the level of the foramen magnum one can clearly see the marked constriction of the spinal cord (Fig. 6.8C).

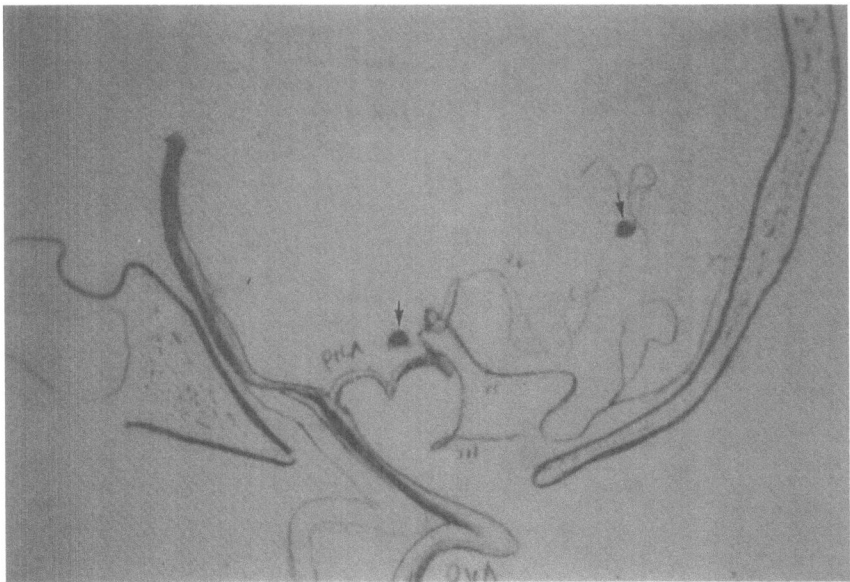

Figure 6.4G. Artistic (Dr. W. Yang) drawing of vertebral artery angiogram in lateral projection reveals two nodular lesions deriving blood supply from posterior inferior cerebellar artery (PICA).

The next case is a patient with rheumatoid arthritis with marked subluxation, synovial changes, partial destruction of the odontoid, and you may observe erosive changes of the end plates at C3-4 (Fig. 6.9). For unknown reasons, these patients, despite showing marked subluxation at C1-2 with associated narrowing of the spinal canal, rarely have symptoms.

The next group are these patients with developmental or congenital lesions of the mid- or lower spinal canal. A large defect is seen in the back of L-5 and S-1 (Fig. 6.10). This is an old examination revealing a cavity filled with pantopaque (Fig. 6.10). The diagnosis in this instance is a meningocele. If you make such a diagnosis of meningocele in some cases in the lumbar and sacral region you must think about neurofibromatosis, or perhaps a forme fruste of neurofibromatosis due to the accompanying enlargement of the thecal sac that may occur with secondary erosion due to pulsation.

In another patient, an MR shows a dilated thecal sac, resulting in the posterior scalloping of L-5 and S-1 (Fig. 6.11). The most common cause of posterior vertebral body scalloping is neurofibromatosis. This is due to the dilated thecal sac and the resultant pulsations that account for the marked compression.

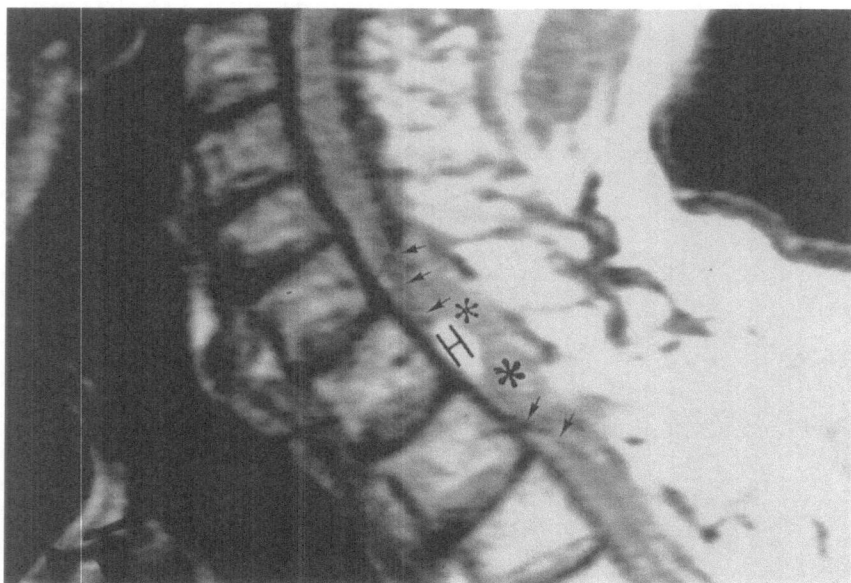

Figure 6.5A. Sagittal T₁ of cervical spine reveals large posthyperintensive epidural hematoma with hemorrhage (H) and fluid (*), with marked cord compression (*arrows*).

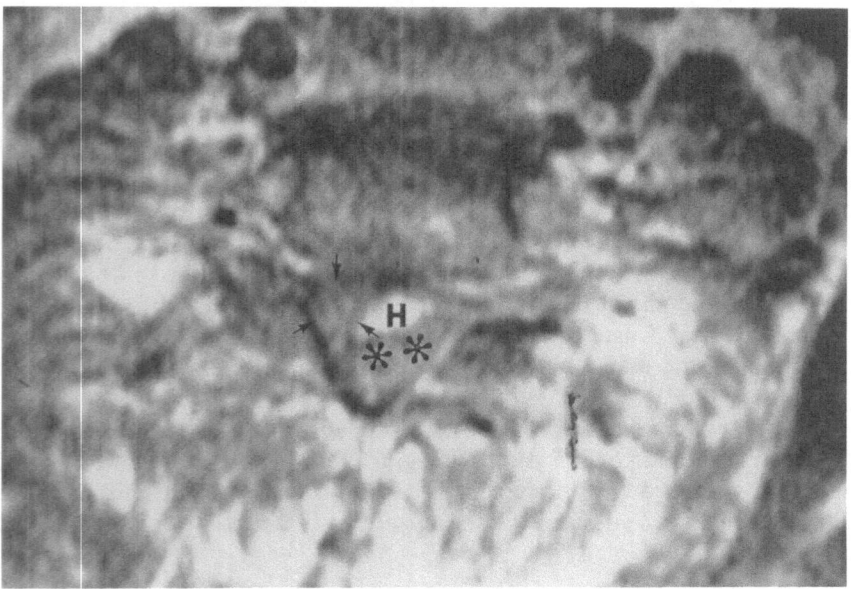

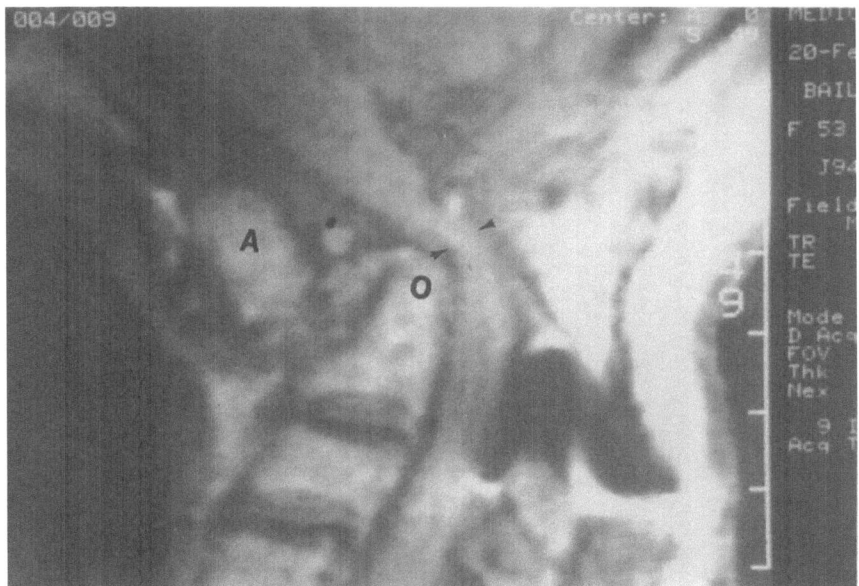

Figure 6.6. Patient with trauma at level of C1-2. Note marked forward displacement of C-1 (A) relative to the odontoid (O). The spinal cord (*arrowheads*) is markedly compressed at this level.

The next patient has diastematomyelia with a classic "butterfly" vertebral body. These changes occur at about the tenth week of life, with the mesenchymal defect as well as formation of Kovalevsky's canal.

At the same time, along with diastematomyelia, neurenteric cysts may be formed. In the case demonstrated, the posterior spur is visible, as well as a split in the butterfly-type vertebral body Kovalevsky's canal and the diplomyelia (Fig. 6.12A,B). On the MR one can see the bone defect, the bony spur, and the fibrous septum in the residual spinal cord. On this view one can also see the splitting of the cord in the axial projection (Fig. 6.12B).

In the sagittal plane the "butterfly" vertebral body and the spur as well as the fibrous septum and the compressed bilobed sac are exquisitely delineated (Fig. 6.12B–D). The advantages of MR in providing detailed anatomical information are demonstrated in these patients (Fig. 6.12B–E).

This next case is an example of a patient with a Chiari 1 malformation with the tonsil extending through the foramen magnum below the odontoid (Fig. 6.13A). Whenever Chiari I malformation is recognized, about 50%

◁ ——————————————————————————————————————

Figure 6.5B. Axial T_1 slice through hematoma reveals similar findings as in **A**, with marked cord compression (*arrows*).

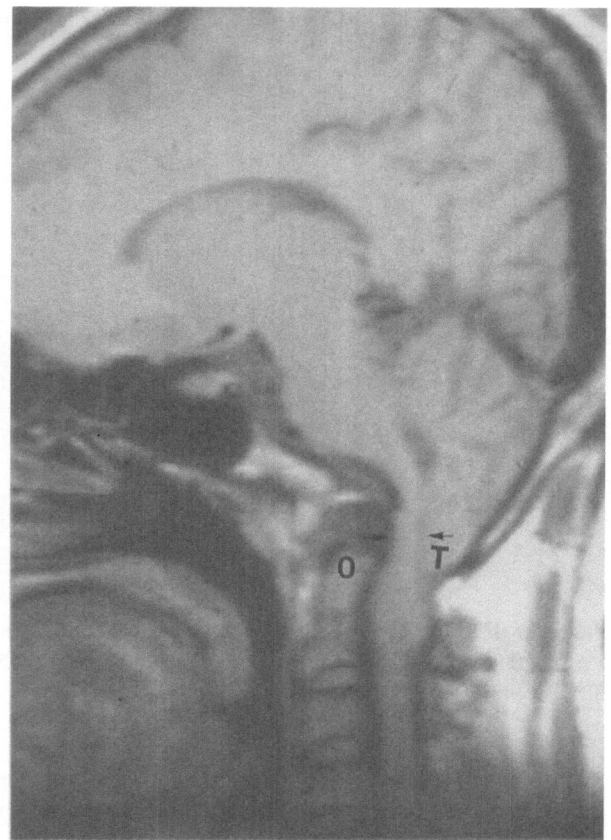

Figure 6.7. The odontoid (O) is elevated "basilar invagination" with resultant compression of the medulla (*arrow*) and tonsillar ectopia (T).

or more will have an associated syringohydromyelia. This patient has a cavity in the cervical region as well as this large central cavity in the lower dorsal region (Fig. 6.13B).

The MRI in this next patient reveals enlargement of the spinal cord. In addition, a focal lesion with a variegated pattern of low and increased intensity is observed. When one observes such a pattern, as in this case, one should think about a cavernous hemangioma (Fig. 6.14). It is interesting

Figure 6.8A. Lateral roentgenogram of cervical spine reveals forward displacement of C1 (*) relative to odontoid (O).
Figure 6.8B. Marked cord compression (C) can be appreciated at the level of the odontoid in the sagittal T_1 image.

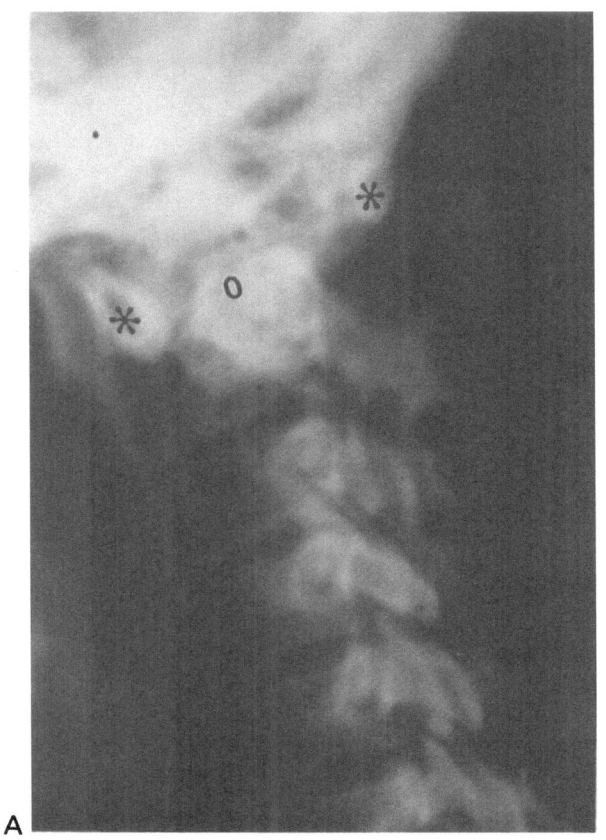

A

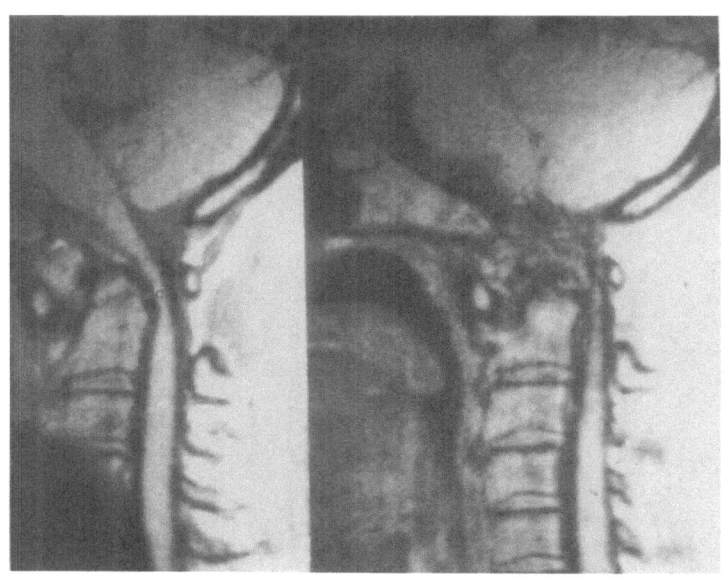

B

151

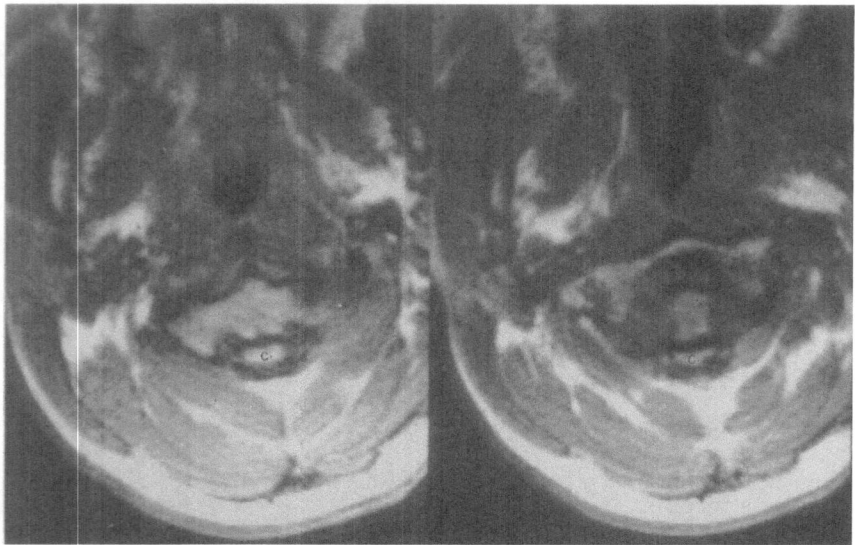

Figure 6.8C. Axial T_1 image at level of odontoid also reveals the marked cord compression (C).

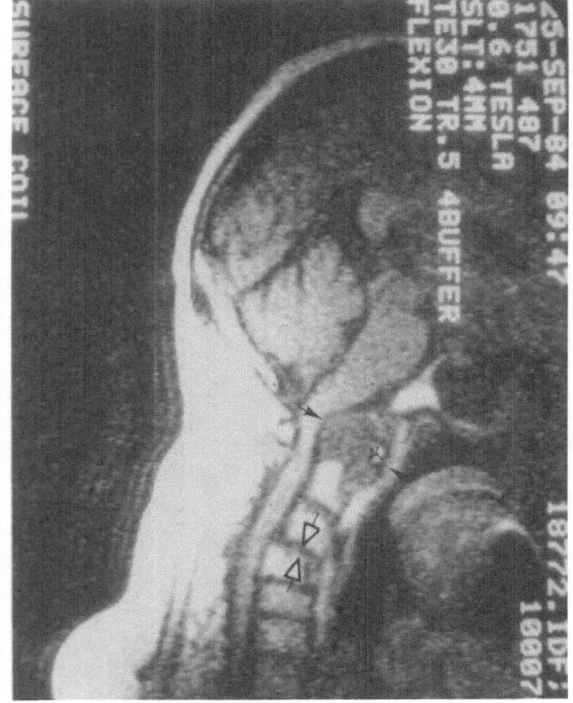

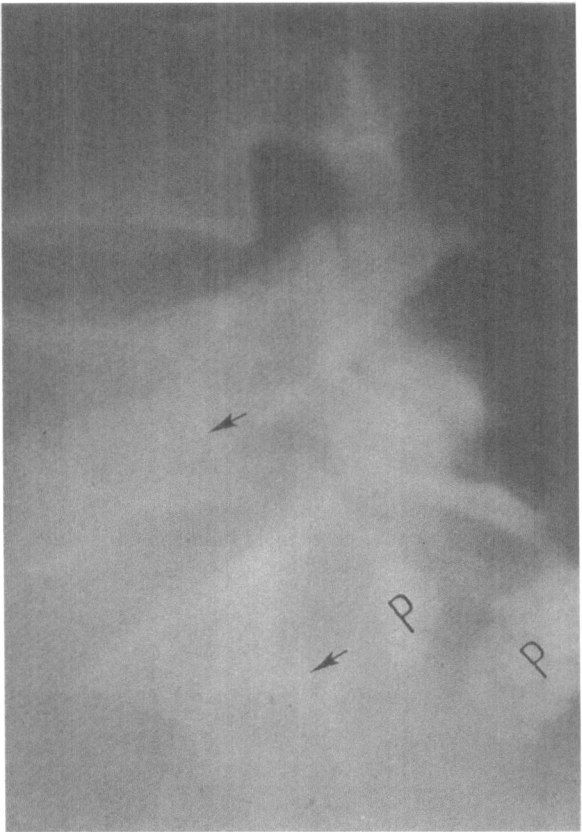

Figure 6.10. Large defects "scalloping" at back of L-5 (*arrow*) and S-1 (*arrow*) due to dilated subarachnoid space or meningocele. Collections of pantopaque (P) within the meningocele.

that this lesion has been recognized with increasing frequency with the advent of MR. This variegated pattern probably represents hemorrhage, hemosiderin, calcium, and so forth.

The disadvantage of CTM (CT myelography) is that often in intradural lesions the displacement of the cord is recognized, but you are often unable to visualize the tumor (Fig. 6.15). It is hard to identify the tumor in comparison with extradural lesions, which distort the cord and thecal sac, as well as intramedullary lesions, which enlarge the cord.

◁───

Figure 6.9. Note marked destruction of odontoid with pannus and synovial changes (*arrows*) with subluxation at C1-2 (*). Erosion of the end plates at C3-4 is also present (*open arrows*), confirming the diagnosis of rheumatoid arthritis.

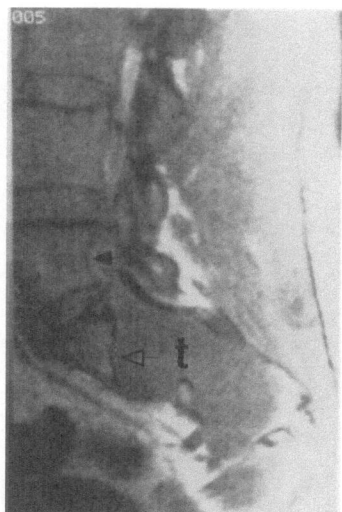

Figure 6.11. Sagittal proton density reveals mild scalloping of L-5 (*arrow*) and marked of S-1 (*open arrow*) due to a dilated thecal sac (T).

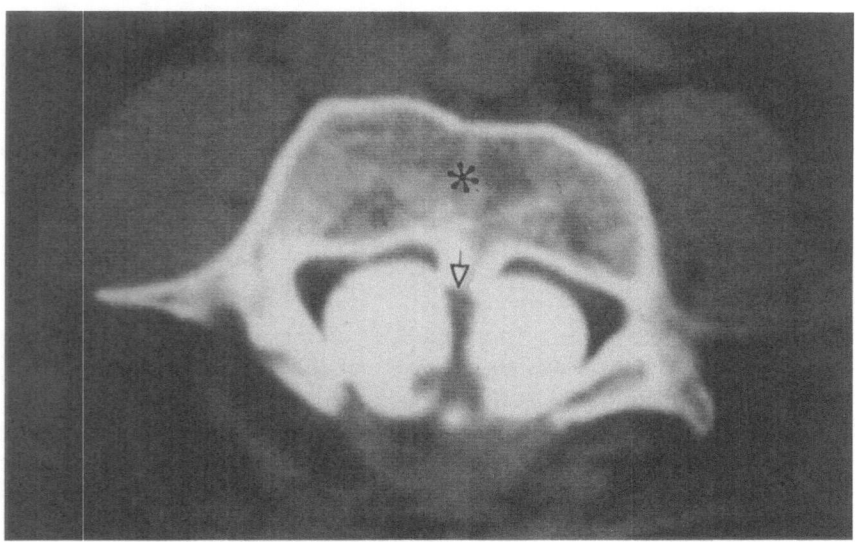

Figure 6.12A. A CT myelogram (CTM) in lumbar region reveals a "butterfly" vertebral body (*), posterior spur (*open arrow*) with fibrous spur (not opaque) causing splitting of the opacified thecal sac.

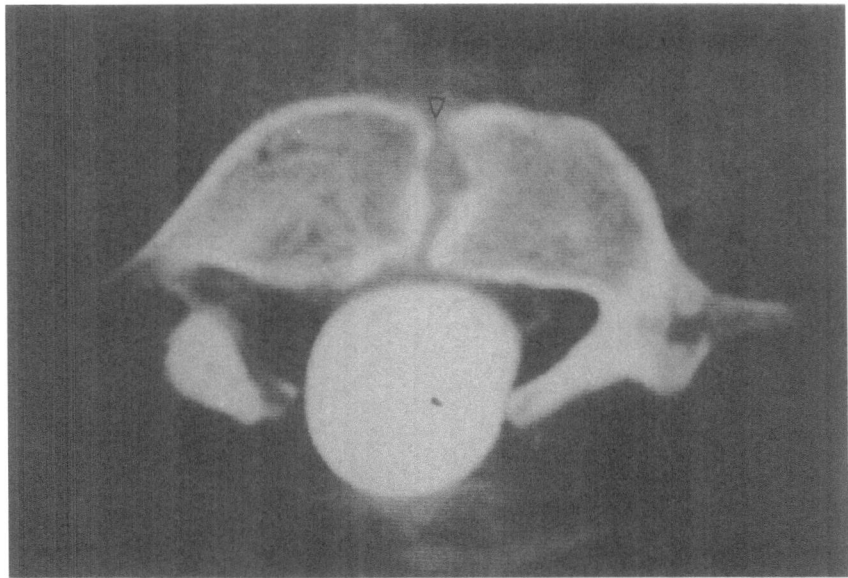

Figure 6.12B. CTM reveals a split in the "butterfly" vertebral body (Kovalevsky canal) (*arrowhead*).

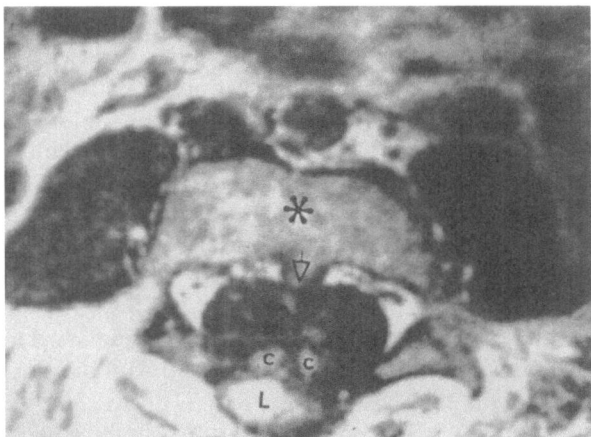

Figure 6.12C. Axial MR reveals similar findings to **A**, but reveals split cord (C) and lipoma posteriorly (L) also.

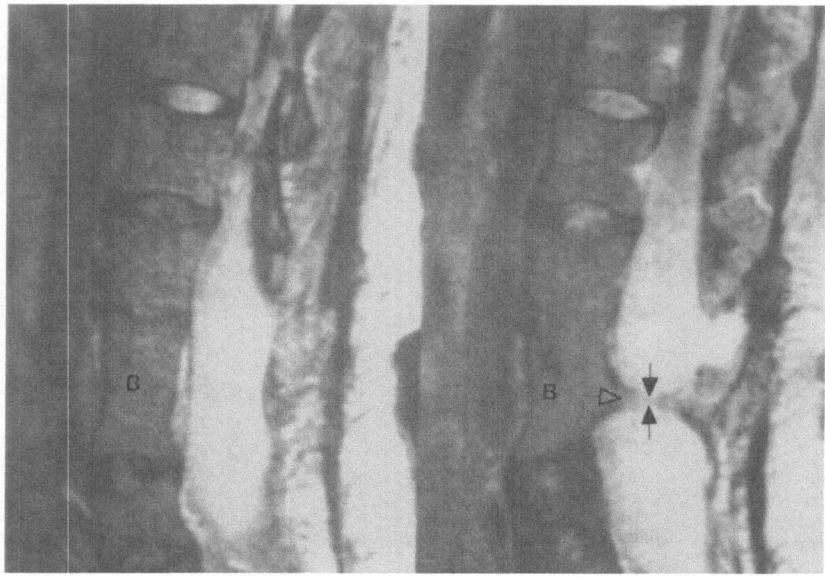

D   E

Figure 6.12D. Sagittal spin echo T_2 to the left of midline reveals "butterfly" vertebral body (B) and intact thecal sac.
Figure 6.12E. Sagittal spin echo T_2 7 mm to right, almost in midline reveals the bony spur (*open arrow*) and fibrous septum (*arrows*) splitting the thecal sac.

We may often identify these lesions, however, with MR. We have the advantage of making the following observations in patients with intradural extramedullary lesions: the expanded CSF on the side of the neoplasm, while it is thinned on the contralateral side. I do not believe any other examinations are necessary (Fig. 6.16).

Meningiomas are almost all ventrolateral because they arise in relationship to the vertebral artery (Fig. 6.17A,B). In this case, a meningioma at the level of the foramen magnum is observed, compressing the spinal cord (Fig. 6.17A,B).

MR is the study to be done first in the study of spinal cord lesions, and if it answers the question raised then one may stop. If it does not answer the question, then other studies are indicated.

In summary, I think what we have heard from our clinical colleagues and from the research is that radiology has a way to go. We are still not on any microscopic level. MR has added significantly and rules out certain things and is an important guide. Certainly I believe if MR spectroscopy proves to be successful it will provide an incredible tool.

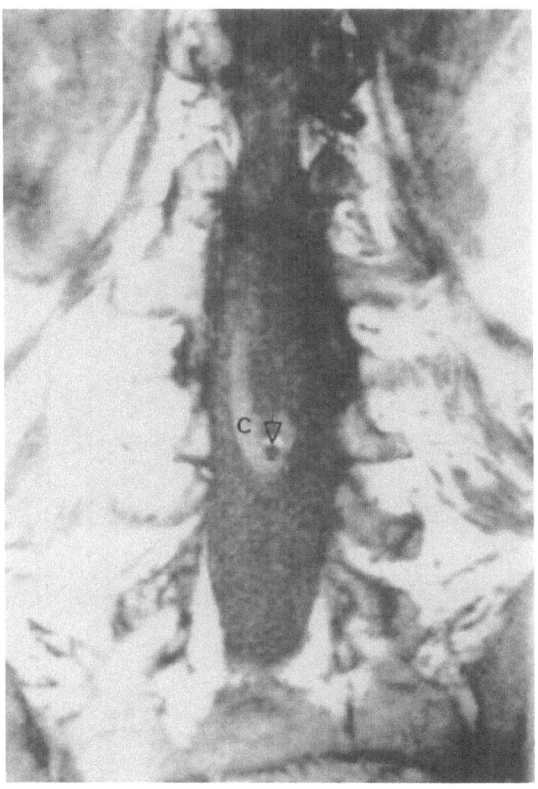

Figure 6.12F. Coronal T$_1$ reveals bony spur (*open arrow*) in midline, splitting cord (C).

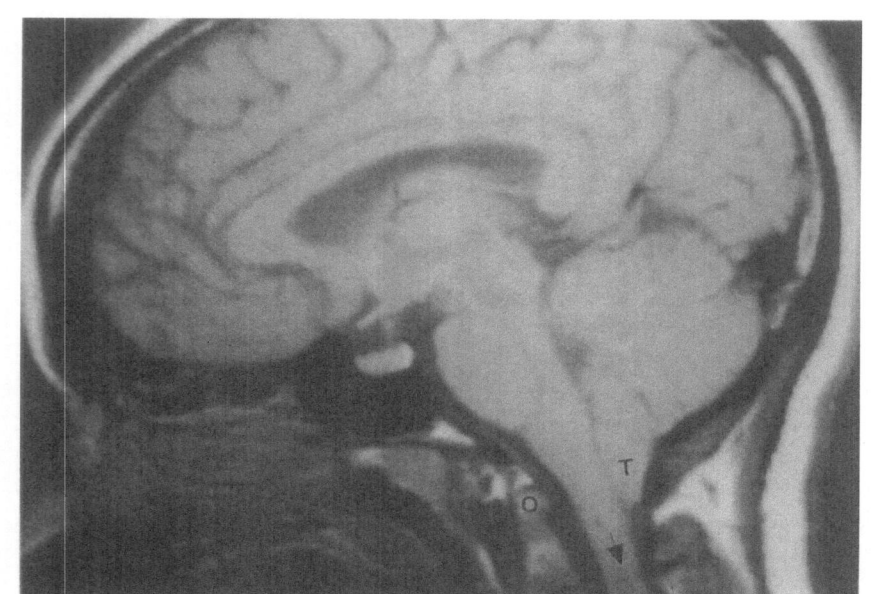

A

B

158

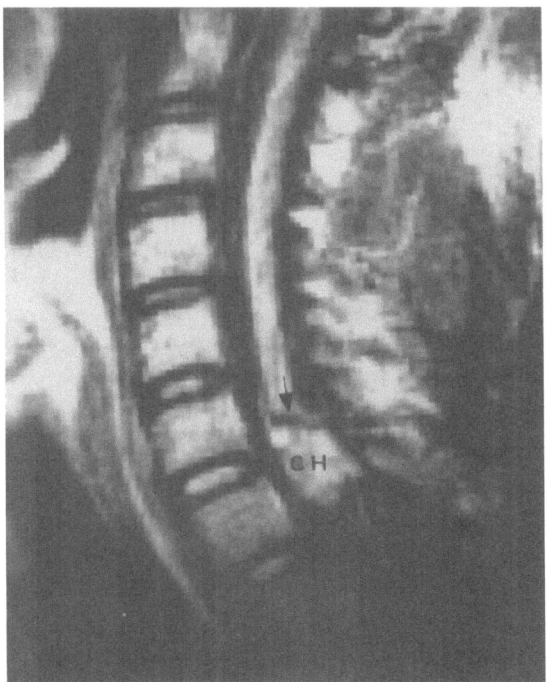

Figure 6.14. On T_1 sagittal spin echo of the cervical spine, a mixed density lesion containing portions of hyper-, iso-, and hypointensity is observed (CH) (*arrow*), characteristic of a cavernous hemangioma.

Figure 6.13A. Sagittal T_1 of brain in midline including upper cervical spine. Tonsillar ectopia is seen extending through the foramen magnum and below the odontoid (O). Faint hypodensity of hydromyelia is observed (*arrow*).
Figure 6.13B. Thoracic T_1 image reveals a localized, enlarged central cavity within the cord (*open arrows*).

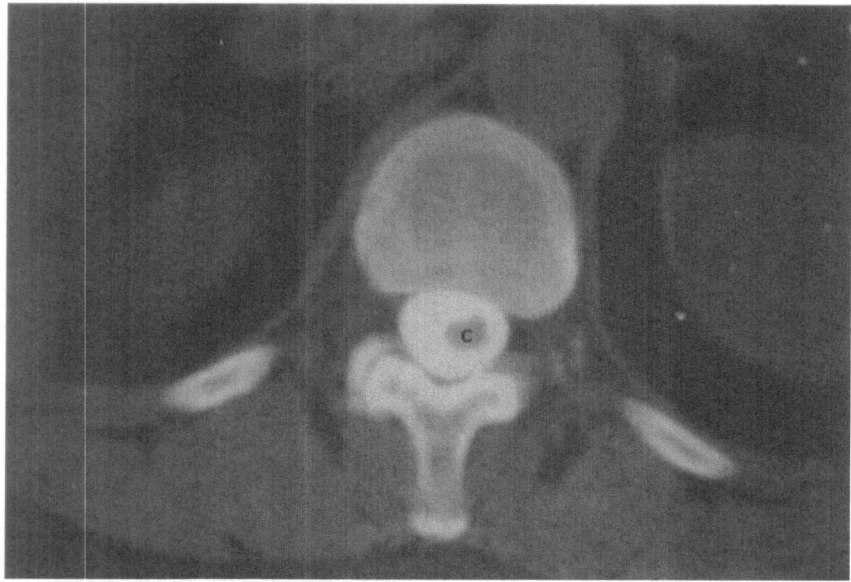

Figure 6.15. CTM in upper lumbar region reveals displaced spinal cord (C) in thecal sac, which is characteristic of intradural extramedullary lesion, although tumor is not identified. ·

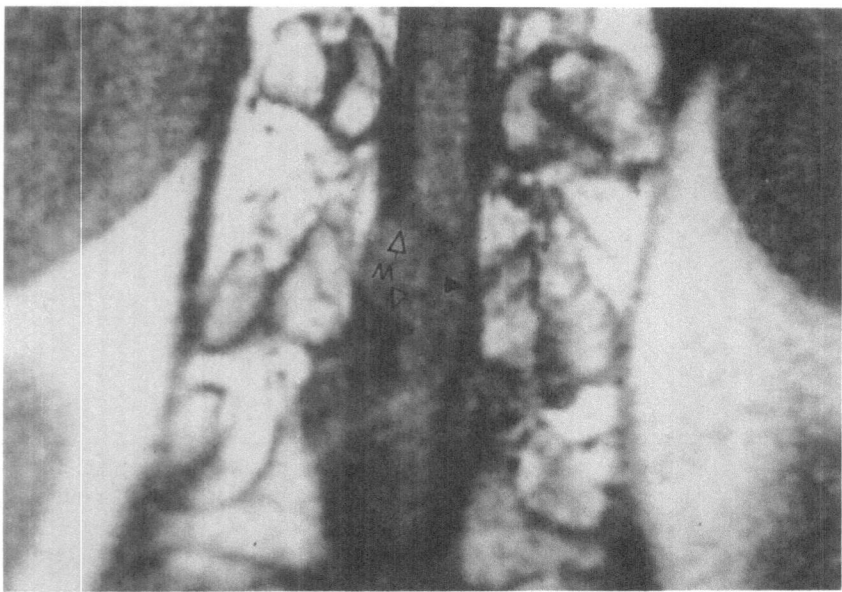

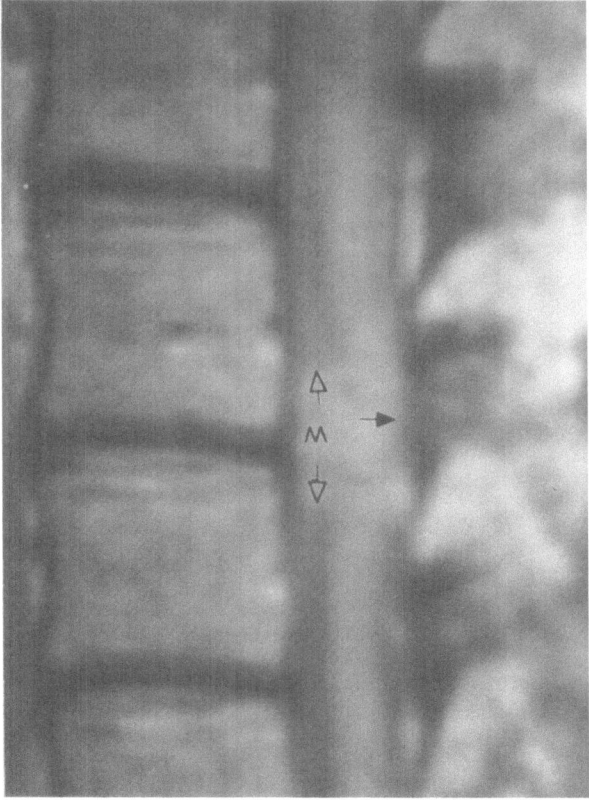

Figure 6.16B. Sagittal T_1 shows similar findings revealing that the tumor (M) is anterior or ventral in location.

Figure 6.16A. Coronal T_1 image reveals dilated subarachnoid space (*open arrows*) encompassing intradural extramedullary meningioma. On the opposite side (*arrow*), the subarachnoid space is thinned.

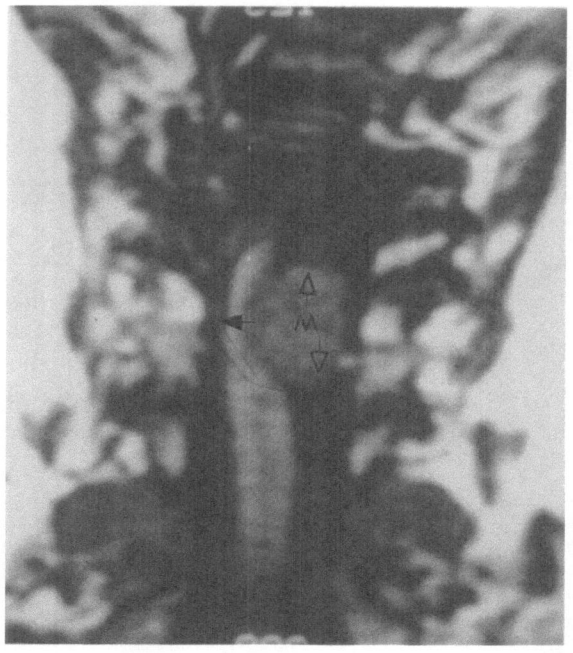

A

Figure 6.17A,B. Coronal and sagittal spin echo T_1 of cervical region again shows ventrolateral intradural extramedullary meningioma with dilated CSF (*open arrow*) on side of tumor, with thin space contralateral (*arrow*) and hyperintense mass (M) on coronal image.

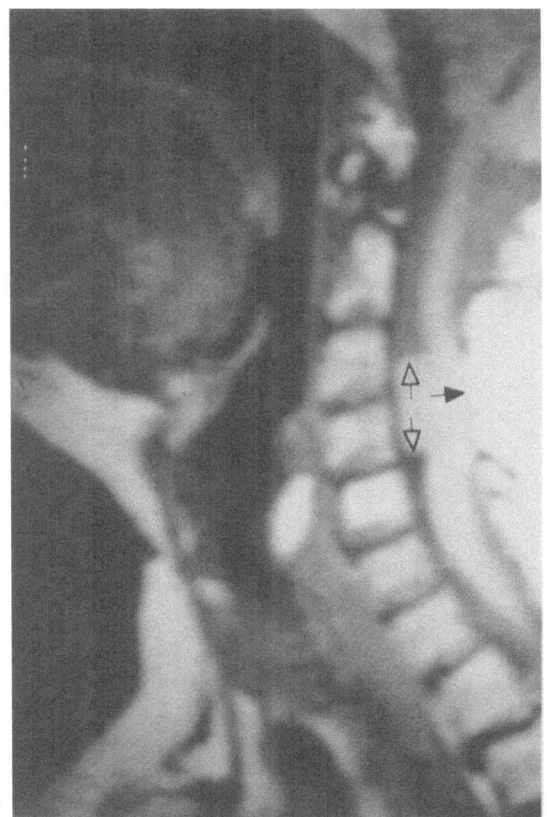

B

CHAPTER 7

Spinal Cord Atrophy

Robert N.N. Holtzman and Wen C. Yang

Spinal cord atrophy represents an irreversible state of degeneration manifested both radiographically and pathologically by a loss of spinal cord substance. It is accompanied by varying clinical states of myeloradiculopathy and is slowly progressive without remissions. There is as yet no significant surgical or medical therapy capable of reversing this process once it has begun. There remains some possibility that a plateau may be reached in the evolution of neurological symptoms by early decompression in instances of mechanical deformation of the spinal cord, and perhaps also by excision lesions capable of producing ischemic disturbances such as intramedullary vascular tumors and arteriovenous malformations.

The concept of spinal cord atrophy is not new. As early as 1858, Dr. Charles Evans Reeves of the University of London and the Faculty of Physicians & Surgeons, Glasgow, devoted a chapter to the subject in his book entitled *Diseases of the Spinal Cord and Its Membranes*. He distinguished between *general atrophy*, which was "sometimes congenital . . . occurred from fluid in the spinal canal . . . with chronic inflammation of the membranes, and is constantly observed in the aged" and *partial atrophy*, which was "excited by tumors pressing on the cord, caries or displacement of the vertebrae or inflammatory deposits in the membranes."[1]

Clinical detection of spinal cord atrophy is difficult and heretofore was based solely on pathological observations. In recent years, with the advent and widespread availability of cross-sectional computed tomography (CT) scanning and water-soluble contrast material for myelography, the diagnosis has been established more readily.

The ensuing discussion is predicated on the need for early recognition of compressive and ischemic processes that can be identified and managed before the evolution of irreversible neurological deficits.

Etiologies of Spinal Cord Atrophy

A review of the neurological and neurosurgical literature yielded a number of categories of spinal cord atrophy, which are listed below:

1. Maturation and Aging   Nordqvist, 1964[2]
2. Congenital Anomalies   Drachman and Banker, 1961,[3]
   Arthrogryposis multiplex   Gibson, 1978[4]
   congenita
3. Hereditary/Neurodegenerative
   Diseases
   Olivopontocerebellar atrophy   Staal et al., 1981[5]
   Spastic paraparesis   Bowman, 1967[6]
4. Demyelinating Diseases
   Multiple sclerosis   Shirare et al., 1971[7]
   Devic's syndrome   Cloys and Netsky, 1970[8]
5. Progressive Necrotic Myelopathy
   Angiodysgenetic
   Idiopathic   Folliss and Netsky, 1970[9]
6. Toxic
   Sodium acetrizoate aortography   Hughes and Brownell, 1965[10]
7. Infections
   Tabes dorsalis   Schiller, 1976[11]
8. Inflammation
   Arachnoiditis   Donaldson and Gibson, 1982[12]
9. Vascular/Ischemic
   Lupus erythematosus   Nakada et al., 1982[13]
   Intramedullary hemangio-   Solomon and Stein, 1988,[14]
   blastomas   McCormick and Stein, 1990[15]
10. Cavitation
    Syringomyelia   Schliep, 1978[16]
11. Trauma with delayed progressive
    myeloradiculopathy
    Penetrating   Nakada et al., 1982[13]
    Nonpenetrating   Komaki, 1976,[17] Jellinger,
    Electrical   1976,[18] Panse, 1975[19]

Assessment of Spinal Cord Dimensions

In the past, measurement of the spinal cord has generated great interest among anatomists and radiologists.[2,20-25] The data obtained from anatomical and radiologic studies have established norms with their respective standard deviations for all levels of the spinal cord. These studies also acknowledge the "normal" variations in spinal dimensions in a given population and serve as the basis for establishing the diagnosis of spinal cord atrophy.

Two types of investigations have been done:

1. post mortem anatomical studies
2. radiologic and neuroimaging studies including:
   positive contrast myelography

gas myelography
post–myelographic CT scanning
ultrasonography[26]
magnetic resonance imaging

In life, spinal cord atrophy is diagnosed by radiologic or neuroimaging techniques. Of all the imaging modalities, we believe that post–myelographic CT scanning is the most accurate method in the assessment of spinal cord dimensions at the present time for the simple reason that it provides the best resolution in cross-section images.

In recent years, non-ionic water-soluble iodinated contrast materials (e.g., Metrizamide, Iopamidol, Iohexl) have been used in myelography with relative ease and minimal side effects. More importantly, this technique allows CT scanning of the spine for a period of several hours after the myelographic procedure to visualize the spinal canal contents. The post–myelographic CT scans thus obtained provide the best anatomical information in cross-section.

When evaluating the spinal cord by post–myelographic CT scanning, it is necessary to recognize that the size of the spinal cord varies according to different settings in window center. The optimum window center is the mean between the contrast medium attenuation number and the cord attenuation number (Fig. 7.1).[20,21]:

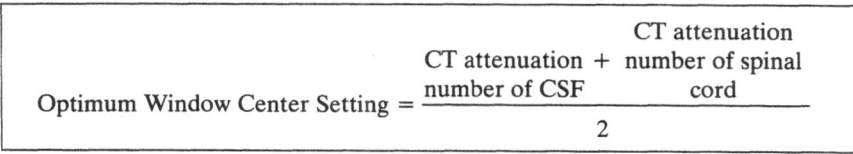

$$\text{Optimum Window Center Setting} = \frac{\text{CT attenuation number of CSF} + \text{CT attenuation number of spinal cord}}{2}$$

Figure 7.1.

Magnetic resonance imaging (MRI) has been proven to be a valuable noninvasive modality to assess the soft tissues within the spinal canal including the spinal cord. It has the advantage of visualizing the spinal canal contents in sagittal and coronal planes. On the other hand, its axial images are suboptimal in the assessment of the spinal cord because of the inherent technical limitation of long imaging time and the recognized distortions caused by truncation artifacts,[22] motion artifacts, and partial volume averaging artifacts.[23]

The methodology of real-time high resolution ultrasonography using transducer frequencies of 5 and 7.5 mHz in patients who have undergone laminectomy so that the bony defect provides, in effect, an acoustic window has been used successfully in the demonstration of spinal cord atrophy[26] and represents an alternative to MR imaging and CT scanning in certain select instances.

Normal ranges for the dimensions of the cervical, thoracic, and lumbar spinal cord, based on previously published data, are seen in Tables 7.1 and 7.2.

Table 7.1. Normal mean frontal and sagittal diameters of the cervical spinal cord based upon CT myelography. (Reprinted with permission of Thijssen et al. Morphology of the cervical spinal cord on computed myelography. *Neuroradiology.* 1979;18:57–62.)[22]

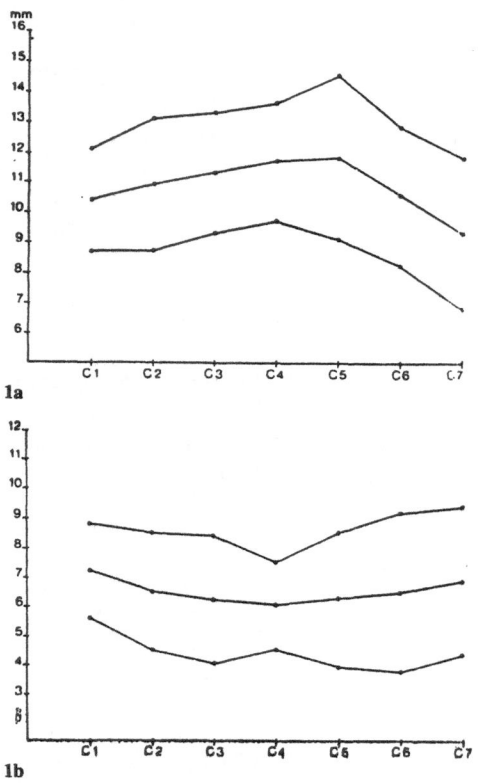

Fig. 1. a Normal frontal diameter of cervical cord; mean value ± 2 SD, n = 20. **b** Normal sagittal diameter of cervical cord; mean value ± 2 SD, n = 20

Table 1. Normal mean frontal and sagittal diameter in mm (± 2 SD) of cervical cord; n = 20

	Frontal diameter	Sagittal diameter
C_1	10.4 ± 1.7	7.2 ± 1.6
C_2	10.9 ± 2.2	6.5 ± 2.0
C_3	11.3 ± 2.0	6.2 ± 2.2
C_4	11.7 ± 1.9	6.0 ± 1.5
C_5	11.8 ± 2.7	6.2 ± 2.3
C_6	10.5 ± 2.3	6.4 ± 2.7
C_7	9.3 ± 2.5	6.8 ± 2.5

H.O.M. Thijssen et al.: Morphology of the Cervical Spinal Cord on CM

Table 7.2. A & B: Sagittal (**A**) and coronal (**B**) diameters of normal thoracic spinal cord in vivo. **C**: Mean CT sagittal and frontal diameters of normal postmortem thoracic cord. **D**: Mean CT sagittal and frontal diameters of normal subarachnoid space in vivo. (Reprinted with permission of Gellad et al. Morphology and Dimensions of the thoracic cord by computer-assisted metrizamide myelography. *ANJR*. 1983;4:614–617.)[23]

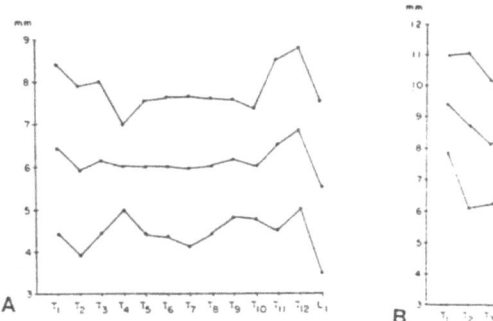
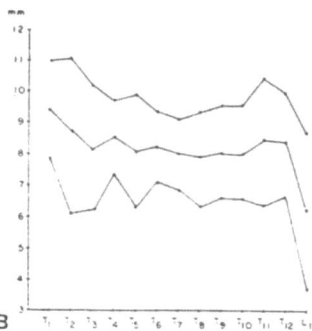

Fig. 2.—CT sagittal (A) and coronal (B) diameters of normal thoracic spinal cord in vivo (*n* = 28). Center line = plot of mean values at each level; upper line = mean + 2 SD; lower line = mean − 2 SD.

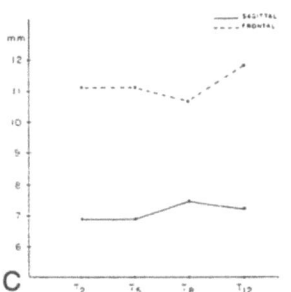

Fig. 4.—Mean CT sagittal and frontal diameters of normal postmortem thoracic cord (*n* = 10) at four spinal levels.

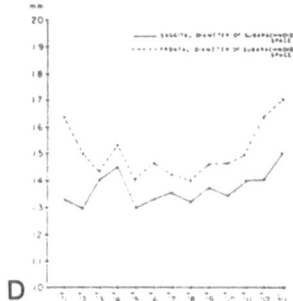

Fig. 3.—Mean CT sagittal and frontal diameters of normal subarachnoid space in vivo (*n* = 28).

TABLE 1: CT Diameters (Mean ± 2 SD) of Normal Thoracic Cord and Subarachnoid Space in Vivo (*n* = 28)

Spinal Level	Diameter of Thoracic Cord (mm)		Diameter of Subarachnoid Space (mm)	
	Sagittal	Coronal	Sagittal	Coronal
T1	6.4 ± 2	9.4 ± 1.6	13.3 ± 2.5	16.4 ± 1.8
T2	5.9 ± 2	8.7 ± 2.5	13.0 ± 2.4	14.9 ± 2.5
T3	6.2 ± 1.8	8.2 ± 2	14.0 ± 2.8	14.1 ± 2.4
T4	6.0 ± 1	8.5 ± 1.2	14.5 ± 2.2	15.7 ± 2.5
T5	6.0 ± 1.6	8.1 ± 1.8	13.0 ± 3.4	13.9 ± 2.8
T6	6.0 ± 1.7	8.2 ± 1.1	13.3 ± 3.2	14.6 ± 2.2
T7	5.9 ± 1.8	8.0 ± 1.2	13.5 ± 3.0	14.2 ± 3.3
T8	6.0 ± 1.6	7.8 ± 1.5	13.2 ± 2.6	13.9 ± 2.7
T9	6.2 ± 1.4	8.0 ± 1.5	13.7 ± 2.8	14.5 ± 2.6
T10	6.0 ± 1.3	8.0 ± 1.5	13.4 ± 2.8	14.4 ± 2.8
T11	6.5 ± 2	8.4 ± 2	14.0 ± 3.4	14.9 ± 3.1
T12	6.8 ± 1.8	8.3 ± 1.7	14.0 ± 3.5	16.3 ± 3.4
L1	5.5 ± 2	6.2 ± 2.5	15.0 ± 3.6	17.0 ± 3.2

TABLE 2: CT Diameters (Mean ± 2 SD) of Normal Postmortem Thoracic Cord (*n* = 10)

Spinal Level	Sagittal Diameter (mm)	Coronal Diameter (mm)
T2	6.8 ± 2.6	11.1 ± 2
T5	6.8 ± 2.6	11.1 ± 2
T8	7.4 ± 2.8	10.5 ± 3
T12	7.2 ± 2	11.7 ± 3.2

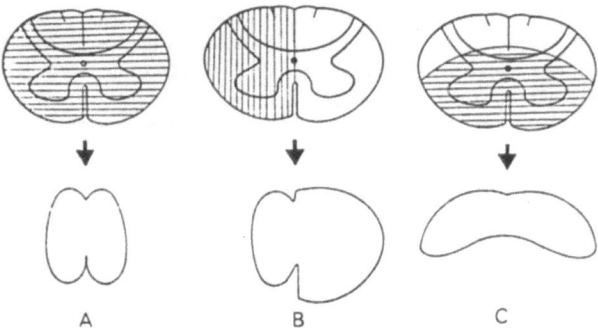

Figure 7.2. Schematic representation of atrophy patterns. ((Reprinted with permission from Nakada et al. Computed tomography of spinal cord atrophy. *Neuroradiology*. 1982;24:97–99.)

Patterns of Spinal Cord Atrophy

Based on the post–myelographic CT scanning studies, there are several patterns of spinal cord atrophy that seem to correspond to fairly definite clinical and pathologic entities.

The first group described by Nakada et al.[13] consists of three types: diffuse atrophy (transverse myelopathy), hemiatrophy (Brown-Séquard syndrome), and anterior atrophy (anterior spinal artery syndrome). (Fig. 7.2)

The second group of patterns described by Mawad et al.[27] characterized the atrophic features with specific disease processes. "In cervical spondylosis (they) . . . included: flattening of the ventral cord surface, central infolding, beaking of the lateral funiculi and wasting of the dorsal surface. Motor neuron disease showed a combination of anterolateral and posterolateral atrophy reflecting the degeneration of anterior horn cells and/or corticospinal tracts. Monomelic motor neuron disease had a striking ipsilateral hemiatrophy of the spinal cord."[27]

Illustrative cases substantiating the above descriptions are presented below with brief case histories:

Case Reports

Diffuse Atrophy

Case 1. A 58-year-old man with luetic meningoencephalitis and residual paraparesis, intractable lumbar, and perineal and rectal pain incompletely controlled with narcotic analgesics. (Fig. 7.3A,B,C)

Case 2. A 70-year-old man with a history of vitamin B_{12} deficiency and progressive myelopathy demonstrates diffuse spinal cord atrophy. (Fig. 7.4A,B,C,D)

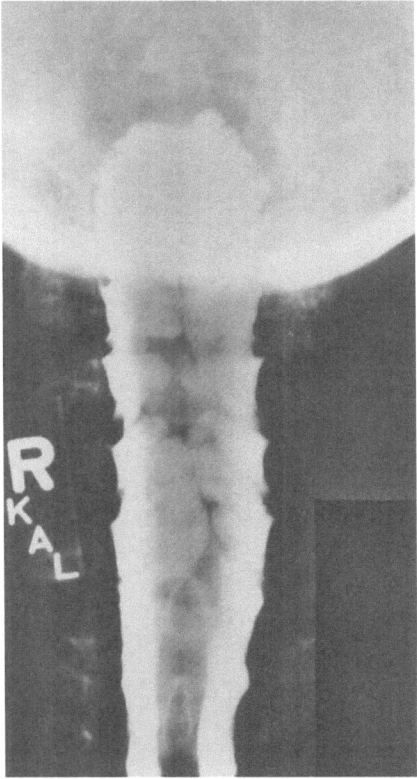

Figure 7.3A. Pantopaque myelogram in posteroanterior view is unremarkable and the spinal cord appears to be normal.

Case 3. A 42-year-old man was stabbed in the upper back 20 years previously and suffered paraplegia from which he made an incomplete recovery and was able to ambulate. In the recent 4 to 5 months he noticed progressive loss of strength in his lower extremities. (Fig. 7.5A,B,C)

Hemiatrophy

Case 4. A 43-year-old man presented with a 6-month history of weakness of the left shoulder, wasting of the left shoulder musculature, and left arm pain. Examination showed left deltoid atrophy and weakness in the biceps and triceps groups. (Fig. 7.6)

Case 5. A 59-year-old woman presented with progressive weakness and paraesthesiae of the right hand for 4 years. (Fig. 7.7)

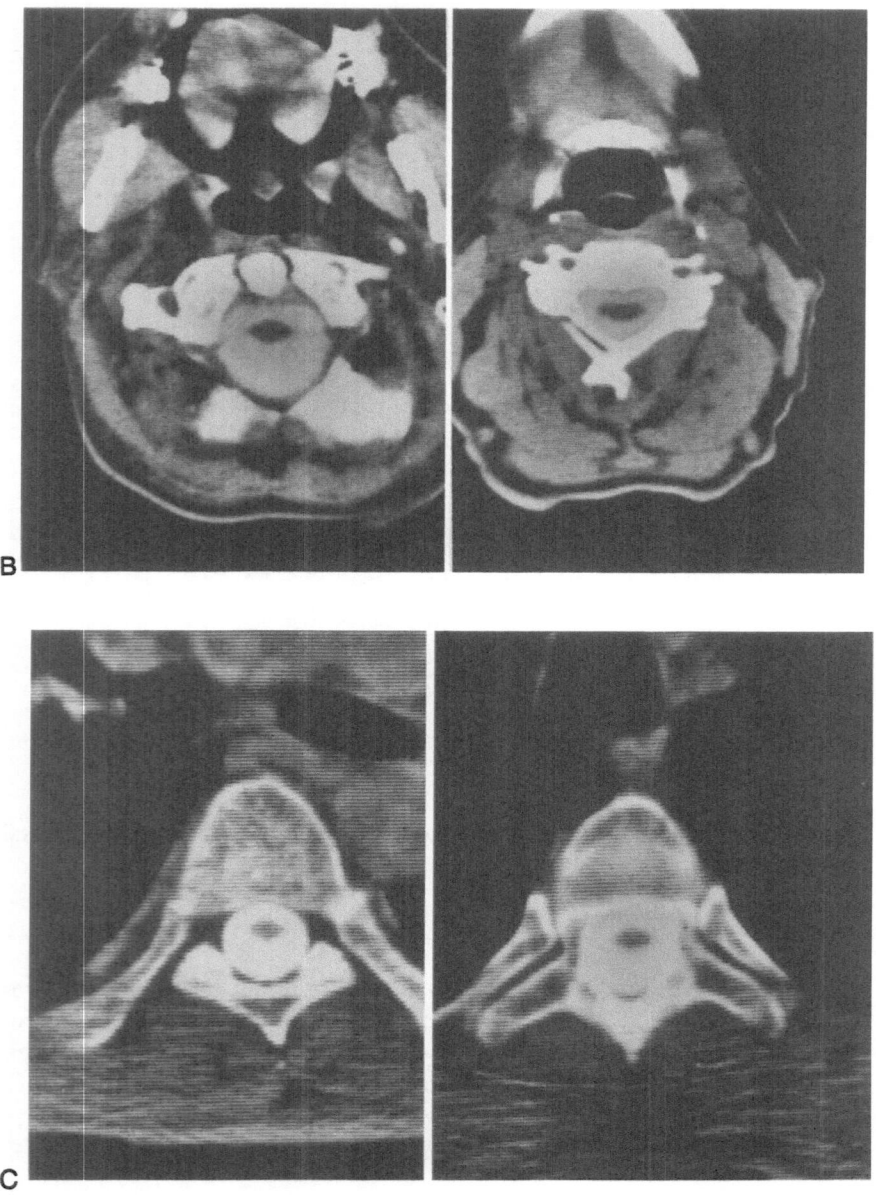

Figure 7.3B,C. CT scan after water-soluble contrast myelography demonstrates diffuse atrophy of the cervical and thoracic spinal cord.

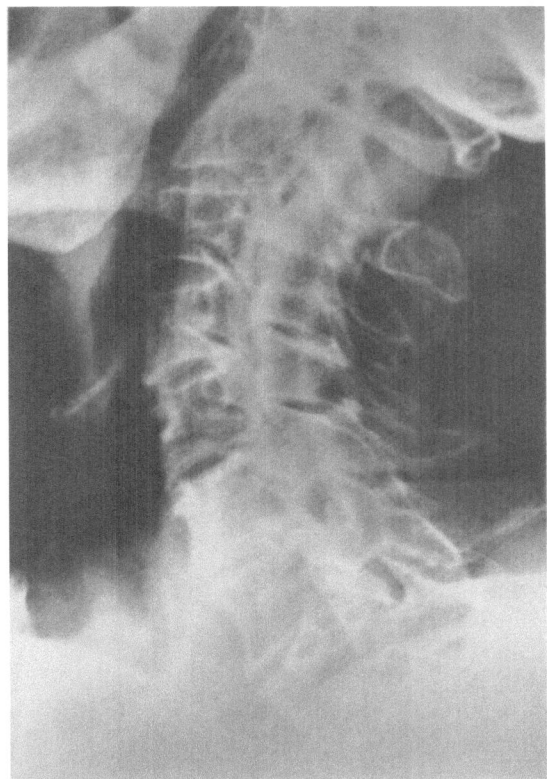

A

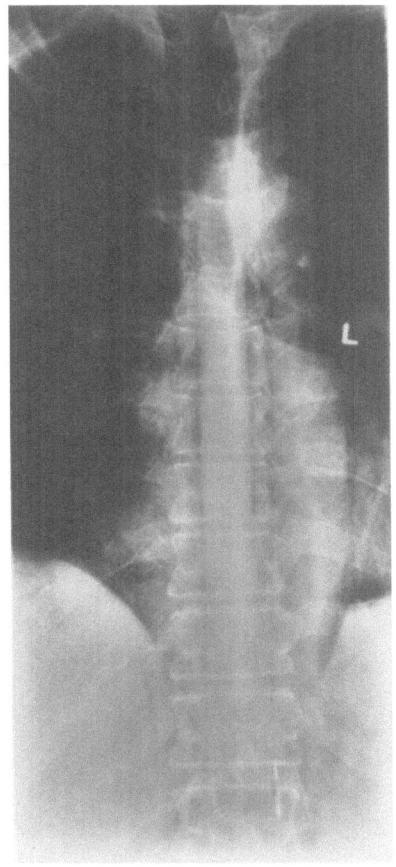

B

Figure 7.4A. Lateral view of the cervical myelogram shows a dilated subarachnoid space and a small spinal cord.

Figure 7.4B. Anteroposterior view of the thoracic myelogram reveals a capacious subarachnoid space. The spinal cord cannot be delineated.

Anterior Atrophy

Case 6. A 68-year-old woman with a history of tuberculosis and arthritis, chronic back pain, urinary incontinence, and deteriorating gait. Examination showed spasticity with a T-3 sensory level and a right Babinski sign. Proximal weakness as evidenced by difficulty arising from a chair. Some response to steroid therapy. (Fig. 7.8A,B)

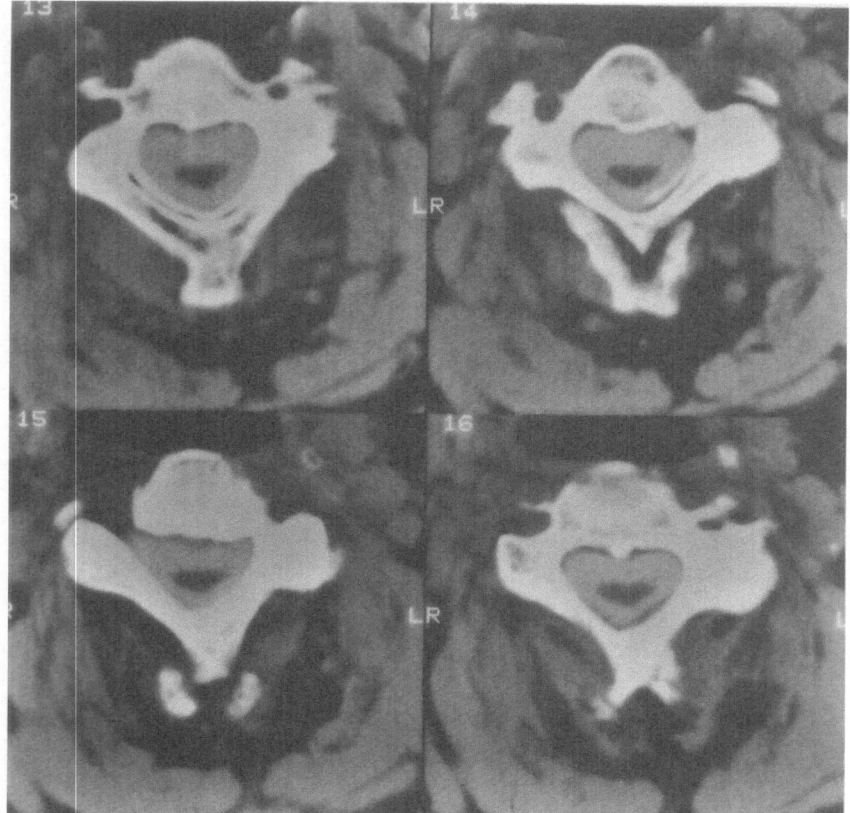

C

Figure 7.4C,D. Representative post–myelographic CT scans of cervical and thoracic levels showing diffuse spinal cord atrophy.

Segmental Spinal Cord Atrophy

Case 7. A 67-year-old woman presented with progressive myelopathy. (Fig. 7.9)

Postsurgical Spinal Cord Atrophy

Case 8. A 71-year-old man underwent cervical laminectomy 10 years previously for cervical spondylosis and spinal stenosis manifested by myeloradiculopathy with progressive weakness and numbness in recent months. Examination revealed areflexic upper extremities and spastic lower extremities. (Fig. 7.10)

Case 9. A 45-year-old man underwent laminectomy and excision of a giant schwannoma located between T-6 and L-3 5 years previously. Now he pre-

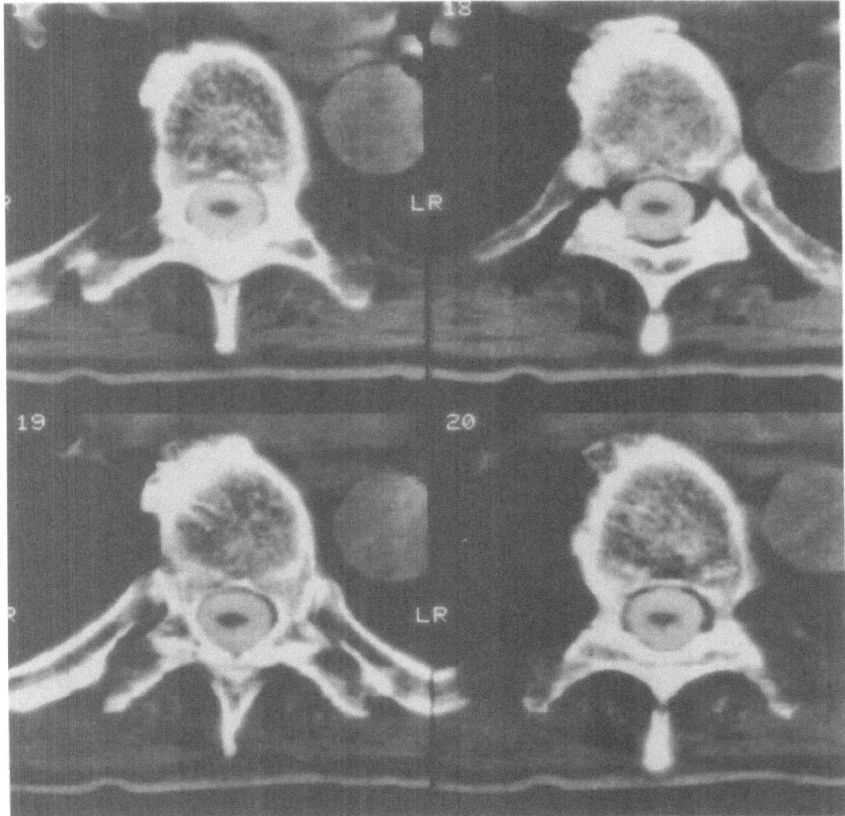

D

sented with increasing gait difficulty and numbness of both feet. Examination showed steppage gait and Babinski signs. (Fig. 7.11A,B)

Case 10. A 48-year-old man underwent laminectomy for Pott's disease 20 years previously. Spastic paraparesis and urinary and fecal urgency progressively worsened over the past 2 years. (Fig. 7.12A,B,C)

Case 11. An 87-year-old woman underwent cervical laminectomy for spinal stenosis and symptoms of myeloradiculopathy. One year later she experienced progressive loss of strength in her lower extremities. (Fig. 7.13A,B,C,D)

Case 12. A 77-year-old man underwent cervical laminectomy 10 years previously with incomplete recovery of upper extremity weakness. He presented with progressive myeloradiculopathy. He was able to ambulate, but suffered marked weakness in his upper extremities and had interosseous muscle wasting. Five years later he was chair-ridden and barely able to care for himself. (Fig. 7.14A,B,C)

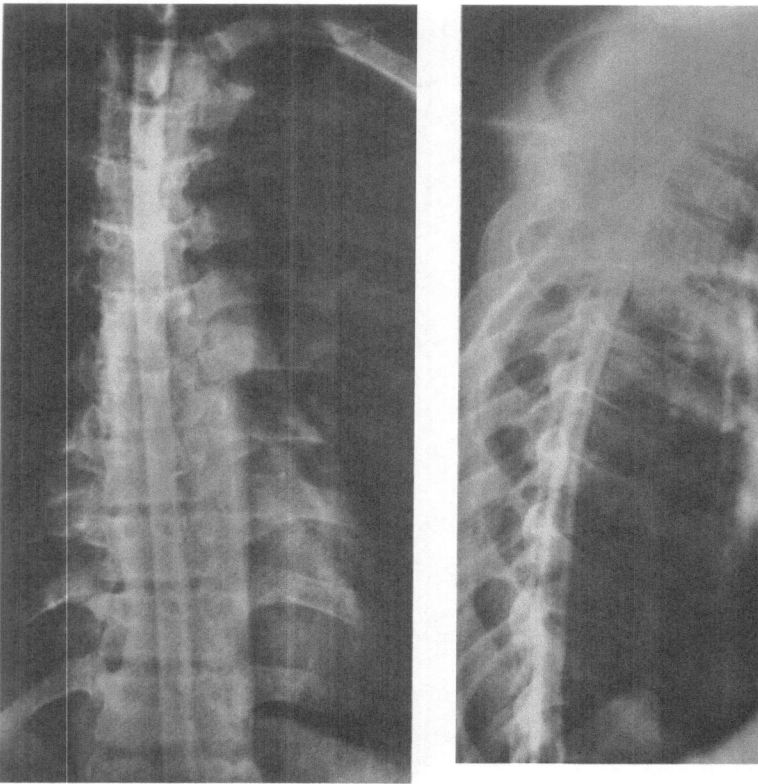

A   B

Figure 7.5A. Anteroposterior view of the thoracic myelogram shows a widened subarachnoid space in the midthoracic region T-6, T-7 and T-8.
Figure 7.5B. Lateral view shows atrophy of the spinal cord in the upper and mid-thoracic levels.

Case 13. A 63-year-old woman suffered severe head and neck trauma at age 16 years with full recovery after 14 weeks of bedrest. At age 51 years progressive difficulty walking and urinary incontinence were noted. Examination showed spastic paraparesis with impaired sensation to pin at the L-1 level. (Fig. 7.15A,B,C)

Discussion

Interest has been aroused in the subject of spinal cord atrophy in recent years, particularly with the advances afforded by CT scanning and MRI. Despite this, the entity and its pathogenesis remain relatively obscure with

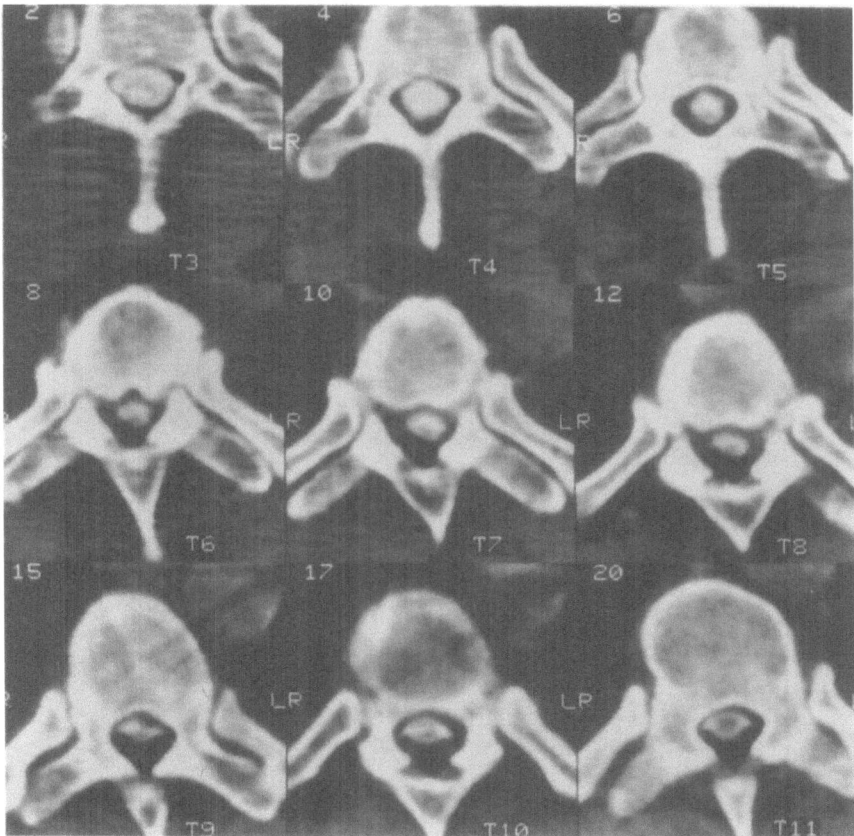

Figure 7.5C. Post–myelographic CT scans suggest hydromyelia at T-3, T-4, and T-5.

most of the descriptive terminology pertaining to radiographic and neuroimaging appearances. The neuropathology of acute spinal injury[10,18] and of maturation and age-associated atrophy[28] has been described, but the slowly progressive clinical profile in spinal cord atrophy is not fully explained by the late stage histologic findings. In essence, there appears to be a chronically evolving process related either to specific disease processes or to trauma, which may have a concurrent or delayed onset with respect to those events resulting in a gradual and irreversible wasting of the spinal cord parenchyma.

From the literature and the group of patients collected in this chapter, several points are notable and worthy of mention: Diffuse atrophy of the spinal cord associated with maturation and aging may not manifest any clinical disturbance.[28] On the other hand, diffuse atrophy associated with

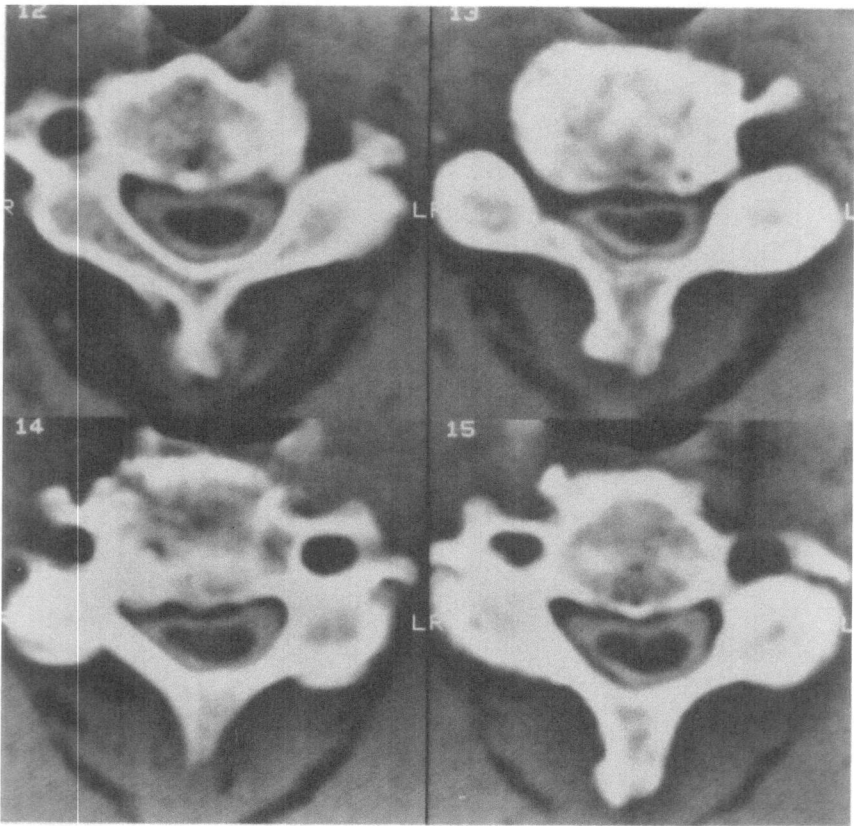

Figure 7.6. Post–myelographic CT scan shows hemiatrophy of the left side of the cervical spinal cord.

infection or resultant inflammation (case 1) and with metabolic or nutrition-al deficiency states (case 2) may have significant clinical sequelae. Second, focal compression and deformation of the spinal cord by extramedullary lesions, particularly those with chronic growth patterns, may give the radiographic appearance of segmental atrophy, yet with uncomplicated ex-cision the existing neurological deficits may remit with or without persisting spinal cord deformation. In case 9 the increase in neurological deficits after surgery implies direct cord trauma or an element of vascular compromise. Factors such as these may trigger a delayed clinical deterioration associated with spinal cord wasting. Third, in intramedullary lesions the appearance of atrophy may be due to intrinsic compressive forces and subsequent atten-uation of the normal parenchyma or there are ongoing degenerative pro-cesses as is seen in syringomyelia,[16] focal cysts such as cysticercus,[29] and

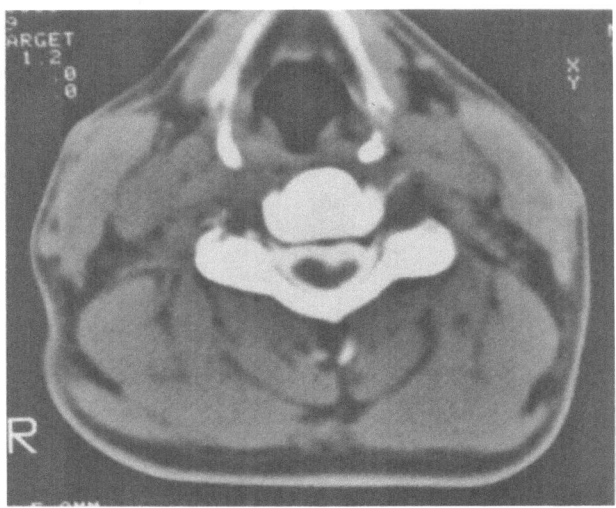

Figure 7.7. Hemiatrophy of the cervical spinal cord at the C-3 and C-4 levels is noted.

tumors such as hemangioblastomas.[14,15] It is suggested that when true atrophy is present and accompanied by clinical deterioration, there is indeed a degenerative process taking place, not simply a mechanical compression or deformation. Fourth, there is the need to give credence to the notion that ischemic events caused by either chronic microtrauma in cervical spondylosis,[30] venous congestion,[14] or perhaps steal phenomena associated with vascular lesions can be implicated in the evolution of a spinal atrophic process.

In reviewing the material, one clinical presentation became especially apparent and that involved patients who had suffered some form of spinal cord injury in the past and then either completely or partially recovered, only to have a progressive and relentless myeloradiculopathy appear years later after a relatively quiescent period. At that time spinal cord atrophy may be documented radiographically (e.g., case 13). It remains to be seen whether this represents a verifiable clinical entity.

In conclusion, it should be emphasized that all compressive lesions of the spinal cord, whether focal or diffuse, as well as inflammatory and even ischemic disturbances eventually may lead to spinal cord atrophy. However, the probability of spinal cord atrophy occurring in any specific setting is unknown at this time, as is the potential for any neural regeneration or recovery. Therefore, we stress the importance of increased awareness among both physicians and patients for the purpose of close follow-up and surgical intervention when there is evidence of spinal cord compression.

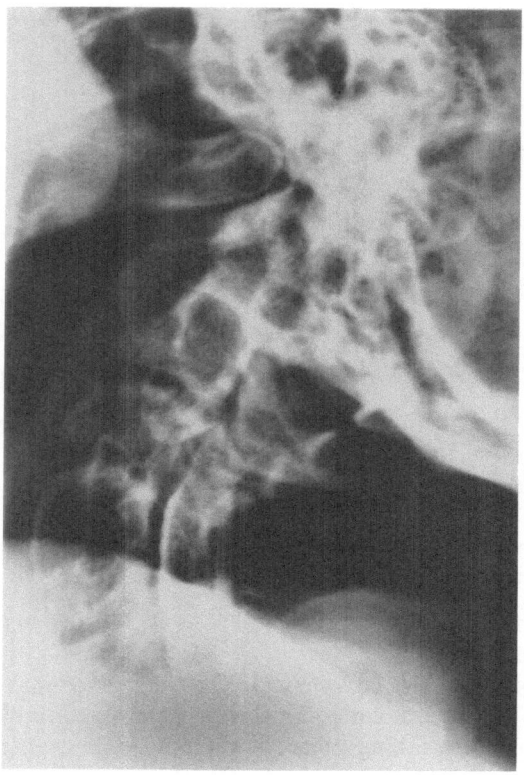

Figure 7.8A. Lateral view of the cervical myelogram shows only minimal anterior extradural defects at the C2-3 and C3-4 levels.

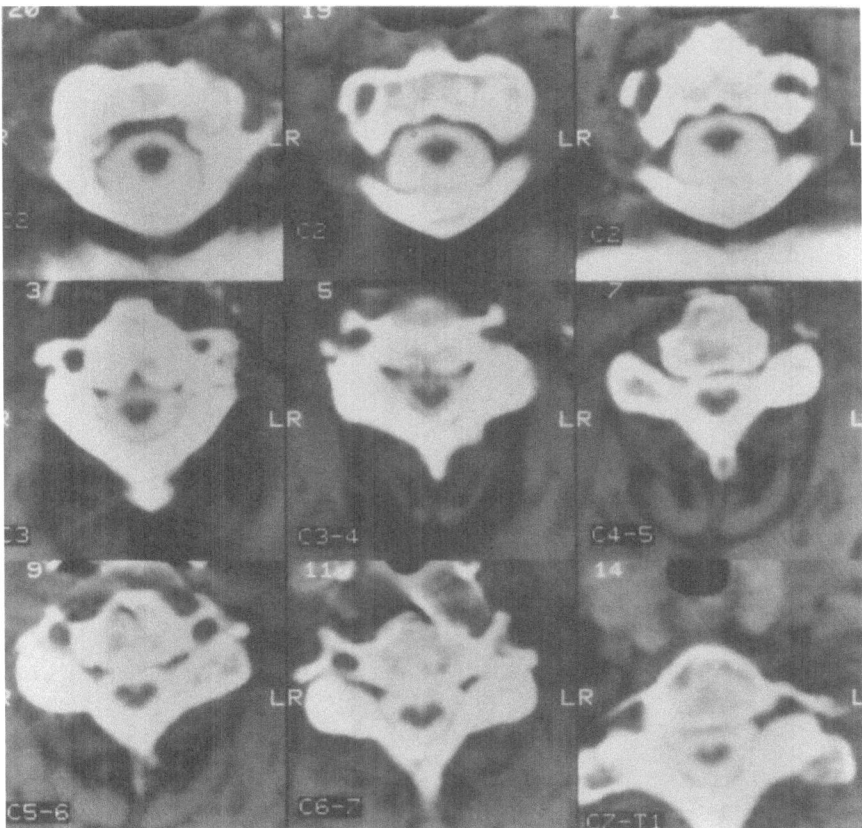

Figure 7.8B. Post–myelographic CT scans at each vertebral level reveal loss of cord parenchyma at all levels and widening of the anterior median fissure most pronounced at C6-7 and C-7–T-1 compatible with anterior atrophy.

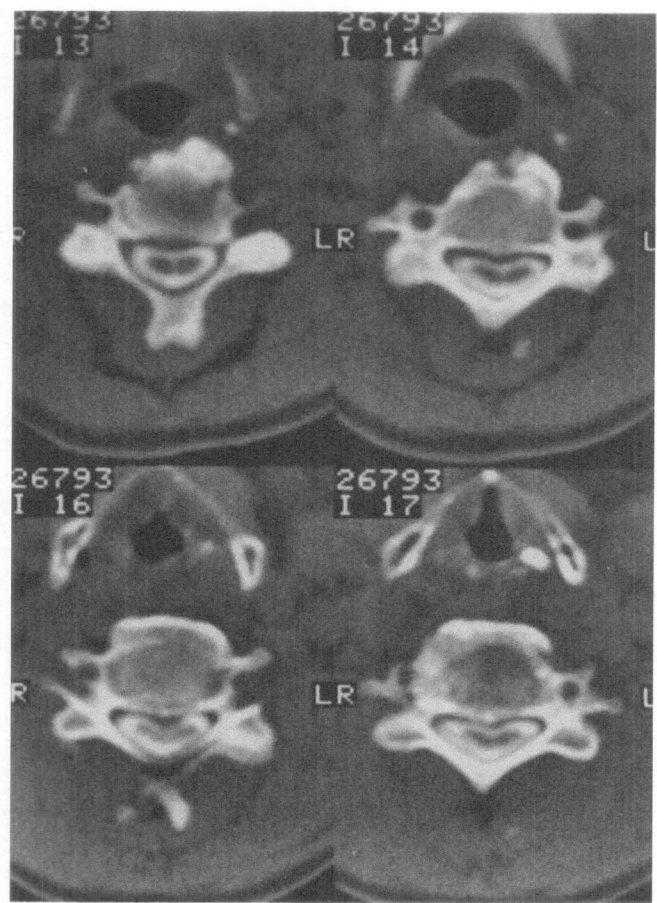

Figure 7.9. Post–myelographic CT shows flattening and thinning of the spinal cord at C-4 and C-5 levels, partly due to narrowing of the vertebral canal.

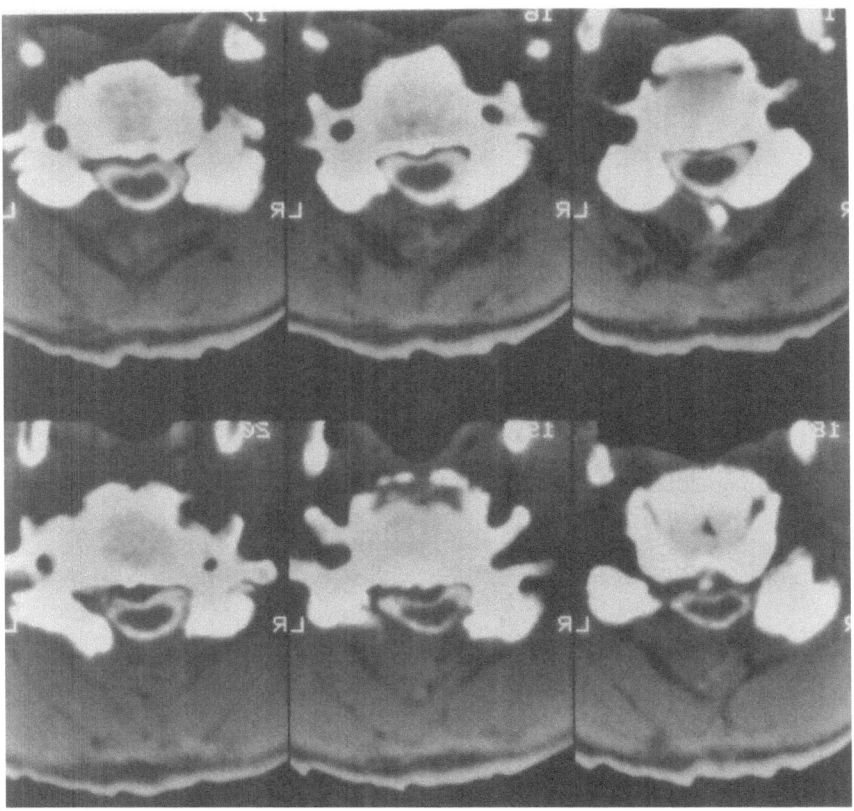

Figure 7.10. Post–myelographic CT shows segmental atrophy of the cervical spinal cord at the C-5 and C-6 levels.

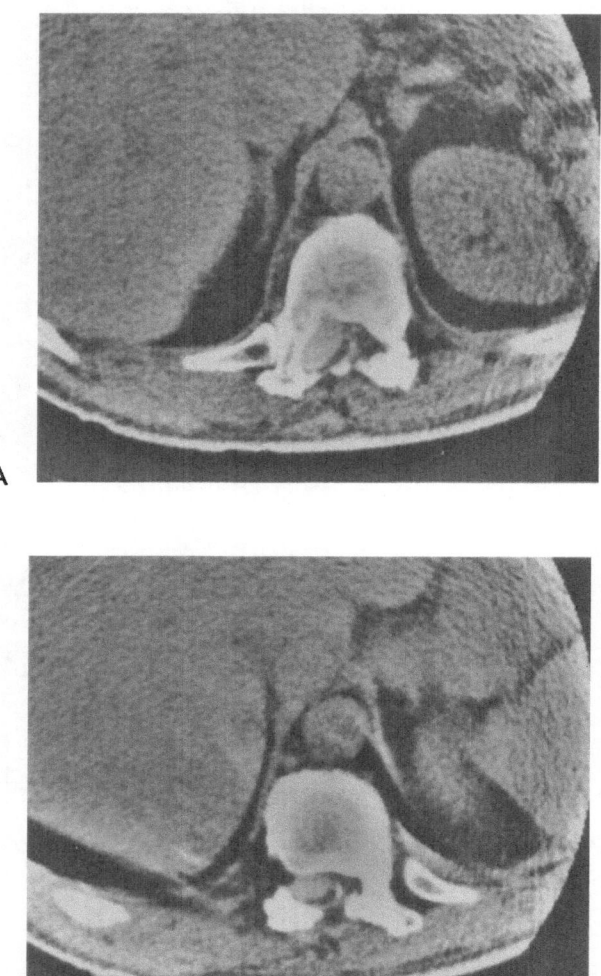

Figure 7.11A,B. Post–myelographic CT scans at T-12 show a crescent-shaped atrophic spinal cord.

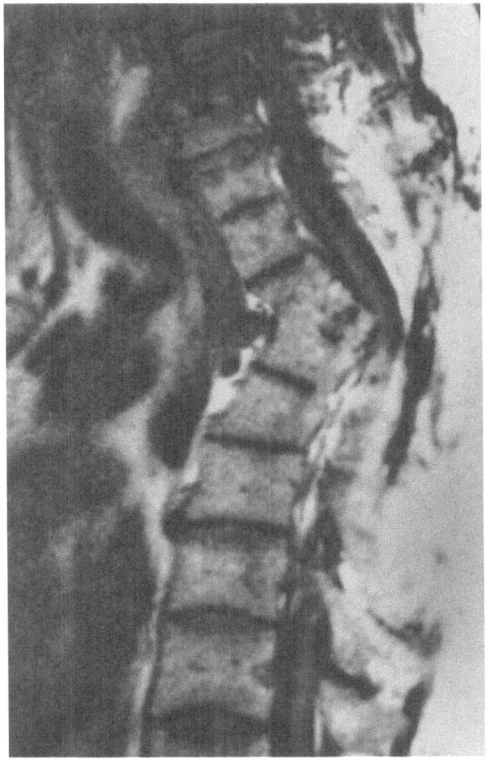

Figure 7.12A. Sagittal T_1-weighted image shows kyphosis at the T-9 level.

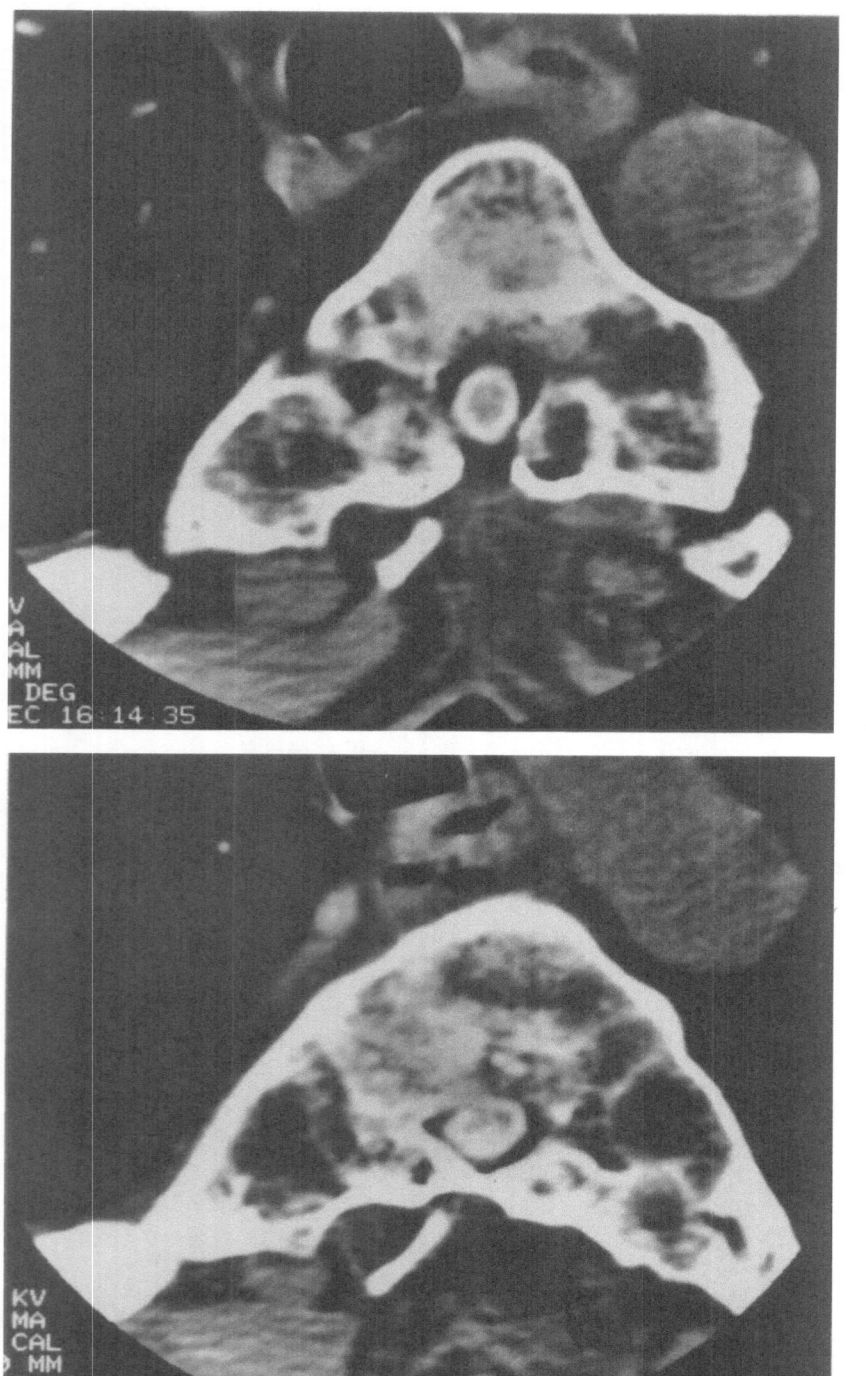

B

C

Figure 7.12B,C. Post–myelographic CT scans reveal spinal cord atrophy at the level of prior laminectomy and adjacent levels where laminectomy was not performed.

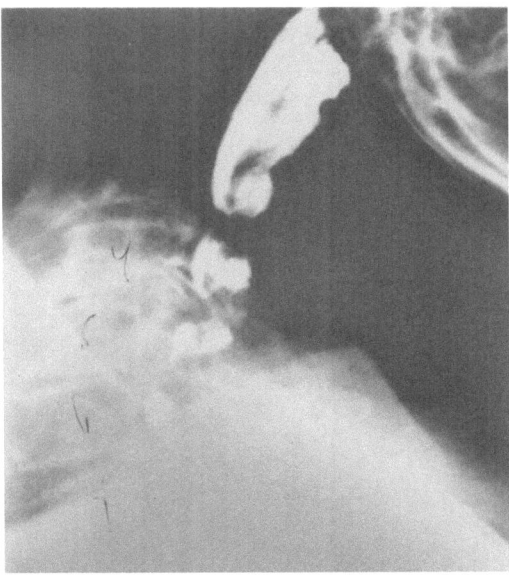

Figure 7.13A. Lateral view of pantopaque cervical myelogram reveals constriction of the thecal sac at interspace levels from C-3 to C-6 preoperatively. The spinal cord is poorly visualized.

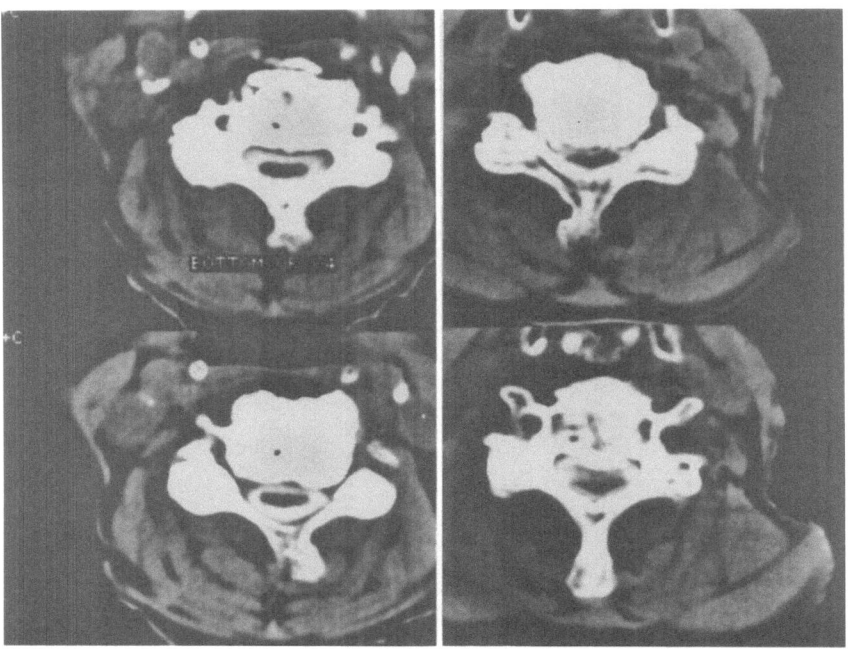

Figure 7.13B. Representative post–myelograpahic CT scans of the cervical spine demonstrate cord atrophy from C-4 to C-6.

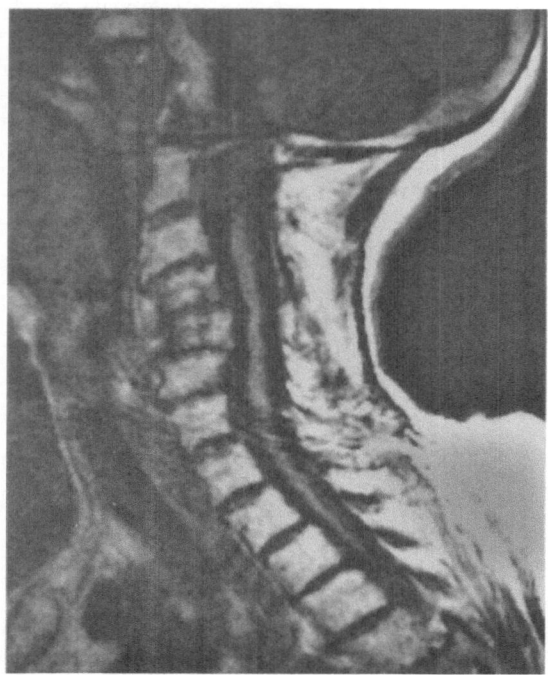

Figure 7.13C. One year later sagittal T_1-weighted images at the C3-4 level show flattening of the spinal cord.

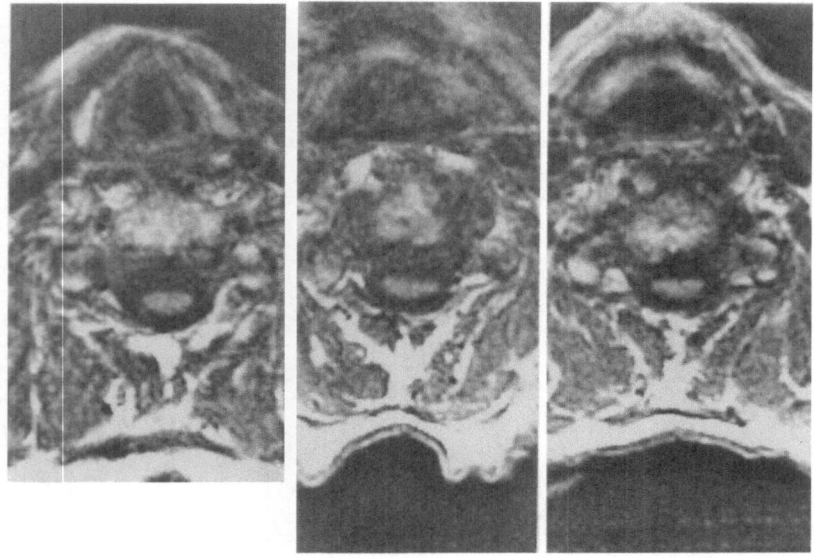

Figure 7.13D.

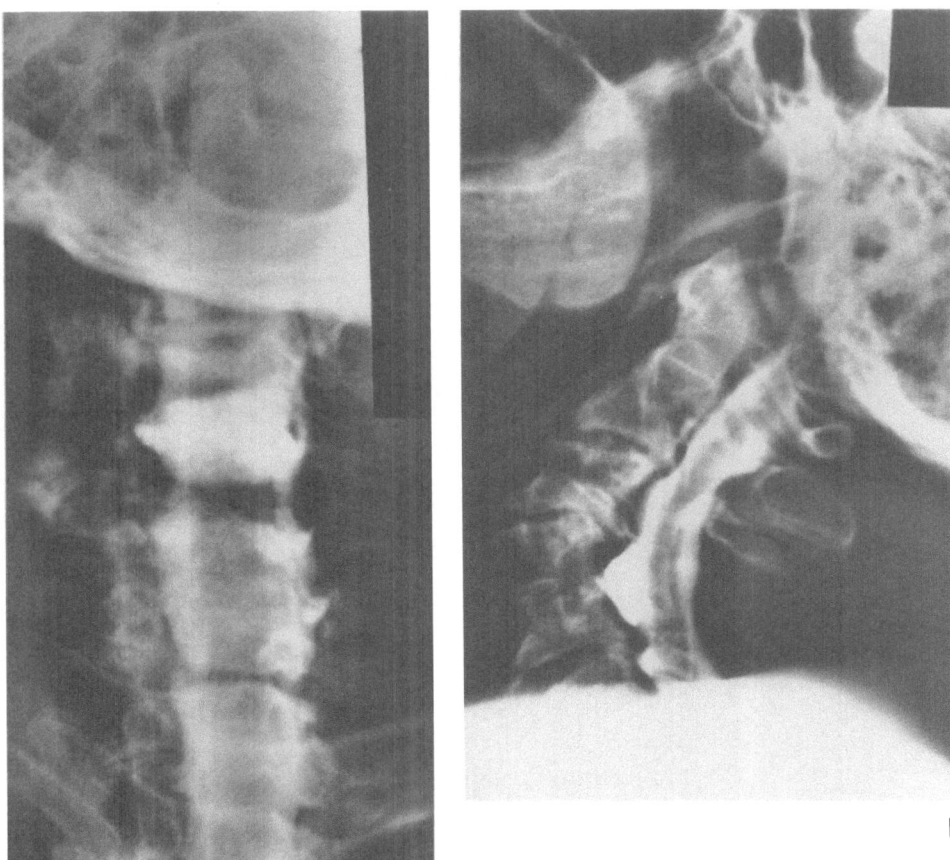

A

B

Figure 7.14A,B. Anteroposterior and lateral views on the cervical myelogram show the width of the spinal cord to be normal. Laminectomy is evident beginning at the C-4 level and continuing caudad.

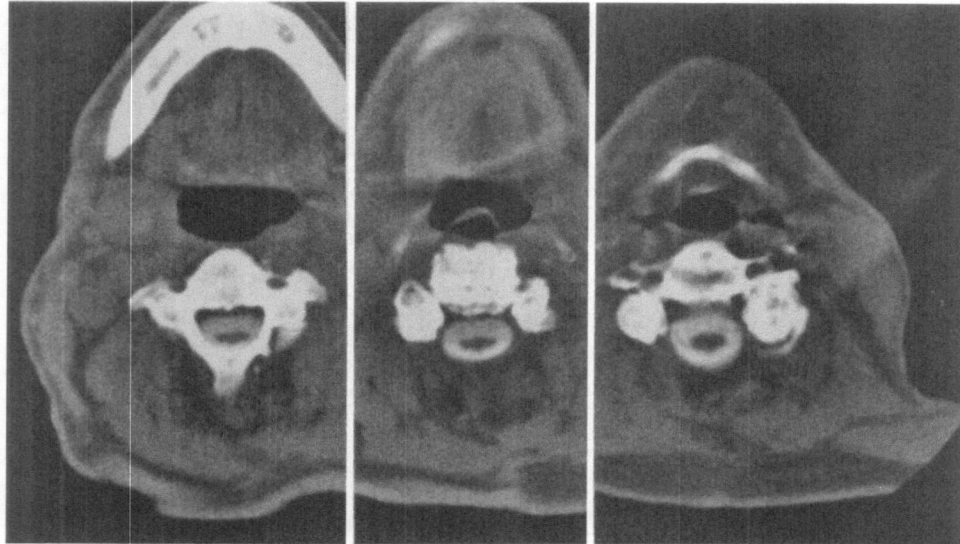

Figure 7.14C. Post–myelogram CT scans show an atrophic spinal cord at the C-3 level.

Figure 7.15A,B. Posteroanterior and lateral views show widening of the subarachnoid spaces at the C4-7 levels with a small spinal cord.

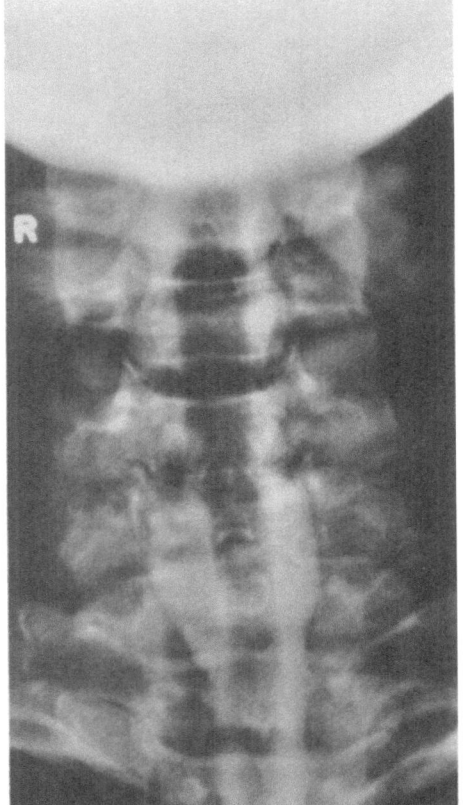

A

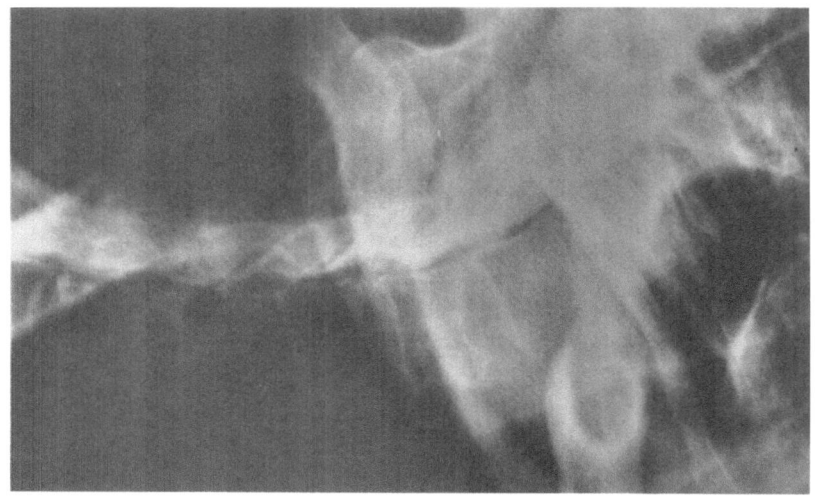

B

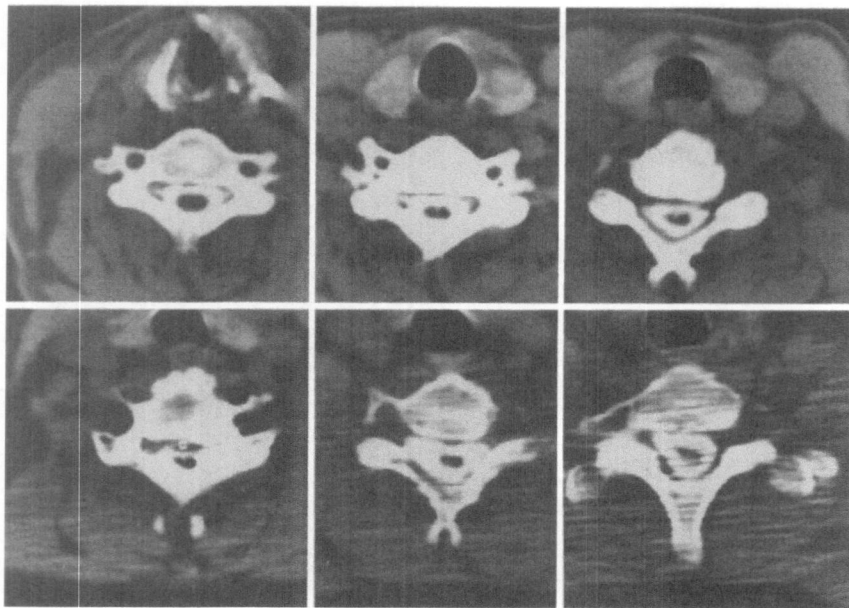

Figure 7.15C. Post–myelographic CT scans confirm the existence of an atrophic cord at the C4-7 levels. At the C6-7 level a posteriorly herniated disc is present, which does not compress the cord.

References

1. Reeves CE. *Diseases of the Spinal Cord and its Membranes.* London: Simkin, Marshall & Co;1858:224–228.
2. Nordqvist L. The sagittal diameter of the spinal cord and subarachnoid space in different age groups—A roentgenographic postmortem study. *Acta Radiol.* 1964;227(Suppl):1–96.
3. Drachman DB, Banker BW. Arthrogryposis multiplex congenita. *Arch Neurol.* 1961;511:89–105.
4. Gibson DA. Arthrogryposis multiplex congenita. In: Vinken PJ, Bruyn GW, eds. *Handbook of Neurology.* Amsterdam: Elsevier/North-Holland Biomedica Press; 1978:511–518.
5. Staal A, Stefanko SZ, Busch HF, Jennekens FG, DeBruin JWC. Autonomic nerve calcification and peripheral neuropathy in olivopontocerebellar atrophy. *J Neurol Sci.* 1981;51(3):383–394.
6. Boman K. Spinal cord atrophy in spastic paraplegia. *Acta Neurol Scand.* 1967;43:180–188.
7. Shirare T, Indue N, Wakisaka S, Yoshida H, Hoshiko M. Case of multiple sclerosis with repeated exacerbations of transverse myelopathy at a single level and severe atrophy of the spinal cord found at autopsy. *Brain-Nerve(Tokyo).* 1971;23(12):1575–1581.
8. Cloys DE, Netsky MG. Neuromyelitis optica. In: Vinken PJ, Bruyn GW, eds. *Handbook of Neurology.* Amsterdam: North-Holland Publishing Co; 1970:452–468.
9. Folliss AGH, Netsky MG. Progressive necrotic myelopathy. In: Vinken PJ, Bruyn GW, eds. *Handbook of Neurology.* Amsterdam: North-Holland Publishing Co; 1970:452–468.
10. Hughes JT, Brownell B. Paraplegia following retrograde abdominal aortography. *Arch Neurol.* 1965;12:650–659.
11. Schiller F. Venery, the spinal cord and tabes dorsalis before Romberg: The contribution of Ernst Horn. *J Nerv Ment Dis.* 1976;163(1):1–9.
12. Donaldson I, Gibson R. Spinal cord atrophy associated with arachnoiditis as demonstrated by computed tomography. *Neuroradiology.* 1982;24:101–105.
13. Nakada T, Kwee IL, Palmaz JC. Computed tomography of spinal cord atrophy. *Neuroradiology.* 1982;24:97–99.
14. Solomon RA, Stein BM. Unusual spinal cord enlargement related to intramedullary hemangioblastoma. *J Neurosurg.* 1988;68:550–553.
15. McCormick PC, Stein BM. Intramedullary tumors in adults. *Neurosurg Clin North Am.* 1990;1(3):625.
16. Schliep G. Syringomyelia and syringobulbia. In: Vinken PJ, Bruyn GW, eds. *Handbook of Neurology.* Amsterdam: Elsevier/North-Holland Biomedical Press; 1978:255–327.
17. Komaki S. Localized spinal cord atrophy: significance of its demonstration. *Radiology.* 1976;121:11–114.
18. Jellinger K. Neuropathology of cord injuries. In: Vinken PJ, Bruyn GW, eds. *Handbook of Neurology.* Amsterdam: North-Holland Publishing Co; 1976:43–121.
19. Panse F. Electrical trauma. In: Vinken PJ, Bruyn GW, eds. *Handbook of Neurology.* Amsterdam: North-Holland Publishing Co; 1975:683–729.

20. Siebert CE, Barnes JE, Dreisbach JN, Swanson WB, Heck RJ. Accurate CT measurement of the spinal cord using metrizamide: Physical factors. *Am J Roentgenol.* 1980;136:777–780.
21. Koehler PR, Anderson RE, Baxter B. The effect of computed tomography viewer controls on anatomical measurements. *Radiology.* 1979;130:189–194.
22. Yousem DM, Janick PA, Atlas SW, et al. Pseudoatrophy of the cervical portion of the spinal cord on MR images: A manifestation of the truncation artifact. *AJNR.* 1990;11:373–377.
23. Curtin AJ, Chakeres DW, Bulas R, Boesel CP, Finneran M, Flint E. MR imaging artifacts of the axial internal anatomy of the cervical spinal cord. *AJNR.* 1989;10:19–26.
24. Thijssen HOM, Keyser A, Horstink MWM, Meijer E. Morphology of the cervical spinal cord on computed myelography. *Neuroradiology.* 1979;18:57–62.
25. Gellad F, Krishna CVGR, Joseph PM, Vigorito RD. Morphology and dimensions of the thoracic cord by computer-assisted metrizamide myelography. *AJNR.* 1983;4:614–617.
26. Braun IF, Raghavendra BN, Kricheff II. Spinal cord imaging using real-time high-resolution ultrasound. *Radiology.* 1983;147:459–465.
27. Mawad ME, Hilal SK, Fetell MR, Silver AJ, Ganti SR, Sane P. Patterns of spinal cord atrophy by metrizamide CT. *AJNR.* 1983;4:611–613.
28. Critchley M. Neurology of old age. *Lancet.* May 23, 1931:1125–1126.
29. Holtzman RNN, Hughes JEO, Sachdev RK, Jarenwattananon A. Intramedullary cysticercosis. *Surg Neurol.* 1986;26:187–191.
30. Breig A, Turnbull J, Hassler O. Effects of mechanical stress on the spinal cord in cervical spondylosis. *J Neurosurg.* 1966;25:45–56.

Discussion

Thoughts on The Etiology of Spinal Cord Atrophy

Dr. Lazorthes said: perhaps this represents an idée fixe, but I give precedence to the role of vascular factors in spinal cord atrophy. From my work there are more than 200 observations of spinal cord atrophy, particularly in the midthoracic spinal cord where vascular supply is dependent on the integrity of the aorta and the iliac arteries. Quite simply, arteriosclerotic changes in the lumen of the aorta influencing flow via the intercostal and lumbar arteries and their radicular branches may significantly impair the irrigation of the spinal cord. I see this as a vascular problem in the elderly population with the presenting symptom complex being spastic paraparesis.

Dr. Leeds commented that we have been too loose with the term "syringomyelia." Myelomalacia can be perceived on neuroimaging studies as central cavitation. Dr. Stein presented cases where the MRI showed long cavities that turned out not to be cavities and Dr. Bello's use of cine to demonstrate pulsations may allow us to diagnose these differences. Even so, not every cavity has pulsations, which makes it difficult to be absolutely certain—we may be jumping to conclusions. For example, in our experience we see large spinal cords, but if you review the literature the majority of spinal cords are reported as atrophic or normal, so a large spinal cord does not necessarily go with a syrinx, although that seems contradictory.

Dr. Schlesinger pointed out that the MRI has shown us, even after very successful surgical decompressions, particularly for spondylosis and narrowing of the foramina, an enormous degree of spinal cord degeneration, cystic pocketing. The literature is indicating more and more the poor results from what we surgeons thought was very good treatment, and this reflects changes that have been going on within the spinal cord concurrent with the extrinsic compression. I agree with Dr. Lazorthes that the vascular supply, from both longitudinal spinal vessels and from the radicular arteries, is often incompletely understood or evaluated in the spinal and foraminal compressions. If we were to visualize the foramina we would find that there is an enormous obliteration of the arterial supply and the venous return. In the same cases where those sort of mammiliform bodies anteriorly are compressing the anterior blood supply we can add motion and vascular sclerotic changes, all of which contribute to the spinal cord degenerative process.

From a clinical and surgical standpoint it has always been my impression that patients who suffered from lateral spinal compression syndromes with interference of blood supply improved more dramatically after adequate decompression and unroofing of the nerve roots than patients who had overt bony compression from midline spondylotic ridges.

I believe that as surgeons we have to be more thoughtful about root decompression and I refer the members of this symposium to the monograph entitled *The Intervertebral Foramen of the Spinal Column** written in 1914.

Swanberg, Harold. *The Intervertebral Foramen: An Atlas and Histologic Description of an Intervertebral Foramen and Its Adjacent Parts.* Chicago: Chicago Science Publishing Co.; 1914.

Dr. Antunes added that there is an experience accumulating now of increasing neurological deficits in patients who suffered poliomyelitis at an early age and 30 to 40 years previously. Some explanation for this may lie in the normal physiological decay of the number of cells in the anterior horns or in the remainder of the spinal cord. This may be pertinent to the cases presented that suggest an initial injury and a delayed deterioration of neurological function. It may reflect a decrease in the original pool of neurons and fibers that accompanies the physiological changes of aging. It may be just the death of normal neurons exacerbating the preexisting state.

European neurologists are attentive to this problem. We thought initially that calcification of the posterior longitudinal ligament was a Japanese disease, but most individuals with cervical spondylosis have calcification of the posterior longitudinal ligament to a certain degree. It may well be that posterior decompression alone is insufficient to protect the spinal cord from delayed changes due to chronic ischemia.

Dr. Leeds added that patients with ossification of the posterior longitudinal ligament (OPLL) have an increased incidence of diffuse idiopathic skeletal hyperostosis (DISH). I reviewed an article from Japan written for our journal and travelled there as a visiting professor. They showed me a Puerto Rican woman with OPLL. Now we see that condition in every ethnic and national group. I cannot believe that it represents a new entity. However, most of these patients have DISH with extensive anterior osteophytes. Often the compression is due to the OPLL, which is often falsely called calcified discs.

I would just like to add one further comment and that is that the venous outflow from the cord may be equally important as the arterial supply and yet relatively little emphasis has been given it.

Dr. Livshitz commented that the problem of spinal cord atrophy is much more extensive than it is currently considered to be. Clearly it is not a problem that will be solved only by decompression of the spinal cord. Attention must be given to repairing the vascular supply to the cord. Some work has been done in this area, particularly by the Chinese who have used omental grafts, but the results have not been sufficiently clear to warrant their general use. I believe in the future we must consider new approaches to restore the circulation to the spinal cord. Perhaps this will prevent the atrophic process.

II-C. CONCEPTS IN BIOENGINEERING AND FETAL TISSUE TRANSPLANTATION

CHAPTER 8

Neurocomputing: The Technology and Some Potential Applications to Neurosurgery

Robert Hecht-Nielsen

The Programming Paradigm

Currently, essentially all automated information processing is based on the "glorified adding machine" paradigm spelled out by John von Neumann in his 1945 consultant's report to the project that developed the first usable electronic digital computer: ENIAC. In this approach, the user defines the problem to be solved and then develops an algorithmic procedure for solving it. This algorithm is then expressed in a software language (e.g., FORTRAN, Ada, C, Pascal, etc.) and run on a computer.

Neurocomputing: A New Information Processing Paradigm

Solving a problem using neurocomputing is quite different from programmed computing. The first step is to consider a list of the known types of neural networks and see if any of them can carry out the type of information processing function required to solve the problem at hand. If one of them can, a network of this type is then configured appropriately (which is done by following rules of thumb that have been developed for each type of neural network) and exposed to an appropriate information environment. The purpose of this exposure is to train the neural network to carry out the desired information processing operation. Rules for constructing an appropriate information environment for training a particular neural network also exist. During the training process the neural network adapts itself to the environment to which it is exposed and, as training progresses, it becomes able to carry out the desired operation.

Comparison between Neurocomputing and Programmed Computing

Clearly, neurocomputing is radically different from ordinary programmed computing. For one thing, it is not necessary to know the algorithm needed to solve the problem. The neural network develops the algorithm by adaptation to the training environment. Further, neural networks obviate need for software, since it is no longer necessary to enter a user-specified algorithm. The implication of these facts is that with neurocomputing we can develop information processing capabilities for which no algorithm can be specified. Also, development cost and time can be shortened dramatically since the laborious and time-consuming process of software development is eliminated.

On the negative side, neurocomputing has the limitation that it is only applicable to those problems that fall into the classes that particular types of neural networks can solve (these are briefly described below). Further, it must be possible to obtain a comprehensive set of examples of the desired information processing operation being carried out. These must be statistically representative of the real-world environment that the neural network will encounter in operational service.

Neurocomputing holds promise, but only in applications for which adequate training examples can be obtained. Examples of application areas in which problems can often be solved by neurocomputing include pattern recognition, control, and data analysis.

Although it may appear that neurocomputing is in competition with programmed computing, this is not the case. In fact, most things that programmed computing does well neurocomputing does poorly or not at all, and vice versa. Experience has shown that these two approaches to information processing are best used in a complementary manner. This has led to the development of neurocomputers (specialized digital coprocessors that can efficiently implement neural networks) that interface directly to standard computers (such as the IBM PC-AT and the Sun 3 and 4 computers). The neurocomputer provides for timely implementation of neural networks (ordinary computers cannot implement neural networks at usable speeds for most applications) under the control of host computer software. In this milieu, neural networks are treated as subroutines or procedures by software running on the host computer, thus providing a simple mechanism for integrating the advantages of neural networks into traditional computing environments.

The details of interfacing between host computer software and the neurocomputer are made invisible to the users by means of a software package supplied by the neurocomputer manufacturer. This package provides simple canned subroutines that the user can call from their software to control the operation of neural networks they wish to use. Typical commands include one that causes a particular neural network to be loaded into the neurocomputer (from a disk file where it is stored), one to put data from the user's program into a specified neural network (neurocomputers typically allow many neural networks to be simultaneously resident), one to activate a selected neural network, one to get output data from the neural network and transfer it to the user's software, and finally, one to save a neural network in a disk file. With the advent of such user-friendly interfaces it has become possible for virtually any scientist, engineer, or systems developer to incorporate neurocomputing into his projects.

Overview of Neurocomputing

Research in neurocomputing has been seriously underway for the last 30 years. Most of the work to date has been carried out by researchers in the areas of electrical engineering, computer science, mathematics, cognitive science, physics, and neuroscience. For all but the last 2 or 3 years this work was carried out by a small but dedicated band of pioneers who were ignored by most of the rest of the world. By 1985 the capabilities of digital electronic technology had advanced to the point where the exciting, but purely theoretical, ideas developed by these pioneers could actually be implemented, evaluated, and confirmed. When the encouraging results that were obtained became generally known, interest in neurocomputing grew explosively.

Neurocomputing, as a discipline, is divided into three main areas:

neural network architecture and theory
neurocomputer design
applications

Today, there are 14 different types of neural network available for use in applications development. Although network theory is a growing area, the growth is limited by the fact that successful contributors must typically be highly skilled analysts, of which there will always be a limited supply.

Neurocomputer design is being pursued by industry, government, and universities. With the exploration of commercial and military applications of neurocomputing quickly expanding, this is an area that is growing rapidly. Many electronic, optical, and electro-optical neurocomputers have already been built and commercial neurocomputers are already being sold. The reason for this interest is the discovery (by several of us during the 1970s) that machines optimized for the implementation of neural networks could carry out those implementations much more efficiently than typical host computers. A simple coprocessor paradigm for interfacing neurocomputers with standard host computers has now been standardized. Software interfaces allow software running on a standard host computer to call neural networks on the neurocomputer as if they were subroutines. Neurocomputing languages (analogous to programming languages such as Pascal and FORTRAN) for expressing neural network configurations have also been developed—which allow networks to be expressed in a simple, machine-portable form. These provisions make it easy to interface computer programs and neural networks.

Applications of neurocomputing are primarily being developed by domain experts in industry, government, and universities. It has been observed that neurocomputing is relatively easy for most domain-expert engineers to learn. Neurocomputing can often be applied profitably in combination with other information processing techniques such as symbolic programming, signal processing, and image processing. The range of industries already attempting to develop practical applications is surprisingly broad. They include defense, entertainment, telecommunications, aerospace, retail franchise, machine vision, finance, automotive, insurance, robotics and industrial automation, securities, general consumer product manufacturing, and industrial inspection.

Neural Networks and their Information Processing Capabilities

Formally, a neural network is a dynamical system with the topology of a directed graph that can carry out information processing by means of its state response to continuous or episodic input. The nodes in neural networks are called *processing elements*, and the directed links (information channels) are called *interconnects*. Each processing element is endowed with some local memory. The processing that takes place in each processing element (this processing is defined by the *transfer function* of the processing element) must depend only on the current values of the input signals and on the values in local memory. The processing elements of a neural network either operate continuously or are *updated* in accordance with a *scheduling function*. Typically, neural networks comprise collections of processing elements called *layers* or *slabs* in which all of the processing elements have the same transfer function (although their local memory values can be different). There are probably at least 30 different types of neural networks currently being used in research and/or applications. Of these, there are 14 types in common use:

Adaptive Resonance (ART): two classes of networks [Adaptive Resonance Theory 1 (ART 1) networks for binary-valued inputs and ART 2 networks for continuous-valued inputs] that form categories for input data with the coarseness of the categories determined by the value of a selective parameter (the vigilance parameter); other capabilities include hypothesis testing and classification decision confirmation

Avalanche (AVA): a class of networks for learning, recognizing, and re-playing spatiotemporal patterns

Backpropagation (BPN): a multilayer mapping network that minimizes mean squared mapping error; the most popular neural network in use today

Bidirectional Associative Memory (BAM): a class of single-stage hetero-associative networks, some capable of learning

Boltzmann Machine/Cauchy Machine (BCM): networks that use a noise process to find the global minimum of a cost function

Brain State in a Box (BSB): a single-stage autoassociative network that minimizes its mean squared error

Cerebellatron (CBT): learns the averages of spatiotemporal command sequence patterns and replays these average command sequences on cue

Counterpropagation (CPN): a network that functions as a statistically optimal self-organizing look-up table and probability density function analyzer

Hopfield (HOP): a class of single-stage autoassociative networks without learning

Learnmatrix (LRN): a single-pass nonrecursive single-stage associative network

MADALINE (MDL): a bank of trainable linear combiners that minimize mean squared error

Neocognitron (NEO): a multilayer hierarchical character recognition network

Perceptron (PTR): a bank of trainable linear discriminants, rarely used today

Self-Organizing Map (SOM): forms a continuous topological mapping from one compact manifold to another, with the mapping metric density varying directly with a given probability density function on the second manifold.

A crucial part of most transfer functions is the *learning law*. This law is an equation that modifies some of the internal memory values of the processing element in response to input signals and transfer function supplied values. The learning law of a processing element allows the response of the processing element to input signals to change with time in response to its input signal environment. There are currently six classes of learning law that have been defined and are in use:

Grossberg: competitive learning of weighted average inputs

Hebb: correlation learning of mutually coincident inputs

Kohonen: development of a set of vectors conforming to a particular probability density function

Kosko/Klopf: formation of representations for sequences of events in temporal order

Rosenblatt: adjustment of a perceptron linear discriminant device via a performance grading input from an external teacher

Widrow: minimization of a mean squared error cost function

Neural networks can use one or more of these learning laws. A few neural networks have no learning law—these networks are usually used for solving fixed problems that can be set up in advance. Neural networks that do use learning are usually subjected to training in accordance with one of three schemes: *supervised training*, in which the network is supplied with both input data and "desired output" data; *graded training*, in which the network is given input data, but is not supplied with the desired output data; instead, it is occasionally given a grading input or performance score that tells it how well it is doing; and *self-organization*, in which the network is only given input data and is expected to organize itself into some useful configuration in response to it.

Neural networks have been shown to be capable of carrying out a number of information processing operations. These include:

Mathematical Mapping Approximation: development of an approximation to a function $f:A \subset R^n \to B \subset R^m$ by means of self-adjustment in response to a set of examples $(\mathbf{x}_1, \mathbf{y}_1), (\mathbf{x}_2, \mathbf{y}_2), \ldots, (\mathbf{x}_L, \mathbf{y}_L)$ (where $\mathbf{y}_i = f(\mathbf{x}_i)$ or $\mathbf{y}_i = f(\mathbf{x}_i) + \mathbf{n}$ and where $\mathbf{n}$ is a stationary noise process) of the mapping's action—BPN, CPN

Probability Density Function Estimation: development of a set of equiprobable "anchor points" by self-organization in response to a set of examples $\mathbf{x}_1, \mathbf{x}_2, \ldots$ of vectors in R_n chosen in accordance with a fixed probability density function ρ—CPN, SOM

Extraction of Relational Knowledge from Binary Data Bases: formation of an aggregate model of knowledge concerning statistically common relationships between fields in the records of a data base by self-adjustment in response to input of the data base records—BSB

Formation of a Topologically Continuous and Statistically Conformal Mapping: self-organization of such mappings based on adaptation to input data chosen in accordance with a fixed probability density function, with the final mapping often exhibiting representations for the similarities between different items in the data space—SOM

Nearest Neighbor Pattern Classification: classification of patterns by comparing them with large sets of stored, preclassified, example patterns; a capability that can be applied to both spatial and spatiotemporal patterns and can use hierarchically stored patterns for compressed storage— ART, AVA, BAM, BCM, BPN, BSB, CBD, CPN, HOP, LRN, MDL, NEO, PTR

Categorization of Data: formation of categories of a selected granularity by means of self-organization in response to data; categories can change, but only a limited number of times, at which point they become rigid; new categories can be formed for any new objects that are not sufficiently close to existing categories—ART

General Applications

It is important to point out that each of the information processing capabilities listed above has important technical limitations. These capabilities cannot be applied at will to arbitrarily chosen problems. In fact, the applications engineering methodology that seems to work best is first to have domain-expert engineers carefully learn the capabilities and limitations of each of the major neural networks and their associated information processing operations. They can then search for potential high-payoff applications within their area of expertise that can be solved within these constraints. This methodology is now being applied by applications developers across a broad range of disciplines. Although it is still too early to predict which, if any, of these projects will succeed, the fact that they are underway is itself significant. Some examples of real-world applications currently being explored by various industries are presented below. Some of these applications (such as real-time translation of spoken language) might take a decade or more to develop, whereas others (such as credit application scoring) are already in daily use.

Finance: credit application scoring, credit line use analysis, new product analysis and optimization, corporate financial analysis, customer set characterization.

Banking: marketing studies, check reading, physical security enhancement, loan evaluation, customer credit scoring

Insurance: insurance policy application evaluation, payout trend analysis, new product analysis, and optimization

Defense: radar/sonar/image processing (noise reduction, data compression, feature extraction, pattern recognition), opposing force models, weapons aiming and steering, novel sensor systems

Entertainment: market analysis and forecasting, special effects, animation, restoration

Automotive: assembly jig control, warranty repair analysis, automobile autopilot

Transportation: waybill processing, vehicle scheduling and routing, airline fare management

Telecommunications: speech and image compression, automated information services, real-time translation of spoken language, customer payment processing systems

Retail franchise: outlet site location selection

Securities: stock and commodity trading advisor systems, technical market/company/commodity analysis, customer credit analysis

Robotics: vision systems, appendage controllers, tactile feedback gripper control

Manufacturing: low cost visual inspection systems, nondestructive testing, fabrication plan development

Electronics: VLSI chip layout, process control, chip inspection

Aerospace: avionics fault detection, aircraft/spacecraft control systems, autopilot enhancements.

Neurosurgical Applications

Initial applications of neurocomputing to neurosurgery will probably be in the areas of improved patient monitoring during surgery and simple prosthetics. These may someday be followed by more exotic developments such as adaptive nerve splice implants and even auxiliary memory devices. Brief descriptions of these concepts are provided below. It is important to realize that even in the cases of initial applications it may require up to a decade of research and development to bring these concepts to the point where they can be applied routinely. The more exotic concepts will probably require multiple decades to bring to fruition.

Patient monitoring is crucial during all surgery, and particularly during noncranial neurosurgery. Factors that must be monitored include the response of patient tissues (particularly the brain) to the oxygen, anesthetics, narcotics, and muscle relaxants used, level of unconsciousness, and changes in reflex arc responses.

Early experiments with two-lead (one per hemisphere with a common ground) on-line electroencephalogram (EEG) systems indicate that this may be a useful way to monitor the activity and health of the brain during surgery. Situations that would otherwise lead to unforeseen necrosis of brain tissue or an awake, but paralyzed, patient can be automatically detected, and possibly predicted minutes in advance, by a neurocomputing-based EEG monitoring system.

Much in the manner of EEG monitoring, it would appear feasible to monitor and/or elicit electromyogram signals during noncranial neurosurgery. This would allow the patency of reflex arcs subserving specific muscle groups to be evaluated as surgery progressed. Such a system would use glue-on electrode arrays, much in the manner of electrocardiogram electrodes. Provisions for dealing with tens of individual muscle groups might be possible. Such a system could also be used for monitoring muscle signals for the activation of electronically controlled motorized prosthetics (e.g., a gripping hand). These would be particularly useful in those cases where unique combinations of muscle activations can be used to cue activation of the prosthesis.

In the distant future, neurocomputing might well make possible nerve splice devices that could be chronically implanted. These would be used in situations where a nerve is severed and possibly shortened. The first step would be, using biological techniques, to cause the severed axons still connected to their neuron cell bodies to grow end caps without branching. The axons that were disconnected from their cell bodies would be stimulated, using similar techniques, to develop new cell bodies. The implant will have biomaterial (i.e., lipid structure) head and tail ends that can interface with these newly terminated nerve elements in such a way as to allow chronic electrical (or chemical) interface without destruction or degradation of the nerve. Provisions for interfacing with hundreds of thousands of individual signals (going in either direction) may well be possible. The nerve splice would have within it a neurocomputing system that would adaptively reconnect the nerve by means of operational testing. The power for the electronic circuits used in the device would be derived from specially bred cells that would convert the biochemical nutrients in the blood (the device would be supplied with a few small blood vessels) to an electric potential.

Given the sorts of chronic nerve interfaces postulated above, it may well become possible to add electronic memory systems to the human brain. The purpose of this memory would not be therapeutic, but "cosmetic." The goal would be to eliminate the problem of forgetting information that was once learned. The presumption here is that neuroscientists will learn enough about how information is stored in the brain to allow such augmentation. Clearly, such developments may take decades, or even centuries. The add-on memory would be housed in an enlargement of the cranium (à la science fiction movies) and would be powered by the same mechanism as the nerve splice. The ability to retain essentially unlimited amounts of information would obviously be of great interest to a variety of people.

In summary, neurocomputing may play an important role in the development of future adjuncts to neurosurgery.

For further information on neurocomputing the reader may consult the references provided after the discussion section below.

Transcription of Dr. Hecht-Nielsen's Talk

Neurocomputing is a subject that goes back to same time period as the development of the computer, namely, the mid-1940s. The idea is that we want to build information processing machines that are more like brains than like adding machines. All of the computers that we are familiar with today are really glorified adding machines. They simply add numbers together, multiply them, subtract them, and do logical operations. They have memory units within them that can store intermediate answers and store the programs that are used to carry out the calculations. That is all they are, from the smallest pocket computer like my little Hewlett-Packard calculator to a Cray 1, a Cray 2, or a Connection Machine. All of these are standard computers that carry out a preprogrammed sequence of steps.

We now have a new type of computing, and that is what I would like to discuss today, and also discuss its implications vis à vis your interests. I'm going to go through only a small portion of this because I want to show you a video tape at the end that I think you will find interesting. It was made at NHK Labs by Kuniniko Fukushima, a Japanese friend of mine, and it is perhaps the best tape ever made in the field.

So I would like to talk about what the subject is and what kinds of information processing we can carry out, and then say a little bit about applications.

One of the characteristics of this field is that it is growing rapidly. Last year we had the first major international conference in the field ever, and we had more than 1500 people. This year, in fact this month, we are having the conference again, and we are expecting 2000 people. It is a subject that has become interesting to a variety of researchers in physics, applied mathematics, engineering, cognitive psychology, and neural modeling. There are a number of other neural network conferences around the world. There was a conference last summer in Japan. There was a conference last month in Europe, Paris, and there will be a major conference next summer in Moscow.

In neurocomputing we deal with computing structures that are, you might say, reminiscent of neurons, but, as I will point out in a moment, are in no way real models of neurons.

What people have done is taken some of the basic ideas that neural modelers have arrived at over the years and simply pulled them out of biology and brought them over into engineering to see if we could do something useful with them. The answer seems to be that we can.

The result of all of this has been a new family of computing structures that have two main properties: one, they are highly parallel, just like the nervous system; and two, you cannot program them. They are not like a standard computer. You can program a computer to do what you want to do. You cannot program these. There is no way to get a program inside of them. There is no way to take an algorithm and enter it into the machine. These neural networks operate by adaptation. They are adaptive in a way that is at least reminiscent of biology. But again, I want to emphasize how simple these are in comparison to biology.

You might think of them as an extremely simplified version of a nervous system. Now again, just as in the nervous system, we have neurons and their axons that connect the neurons together. Here we have what amounts to an axon branching out into collaterals, and other axons arriving at this processing element.

We call the analogs of axons *connections* rather than *axons*, and we call the analogs of neurons *processing elements* rather than *neurons*. That is terminology. All of the processing that goes on inside a processing element is localized, just as in biology.

Now, just as in biology, neural networks are made up of groups of processing elements called slabs or layers, in which all of the elements in a group have similar processing functions. They are not the same: they are similar. Just as you have the primary visual cortex and primary motor cortex, each of which has a slightly different functional characteristic or the cerebellum, which is radically different.

We have structures that are made up of large numbers of these little processing elements that are connected together and that carry out a function. One of the first things that happens when people hear about this subject is an immediate assumption that this is an entirely empirical subject. In other words, we build these little things and we play with them and they do something, but we do not really know what it is. That's not true. That's neurobiology. In neurobiology nobody knows how neurons work. Nobody knows how neural structures function in detail. Here we do. Here we have definitive detailed mathematical theories that tell us exactly how these work. This makes neurocomputing a lot more enjoyable than neuroscience because we can readily expand the range of theories that we have in order to encompass new and more useful structures.

Each processing element has within it two things. One is a transfer function that defines the input–output relationship and the learning. The other is a local memory in which values can be stored, just as you can have adaptation in the nervous system, and somehow memory of that adaptation is stored biologically. We have local information storage inside these processing elements.

These neural network structures are organized according to certain designs, called architectures. These designs allow us to understand the mathematical capabilities of these structures in terms of what kinds of information processing they can carry out.

We view a neural network as what might be called a mathematical subroutine, just like in computer science. In fact, we can put computers and neural networks together via this interface. The computer generates an array of data that is then sent to the neural network as if it came from another neural network. The neural network then carries out its processing and ultimately produces output signals that then leave the network and go back to the user's software. By this means, we can have a neural network interact with standard engineering software in an effortless fashion. It is very easy to combine the two technologies, and that is the main theme of how engineers are applying these new ideas.

How many different neural network architectures do we know about? Well, we know about 50. But of those, only about 14 are in common use today. Each type of architecture can carry out a small set of information processing operations. However, this is a new subject and new architectures are being discovered every year.

Again, neurocomputing is an entirely new *style* of computing. Up to now, for the last 40 years, all we have had is programmed computing. In other words, somebody writes down a computer program and runs it in a computer. It does not matter if it is a parallel computer or a single processor computer or a big one or a small one, it is all the same. This standard approach is called programmed computing, and that is all we have had. Basically it goes back to John von Neumann's 1945 idea of a glorified adding machine.

Now we have a new style of computing, called neurocomputing, that has the property that you select an appropriate neural network and expose it to a statistically exhaustive set of data, to which it adapts. Eventually it will be able to carry out an interesting and useful information processing operation.

Let us examine a specific example of how neurocomputing can solve a real-world problem. At HNC we have a customer—a financial company. They make personal loans. When someone comes in to make a loan, they fill out an application form and this application form asks data about the person, for example, their salary, what kind of home they have, how long they have lived in the home, the information that the federal government allows loan companies to ask.

This information is then typed into a computer and run through a computer program. The program takes that information and from it makes a prediction of how good—how creditworthy—the applicant is. In other words, it actually makes what is called a yield score, which is the projected number of dollars of profit made per dollar loaned per year of term. If that score is high enough, they make the loan. Now the current systems that loan companies use are based on two different approaches. One is statistical modeling. The other one is rule-based systems, where they interview loan officers and pick up rules for making judgments about loans.

What we do is we take a particular neural network structure, and we put in at the bottom of the network the loan application data. We take that data and form it into a long data vector and we put that into the processing elements—or neurons, if you want to call them that—at the bottom.

The processing elements take that information and make output signals out of it, which go to the next layer, which go to the next layer, and so forth, and eventually out comes the score. In other words, the data "bubbles up" through the network and the result is a score.

The score that the network gives you at the beginning of training is completely wrong. It is almost a random number. So what you do is, after it has given an estimate of the score, you tell it what the correct score is. Now, how can you do that? Well, you only train it on loans that have already been paid back or defaulted, so you have ground truth data.

So you take its output signal, and give it the correct output signal; then the error bubbles down through the network and causes changes to occur in the computing structure. We can prove mathematically that as you continue to do this—putting in another example, having it bubble up, letting it make an estimate, giving it the right answer, the errors bubble back down and everything adjusts itself—over a period of time for a given class of transformations, this network will get better and better and better at making a good estimate. In fact, in this real-world application we make an estimate that is 24% to 27% better than the statistical model the rule base system is intended to replace.

It is an approach that has many of the flavors of biological computing, but is also quite different. Of course, there is an algorithm inside these processing elements, in the neural network, but we do not know what it is. We do not have to know what it is in advance. With von Neumann computing, you have to know the algorithm in advance and program it into the machine.

So these neural networks are adaptive systems that actually learn by looking at examples or by other means. There is another type of training or learning called *graded training*, where you do not tell it the right answer at the top, but rather tell it how well it has been doing. For example, we have a machine that can balance a broomstick, just like a human would, only we do not tell this neural network how well it is doing because we do not know. This is a complicated mechanical system, and we do not actually know what the correct control inputs are. We can, of course, measure how well it keeps the broomstick balanced, and how well it keeps it in the center of the playing field, where it can move. Every once in a while we will simply tell the network how well it is doing and that is enough. It learns to do a very good job of balancing.

There is a third approach to learning, which is called *self-organization*, and that is what we are going to see in the movie. This approach is quite startling, because there you do not tell it anything, you just give it examples.

One question you might ask is: how does all this compare to biology? Ted Bullock at UCSD has identified 46 attributes, or changeable characteristics, within actual biological neurons. In other words, this is a reflection of the complexity of biology. Remember now, we heard an excellent talk earlier this morning that actually showed a number of different neuron structures. For example, the dendritic processes of neurons, which themselves carry out localized information processing before any of that gets to the actual cell body and the axon hillock.

There is a tremendous amount of processing that goes on in one single neuron. This is a list of all of the elements that can be involved in that processing, 46 of them. In a typical processing element in neural networks we use in engineering, there are two. So we are comparing here a biological neuron that has 46 characteristics to determine its functional behavior, and an engineering neuron where there are two characteristics. Obviously we are dealing with an extremely simplified situation, and yet we can do very interesting things.

Two processing elements by the way are typical, but there are some neural networks that have five or six. Still, in terms of the comparison to biology, there *is* no comparison.

Although this is a subject that is rather mathematical, there are people who work in this field who are highly experimental, who do not know a lot of mathematics necessarily, but who do lots of experiments and have discovered some amazing new principles. Some of these new discoveries may actually be able to go back into biology to help explain how biological systems function, at least some parts of them.

One of the results, which I will focus on, is due to the Soviet mathematician, Kolmogorov. We can take one of his most famous theorems and reinterpret it as a theorem about these neural networks.

What this theorem says is that any continuous mapping between some compact interval in n-dimensional space, to n-dimensional space (like our loan application scoring application, for example), no matter how complicated or simple it might be, can be implemented exactly with a three-layer neural network structure.

Kolmogorov does not tell us how to find that network, but he proves that it exists. There is a whole class of networks called mapping networks that can approximately carry out this function, like the one for loan application scoring or the one for the broomstick balancer. There are many others.

For example, there are two automobile companies, one in America and one in Japan, who are looking at the application of this technology to what is called active suspension, where instead of having a spring and a shock absorber on each wheel of a car, you now have a hydraulic cylinder so that you can actively control the position and force on each wheel. As you drive down a bumpy road, the car will "walk" over chuck holes, and you will have a smooth ride, even on a bumpy road. This looks like a successful technology for that.

In summary, in order to implement the architectures I have been discussing, in hardware it turns out that ordinary computers do not do a good job. So we have developed a new class of computers called neurocomputers, which implement these simple neural network structures efficiently and cost-effectively. A surprising number of these have already been built, some of them built in optical hardware, many of them electronic. In fact, our company sells a whole line of these new types of computers specifically intended for running these neural networks.

Of course, with these new computers, you have to have a way of describing a neural network in formal language. This is called *neurosoftware*—the neurocomputer equivalent of software such as you use to describe an algorithm or computer program.

Many applications of this technology are in fact being explored today. Some of them have even gone so far as to go to field testing, where they are being used on a daily basis; but only a few have reached this phase: The credit application scoring is one of those. In the medical applications area, we are working with the UCSD Medical School and with another company on an EEG monitor for surgery. The idea is to predict the potential onset of brain ischemia 5 to 7 to perhaps 10 minutes in advance.

There are very subtle trends in the EEG that would allow you (if you could use them as a predictor) to predict the onset of a dangerous condition. We are having quite a bit of success with this area. Some potential applications are very remote at present, but they are being investigated nonetheless.

I did want to address some remarks about your interests, and in particular about the spinal cord that might be, in one way or another, relevant.

First of all, let me relate what I just told you to the present subject of interest here. It is very important to understand that in neurocomputing we do not have grandiose expectations. We expect to draw knowledge from neuroscience, from medicine, from psychology over many, many decades before we really can do much at all. The capabilities that we are able to exhibit today are extremely modest.

However, the future looks bright. It looks as if we are going to be able to make continual progress from here on out, and have the hardware in order to use those new discoveries in practical applications. I will make a prediction here that we could possibly exceed the capabilities of a frog, which actually is pretty impressive, if you really think about that.

One of the things that I have learned in my career is that sometimes it is valuable to be extremely presumptuous. Instead of saying that a problem is totally beyond solution, instead think about a problem as if you were not convinced you could not solve it, and just say whatever you could say about it.

Let's say, for example, there is a traumatic injury to a spinal cord. What I am suggesting here is that perhaps under certain circumstances the patient's own tracts could be the source of cells that could assist with the regeneration process.

Let's go on to the next idea. The next step would be to operate and remove the damaged area. What I am suggesting here is that, as stated many times this morning, one of the main blockades to regeneration is the existence of scar tissue and other forms of material that occur as a result of the injury, so a thought is: why not go in and simply remove all of that material by making extremely careful cuts to establish a prepared surface in a known condition.

Now, immediately, instead of having a delay of hours between the trauma and the time any attention is available, after these cuts are made one could insert a microchannel plate in less than a minute, so that many of the results of trauma that are processes that take minutes or hours to evolve would never have a chance to evolve. The idea of this is that you would use something like a cyanoacrylic cement and the microchannel plate would be literally cemented on, on a small-scale basis, to the tissue to create a completely closed surface. (There is a technology in electronics for building plates, or actually cylinders, of any size, with holes in those cylinders of sizes ranging from one micron up to hundreds of microns if you want, virtually any size holes you want, and these can be made relatively inexpensively and can be cut and machined.)

Then you finish the repair, immobilizing it and so forth, and of course the idea is that the insides of these tubes have been cultured with Schwann cells, but perhaps astrocytes are more useful so that the physical and chemical medium that would promote axon growth is there.

The main concomitant of the use of this is that any gray matter connections within this region are eliminated forever. There is no hope of restoring those, but at least there is some possibility of having fibers transit the region.

References

1. Amari S, Arbib MA. *Competition and Cooperation in Neural Nets*. New York: Springer–Verlag; 1982.
2. Anderson DZ, ed. *Neural Information Processing Systems*. New York: American Institute of Physics; 1988.
3. Anderson JA, Rosenfeld E, eds. *Neurocomputing: Foundations of Research*. Cambridge: MIT Press; 1988.
4. Denker J. *Proc. Second Annual Conference on Neural Networks for Computing*. New York: American Institute of Physics, Proceedings Vol. 151; 1986.
5. Grossberg S. *Neural Networks and Natural Intelligence*. Cambridge: MIT Press; 1987.
6. Grossberg S. *The Adaptive Brain*. vols. I, II. Amsterdam: North Holland; 1987.
7. Grossberg S, Kuperstein M. *Neural Dynamics of Adaptive Sensory-Motor Control*. Amsterdam: North-Holland; 1986.
8. Grossberg S. *Studies of Mind and Brain*. Reidel; 1982.
9. Hecht-Nielsen R. *Neurocomputing*. Addison-Wesley, Reading, Mass.; 1991.
10. Hinton GE, Anderson JA, eds. *Parallel Models of Associative Memory*. Hillsdale, N.J.: Erlbaum, 1981.
11. Kohonen T. *Self-Organization and Associative Memory*. 2nd ed. New York: Springer–Verlag; 1987.
12. Kosko B. Bidirectional associative memories. *BYTE Magazine*, September 1987.
13. Rosenblatt F. *Principles of Neurodynamics*. Spartan Books; 1961.
14. Rumelhart DE, McClelland JL. *Parallel Distributed Processing: Explorations in the Microstructure of Cognition*. vols. I, II, III. Cambridge: MIT Press; 1986, 1987.
15. Steinbuch K. *Automat und Mensch*. 2nd ed. Berlin: Springer–Verlag; 1963.
16. Szu H. ed. *Optical and Hybrid Computing*. *SPIE Proc*. 1986; 634.
17. Widrow B, Stearns SD. *Adaptive Signal Processing*. Englewood Cliffs, N.J.: Prentice-Hall; 1985.

Discussion

Use of the Neocognitron in Prosthetics

Dr. Holtzman asked if it were possible to give the neocognitron information from striated muscle intrafusal fibers via Ia afferents allowing it to feed information back to the muscle via gamma efferents and alpha motor neurons, could it facilitate the preservation of muscle integrity in the face of spinal cord transection? Dr. Hecht-Nielsen felt that that was not out of the question. I believe that the applications of this technology to prosthetics in general and the kind of situation you just mentioned look hopeful. The main thing that we in the engineering community lack is first of all an understanding of the kinds of problems that are in a position to be attacked today and second where it is possible to have a good interface with biological systems.

One of the difficulties we were discussing is the problem with chronically implanted electrodes. There have been a number of successful systems developed, for example, for the visual cortex and the cochlea. There are, however, many other situations where it would be problematic to envision a chronically implanted electrode array that would have sufficient spatial resolution to make a patent connection to the neurons. For example, in the spinal cord at the site of damage there are no cell bodies and you somehow have to have an axonal connection.

The Importance of Spinal Segments

What are the thoughts on the importance of any given spinal segment? Dr. Holtzman further inquired what if the gray matter of a segment is absolutely required for the functioning of the surrounding white matter in that segment. Dr. Hecht-Nielsen responded that his thoughts on this matter would be to sacrifice whatever functionality the gray matter within the damaged segment was carrying out and to try to reestablish the long tracts so that the segments above and below would still remain functional.

My understanding of the problem is twofold. One is getting the axons that are connected to the cell bodies to want to grow, and some of those factors were discussed this morning, and the second is to guide that growth. My thought was having astrocytes or Schwann cells cultured in this microchannel plate before it is inserted. You have a quarter of a million holes all larger than Betz cell axons that could be coated. The microchannel plate could then be precision cut and "glued" in place. I think that over the long haul there promises to be a lot of useful interaction between this subject and medicine and I am hoping that by making you aware of its existence you will begin to think about it.

The Basic Design of Neural Circuits

Dr. Kliot inquired if we can go backward. If you understand the input–output relations of something, can you infer what the layering structure might be and therefore determine circuitry? I am thinking of a structure like the retina. Would it be possible if you understood input–output? Would these layers correspond to the cell layers? Is there any hope for that?

Dr. Hecht-Nielsen responded that there is, and in fact Carver Mead at Cal-Tech has dedicated his career to building neural networks directly in silicon. He has built silicon retinas. They are extremely small and perhaps have the equivalent of 20 rods, but they do contain functional elements that correspond to virtually every cell in the retina and have functional properties that are similar to those of the retina.

Dr. Kliot continued, in going from layer to layer and as the machine learns is it adapting to Hebbian laws?

Dr. Hecht-Nielsen pointed out that the Hebbian approach is one of about six approaches. There are six different adaptation principles that are used in all these networks. Each network uses one or more of them and the *Hebb law* is sort of the special case of all of them. They are all more general than that. For example, there is one neural network type that is not really in common use so it was not on the list that has actually exhibited every known form of classical conditioning that one would see in a psychology laboratory. We have actually been able to demonstrate all 16 types of classical conditioning with this neural network, so the learning processes are fairly sophisticated, but again I have the feeling that they are nothing but mere shadows or small replicas of what we see in biology.

Dr. Oldfield asked how expensive are these units you are speaking of? Dr. Hecht-Nielsen replied that the two models we sell cost about $7000 and $15,000 and those are circuit boards that fit into an IBM PC-AT type computer. People will take that and then apply it to a specific problem such as loan application scoring or pattern recognition or retinal modeling so it functions as a general purpose tool. It's really a tool rather than a specific application.

Dr. Oldfield asked if there is auditory input yet. It would seem that this would make it possible for deaf people to receive telephone calls and hear what was being said to them. Dr. Hecht-Nielsen said that it simply has not been done. The closest thing is work with dolphin utterances. Dolphins have both hearing and speech or sound production between 10 kHz and 150 kHz so they are effectively above the human hearing range. There have been some systems designed to take a sound stream in that frequency range, compress it, and bring it down to the human range so that all those sounds come down to between 300 and 3000 Hz so we can hear them perfectly. I think that some of the same processing principles that are used in that technology could be readily applied and to considerable advantage, but that work has not been done yet.

Dr. Friedman asked if Linás' work on a model of the cerebellum fell in your area of neurocomputers. Dr. Hecht-Nielsen said, yes, very much so. There was mention of Marr and Altis and Linás' work. The cerebellum, in some senses, is the most well understood structure in the brain in terms of its microscopic cellular neuro-anatomy and physiology. The big mystery is how does it fit into the overall actions of other parts of the brain.

We have some astounding cerebellar models. We have a neural network that can take a multijointed arm with as many joints as we wish and move the fingertip through an arbitrary trajectory with all of the joints articulating appropriately to allow the movement to occur with minimal energy and that is a cerebellar model. It is the equivalent of Purkinje cells and climbing fibers and it is marvelously effective.

In summary, there is a great deal of belief that the structure of the brain is becoming understood in detail and we can see lots of applications to robotics. That too is an exciting area that we are starting to work in. Unfortunately there have not been a lot of payoffs yet.

CHAPTER 9

Fetal Tissue Grafts for Cerebellar Atrophy in Humans: A Preliminary Report

Wu Cheng-Yuan, Bao Xiu-Feng, Zhang Cheng, and Zhang Qing-Lin

Studies of neural grafting by a number of investigators[1-8] have demonstrated survival of fetal neurons in host brains. Lund et al.[9] have demonstrated point-to-point synapse integration of neural grafts.

Recent studies have provided strong evidence that grafts can correct some of the behavioral impairments, resulting from damage to the adult host brain.[10] Lack of lymphatic drainage renders the central nervous system (CNS) relatively immunologically privileged.[11,12] Allogenic embryonic mammalian brain grafts can survive in the nervous system without immunosuppression for prolonged periods of time.[13]

In 1982, Backlund et al.[14,15] performed the first autograft of human adrenal medullary tissue for Parkinson's disease. Madrazo et al. have reported transplantation of fetal substantia nigra and adrenal medulla to the caudate nucleus in two patients with Parkinson's disease. In both patients there was objective symptomatic improvement.[16]

Experimental Evidence

Zhang Hai-Qi and Liu Yu-Mei, at Shandong Medical University, have studied cerebellar grafting since 1964.[17] Zhang Hai-Qi reported in 1986 that cerebellar tissue from newborn Wistar rats grafted into the injured cerebellum of adult Wistar rats can promote the mitosis of Purkinje cells in the host cerebellum and improve the ataxia that results from the injury[18] (Fig. 9.1a). Wu Cheng-yuan et al. at Utah University Medical Center did experiments in mice with monoclonal antibody staining of the nuclear membrane of donor Purkinje cells from embryonic grafts and confirmed graft viability (Fig. 9.1b).

Patient Selection

Six patients with cerebellar disease associated with severe symptoms were treated surgically with fetal cerebellar tissue grafts to the diseased cerebel-

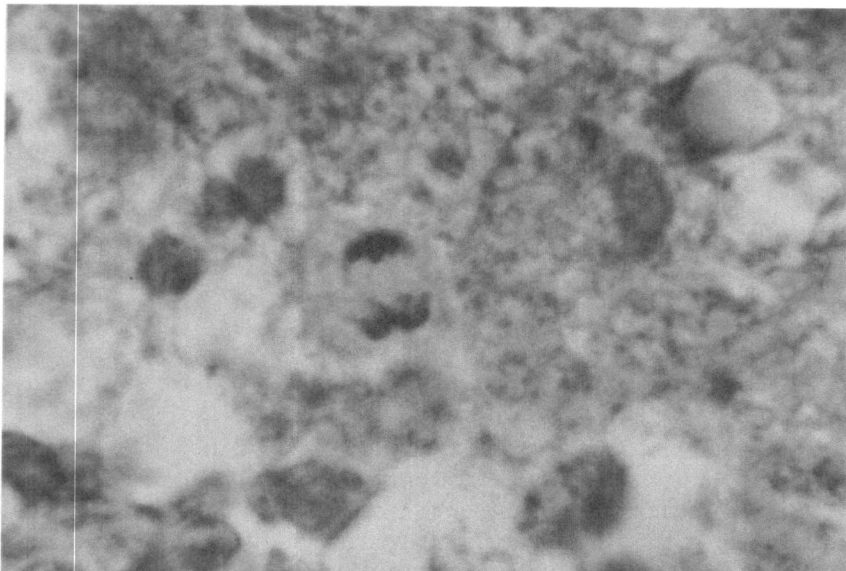

Figure 9.1A. Mitosis of Purkinje cells after the implantation of solid pieces of cerebellar primordia of adult Wistar rats (late stage).

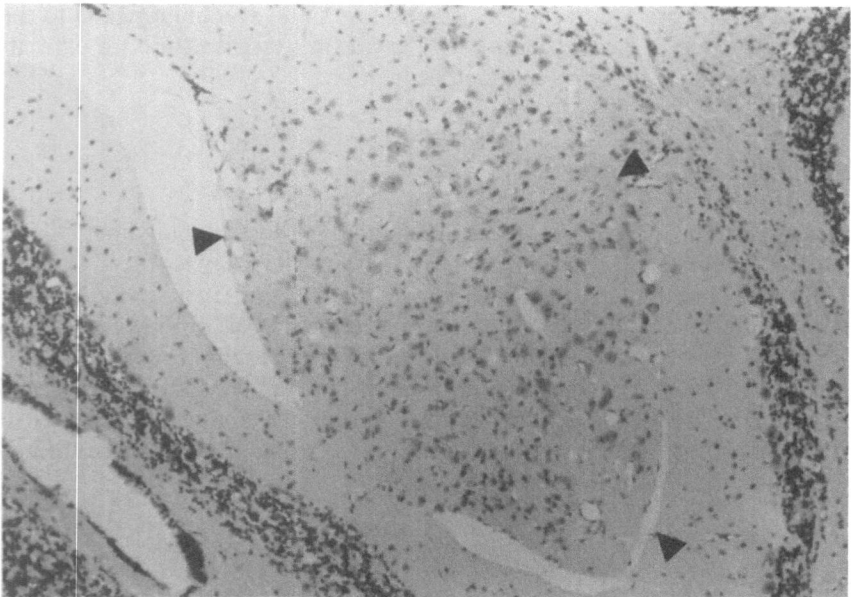

Figure 9.1B. Graft of donor's embryonic cerebellum (arrows) showing survival in the cerebellum of the host. (Hematoxylin-Eosin ×150).

Table 9.1. Summary of data in six patients.

Case no.	Sex	Age	Surgery date	Duration of symptoms	Clinical diagnosis	CT scan findings
1	M	58	4/7/87	7 yrs	Heredodegenerative ataxia	Cerebral/cerebellar atrophy
2	M	60	5/15/87	5 yrs	Cerebellar atrophy	Cerebral/cerebellar atrophy
3	M	12	7/11/87	12 yrs	Cerebellar atrophy	Cerebellar atrophy
4	F	49	8/12/87	2 yrs	Heredodegenerative ataxia	Cerebellar atrophy
5	M	29	9/29/87	9 yrs	Heredodegenerative ataxia	Cerebellar atrophy
6	F	44	10/30/87	4 yrs	Heredodegenerative ataxia	Cerebellar atrophy

lum. The clinical data are summarized in Tables 9.1 and 9.2. There were four men and two women with an age range of 12 to 60 years, averaging 42 years. The main symptoms were progressive ataxia and dysarthria. The disease process varied in time from 2 to 12 years, with an average period of 6.5 years. Three patients with severe dizziness were chronically bedridden, two patients had diplopia, five of them had difficulty eating and writing, and one had bowel and bladder incontinence. The major signs were ataxia in all six patients. Four had severe hypotonia. Superficial and deep sensation was normal in all patients. One patient (case 5), bedridden with severe ataxia and dizziness, was depressed and suicidal.

The diagnosis of cerebellar disease and documentation of failed preoperative medical treatment was confirmed by independent neurologists. Medical treatment over several years was ineffective in all cases.

Institutional approval was obtained from the civil, and research committees of Shandong University Hospital and written consent was obtained from the patient's relatives. The fetuses of 10–12 weeks (except one) were from spontaneous or induced abortions in patients with toxemia of pregnancy or other diseases. Fetal death was certified by two physicians who were not part of the neurosurgical team.

Surgical Technique

Preparation of Cerebellar Implant

Embryonic cerebellar tissue was obtained from fetuses after spontaneous or induced abortion. The fetal nonviability was documented by at least two physicians. The scalp of the fetus was prepared, after which the skull was opened along the sagittal and the coronal sutures using sterile technique. The dura was opened and the cerebellar hemisphere, with brain stem, was carefully removed. Grafts of 0.5 to 1.0 mm^3 were harvested from the cere-

Table 9.2. Summary of signs and symptoms in six patients.

Case no.	Preoperative						Postoperative					
	Dysarthria	Ataxia	Bedridden	Nystagmus	Diplopia	Hypotonia	Dysarthria	Ataxia	Bedridden	Nystagmus	Diplopia	Hypotonia
1	+	+	+	–	–	+	+/–	+	–	–	–	+/–
2	+	+	–	–	–	–	+/–	+/–	–	–	–	–
3	+	+	–	–	–	–	+/–	+/–	–	–	–	–
4	+	+	–	+	+	+	+	+	–	–	–	+
5	+	+	+	+	+	+	+/–	+/–	–	–	–	+/–
6	+	+	–	–	–	+	+	+	–	–	–	+

+, present; –, absent; +/–, present but improved.

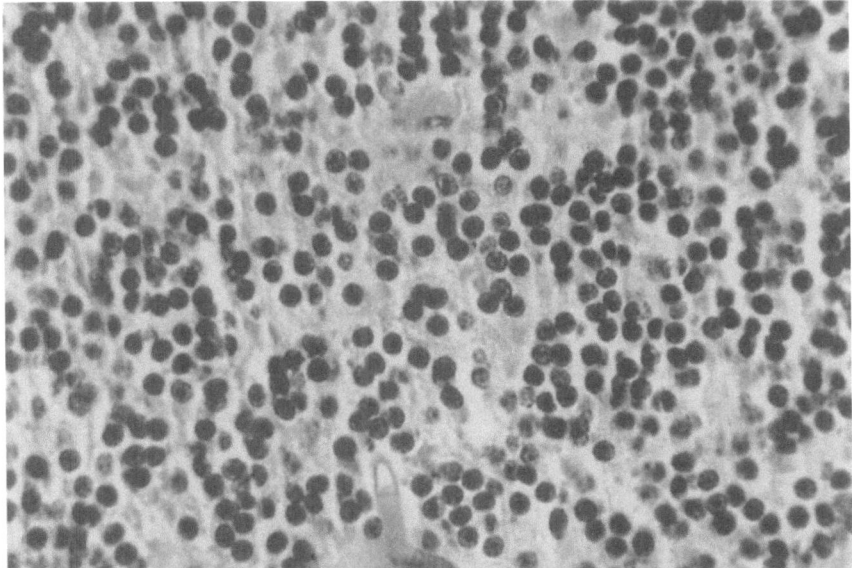

Figure 9.2. Histologic features of human fetal cerebellar cells (13 weeks).

bellar tissue (cortex, vermis, flocculonodular lobe) and placed in lactated Ringer's solution preparatory to transplantation (Fig. 9.2). Craniectomy for cerebellar grafting was performed simultaneously in recipient patients.

Operative Procedure

The patient was placed in the left lateral position to approach the right cerebellar hemisphere. After sterile preparation, a 6-cm right paramedian incision was made and a right suboccipital craniectomy of 3 cm in size was performed. The dura was opened in a semicircular fashion. The cerebellar hemispheres were all small and atrophic secondary to the disease process. A cerebellar cortex biopsy was performed in each case to confirm the diagnosis (Fig. 9.3).

Solid pieces of fetal cerebellar tissue were injected into the target site using a special tissue grafting cannula designed by the authors (Fig. 9.4). With this method, multiple grafts ($0.5-1 \text{ mm}^3$) can be implanted into target areas of the anterior superior vermian and flocculonodular lobes. Using this injection technique, grafts were introduced into multiple sites, with a minimum of brain tissue disruption. After completion of the grafting procedure, the dural edges were reapproximated and the incision was closed in layers.

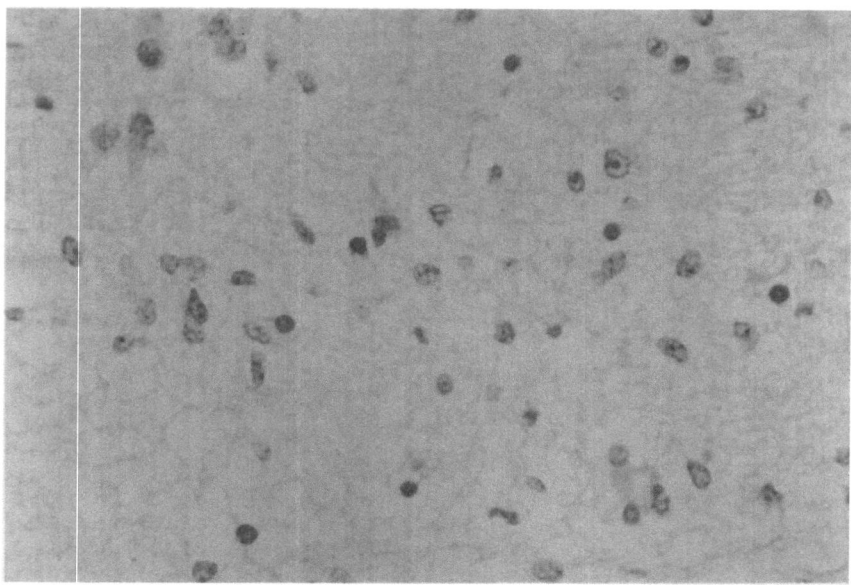

Figure 9.3. Surgical biopsy (case 2) showing marked cerebellar atrophy.

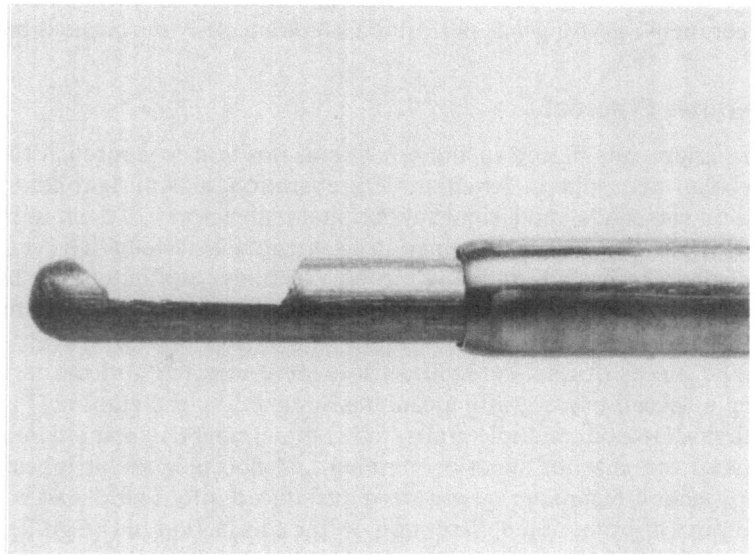

Figure 9.4. Specially designed cannula for implantation of brain tissue.

Postoperative Care

Prophylactic antibiotics were routinely used in the perioperative period. The patients were maintained on intravenous dexamethasone 20 mg per day for 2 weeks and then oral dexamethasone 0.75 mg BID on a daily basis through follow-up. There were no postoperative infections or bleeding complications in any of the six patients.

Clinical Results

The clinical results are summarized in Table 9.2.

Clinical Course

Postoperatively, two of the six patients showed marked resolution of symptoms. Three showed moderate improvement. One improved during the initial 2 months after implantation but then gradually deteriorated. However, his symptoms were still better than preoperatively.

Before surgery all six patients had symptoms of dysarthria and ataxia. Postoperatively four patients with dysarthria and three patients with ataxia markedly improved.

Two patients with diplopia preoperatively had complete resolution after

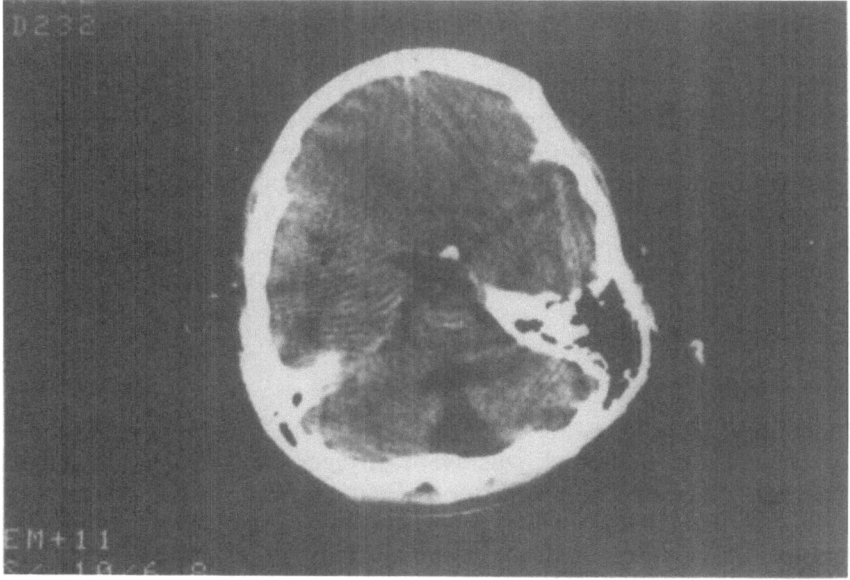

Figure 9.5. CT scan (case 3) demonstrating cerebellar atrophy (preoperative).

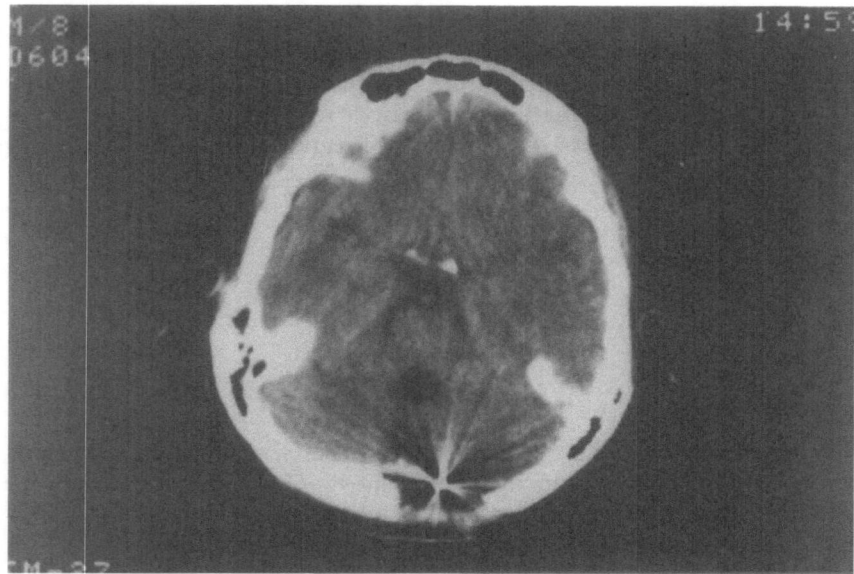

Figure 9.6. CT scan (case 3) demonstrates the postoperative state of the cerebellum.

surgery. The two patients who were bedridden before surgery, within 2 to 3 months postoperatively, were able to ambulate with minimal support.

At 2 to 8 months after surgery, none of the patients has had any complications. Two of the six patients (cases 3 and 5) have shown marked improvement after the implantation. Three patients (cases 1, 4, and 6) have moderate improvement. One (case 2) improved within 2 months postoperatively, then deteriorated but not to his preoperative state.

In general, all six patients had improved symptoms and signs, especially with regard to their speech.

Laboratory Results

Immunological Markers

Immunoglobulins were determined both pre-operatively and postoperatively in five of the six patients. None of them showed marked immunologic changes before 4 months after grafting. However, in one patient (case 2) the immunoglobulin level became elevated 4 months after grafting. At 6 months after grafting the level of immunoglobulin was normal using both spectrophotometric and immunofluorescence staining techniques (Table 9.3 and Fig. 9.7).

Table 9.3. IgG, A, M in the blood of six patients.

Case no.	Preoperative			1–2 Months postoperative			4–5 Months postoperative		
	IgG	IgA	IgM	IgG	IgA	IgM	IgG	IgA	IgM
1	837	166	112	1230	247	150	1256.8	328.7	187
2	1283	233	32	1640	293.4	190	2460/ 1610	220.7	115
3	1229	199.8	86	1372	157.2	140.5	1372	157.2	140.5
4	1150	262.5	125	1150	233.3	86	—	—	—
5	1339	145.9	147.6	1488	155.1	172.8	—	—	—
6	1600	249.8	82.5	1580	268.7	156	—	—	—
Normal con- centration level	76– 1660 mg%	71– 335 mg%	48– 212 mg%						

Ratio of Lymphocyte Transformation in Mixed Culture of Fetal Brain Suspension and Patient's Lymphocytes

There were no marked differences between the implant group and the control group.

Testing of Anti–Fetal Brain Antibody and Anti–Nucleus Antibody

Both tests were negative in three cases using immunofluorescence technique and counter-immunoelectrophoresis.

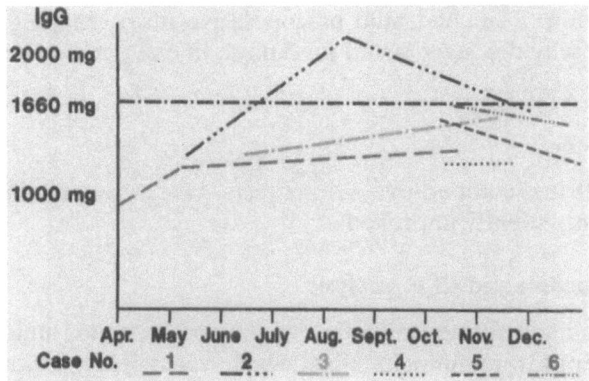

Figure 9.7. Serial serum immunoglobulin levels demonstrating normal levels in five patients and transient elevation in single patient (case 2).

Trace Element Analysis of the Blood and Cerebrospinal Fluid

In one patient these analyses included zinc, manganese, iron, lead, copper, and magnesium. The values were normal and there were no differences before and after surgery.

Brain Stem Evoked Potential Testing

Three cases were tested. There was no difference in preoperative and post-operative patterns.

CT Scanning and Biopsy

All six patients were examined with computed tomography (CT) scans preoperatively and postoperatively. Cerebellar atrophy was diagnosed preoperatively and was confirmed with histologic examination of the biopsy at the time of implantation (Figures 9.3, 9.5, 9.6 and Table 9.1).

Routine Blood Counts and Urine Analysis

The results were within the normal range preoperatively and postoperatively, without any significant change. Absolute lymphocyte and poly-morphonuclear leukocyte counts were unaffected by the transplantation procedure.

Liver Function Tests and Renal Function Tests

All patients had normal SGPT, SGOT, ZnTT, and so forth. One patient was HBSAg positive at 1:256.

Vital Signs

Blood pressure, respiration, and pulse showed no differences before and after operation. Four had mild postoperative fever, ranging from 37° to 38° C. Generally the fever lasted for 3 days; in one patient the fever lasted for 6 days.

Writing Ability

Two patients had comparative writing tests. One was much improved, the other was only slightly improved.

Lumbar Puncture and CSF Analysis

One patient had routine evaluation of the cerebrospinal fluid, which was normal except for immunoglobulins, which were slightly elevated.

Discussion

Cerebellar atrophy occurs mainly in cerebellar system degeneration, such as hereditary ataxia and rarely as a sequela of trauma, intoxication, alcoholism, inflammation, and cerebrovascular disease. Heredodegenerative ataxia is a disease of chromosome inheritance.

Many of the diseases are characterized by progressive deterioration of cerebellar neurons, leading eventually to death and disappearance of these neurons.[20] There are various proposed etiologies including defective enzyme systems, exogenous toxins, or autoimmune diseases. The cerebellar abnormalities involve Purkinje and granule cells, which show degenerative changes. In the case of parenchymatous cerebellar degeneration, there is absence of Purkinje cells.[20,21]

In recent years, basic animal studies on brain tissue transplantation have demonstrated that immature neurons transplanted into the brain of an adult host cannot only maintain viability but also maintain their characteristics of neurological function including synthesis of neurotransmitters.[1–10,22,23,24]

Bjorklund showed that in the first 2 weeks after grafting, solid septal grafts underwent a reduction in size to about half their original volume.[24] Between 1 and 4 months after grafting, however, they grew approximately threefold to reach a final size that was about 50% larger than that of the initially implanted pieces. By 4 months a new cholinergic innervation had been established up to a distance of about 6 to 8 mm from the graft. Electron microscopy investigations, combined with immunocytochemistry, have shown that the ingrowing cholinergic axons from the grafts form abundant synaptic contacts with neuronal elements in the host dentate gyrus.[24–26]

Electrophysiological experiments demonstrate that embryonic Purkinje cells from the graft can completely differentiate in the adult host cerebellum and establish specific synaptic contacts with the presynaptic elements previously impinging on missing neurons of "Purkinje cell degeneration" mutants. This process may lead to a qualitative functional synaptic restoration of the cortical cerebellar network.[27]

A major consideration in selecting the cerebellum as a transplantation site stems from the fact that this structure develops largely postnatally, exhibiting extensive neurogenesis for several weeks into postnatal life of the animal, and the efferents of the cerebellar cortex consist entirely of axons of Purkinje cells and categorized as corticonuclear fibers or corticofugal fibers. Generally, the entire cerebellar cortex provides efferent fibers to the deep cerebellar nuclei whereas the corticofugal or corticovestibular fibers originate from vermal regions and the flocculonodular lobe. This system thus provides a relatively uncomplicated and well characterized set of outputs that simplify the study of changes resulting subsequent to transplantation into the cerebellum.[28]

We have histologic evidence that mitosis of the Purkinje cells may be substantially increased by biologic transplantation of embryonic cerebellar tissue and the implants of fetal tissue can enhance recovery of cerebellar function in Wistar rats.[19] Immature fetal neurons have strong vitality and striking plasticity in the adult brain, especially with immunosuppressive agents such as cyclosporine-A.[1–10,28]

For these reasons, we elected to evaluate human fetal cerebellar tissue as donor tissue in severe heredodegenerative ataxia and cerebellar atrophy, which are otherwise untreatable diseases leading eventually to death.[20]

Considerable evidence now indicates that transplanted brain tissue can indeed survive, differentiate, and innervate in the host. However, many important issues remain in dispute such as the functional nature of transplanted tissue and long-term therapeutic value of the procedure for treating some neurological degenerative diseases.[29,30]

Crain showed the capacity of fetal central nervous system (CNS) neurons to establish appropriate interneuronal relationships with host CNS tissue.[31] Migration of neurons from transplant into host tissue, extension of processes, and synaptic contacts in the hosts are some of the types of integration thought necessary.[10,32] The role of stimulation of trophic factors such as nerve graft factor is poorly understood. Stein and Mufson point out that cell suspensions can enhance recovery when they have been chemically and mechanically dissociated and then injected into the cerebral ventricles. Systemic or intracerebral administration of trophic substances, such as GM-1 gangliosides or nerve growth factors, may enhance establishment of contacts.[10,31,32,33,34] Recent work reported by Nieto-Sampedro and Cotman has shown that injury-induced neurotrophic factors or implants of purified and isolated glial cells can enhance behavioral recovery.[35–37]

Nieto-Sampedro et al. confirmed that the traumatized brain of the host produces a substance that could promote the growth survival of the grafts.[12,34,35] This substance that influences the growth and survival of transplant in vivo can also be documented in tissue culture studies.[12,36,37]

The symptoms in this series of patients were improved 4 days after surgery. At this time, the neuron integration between the graft and the host could not have formed. The rapid improvement of neural function must result from stimulation of biochemical substances, growth factors, and neurotransmitters rather than reinnervation.[29,34] Animal experiments have indicated that the behavior of the host may change as early as 4 days after cerebral cortex grafting.[36] Function may improve before possible synaptic integration of the donor tissue and the host.

Cerebral transplantation techniques are well established in neuroscience. The surgical procedure of fetal cerebellar implantation is straightforward. However, transplanting the immature cerebellar tissue into the multiple target sites within the cerebellum without injuring the graft can be quite difficult. The specially designed cannula for grafting the brain tissue is helpful (Fig. 9.4).

Recently, some authors have proposed performing the implantation procedure in two stages. The first stage would be to create a bed for the graft in the brain tissue. After several weeks, when vascularization has developed, the transplant would be placed in the bed.[12]

Injection of fresh fetal brain tissue grafts of 0.5 to 1 mm^3 in size through the special implant cannula into the brain parenchyma has the advantage of minimal injury to the brain and the transplants can be placed in many sites where they have more ability to survive.

In our group of six cases of cerebellar transplantation, all showed continued symptomatic improvement, except one patient whose improvement did not last more than 2 months. Deterioration may be associated with several factors. This patient, at 60 years of age, was the oldest of the group. Tissue may integrate better in younger hosts. The fetal brain transplants of this case were taken from comparatively mature fetuses of 5 months. The survival of less mature neurons transplanted into the brain is better than older neurons. Immunoglobulin levels were elevated preoperatively. Four months postoperatively, the immunoglobulin levels were IgG 2460/1610 mg%, IgA 220.7 mg%, and IgM 115 mg% in his blood. This suggests that the grafts may have been rejected. The patient was the only one not given dexamethasone postoperatively. Although the rejection response associated with brain transplantation is not as strong as in other organs, the adequate use of immunosuppressive agents such as dexamethasone and cyclosporine-A might promote improved survival of the graft.

Summary

Animal models have shown that surgical injury to the right cerebellum with resultant ataxia can be functionally corrected by implantation of embryonic cerebellar tissue into the injured cerebellum of rats and mice. The surgically induced ataxia resolves more rapidly in the cerebellar implant group than in the control groups. Histological examination of the cerebellar tissue reveals that embryonic grafts can survive and that mitoses of the host Purkinje cells of the implanted group were increased substantially over the control groups. Monoclonal antibody staining of the nuclear membrane of mature donor Purkinje cells from embryonic grafts confirmed graft viability.

Based on this experimental evidence, we applied a similar technique in six medically intractable patients with severe hereditary cerebellar degenerative ataxia. The preliminary results show two patients with marked improvement and three with moderate improvement. One patient showed improvement for two months followed by mild deterioration, however, his condition remains better than prior to implantation. Examination of his immunological markers in the blood revealed changes compatible with graft rejection. Further evaluation of both experimental animals and human subjects is indicated.

Embryonic cerebellar grafts can survive, differentiate and integrate in the cerebellum of the host animal; and fetal grafts have a strong potential to correct disorders of cerebellar degenerative diseases in humans.

Acknowledgments. The authors acknowledge the assistance of Herman F. Flanigin, M.D., M. Peter Heilbrun, M.D., Joseph R. Smith, M.D., Marshall B. Allen Jr., M.D., Thomas R. Swift, M.D., J. Richard Baringer, M.D., Farivar Yaghmai, M.D. and Frances M. Huey in reviewing and revising the manuscript and also acknowledge Richard J. Mullen, M.D. and Mark Reichman, M.D. for their assistance with the research project.

References

1. Dunn EH. Primary and secondary findings in a series of attempts to transplant cerebral cortex in the albino rat. *J Comp Neurol.* 1917;27:565–582.
2. May RM. La graffe dans l'oeil de rat blanc adult du tissue cerebral de rat nouveau-ne. *Arch Anat Microsc.* 1930;26:433.
3. Le Gros Clark, WE. Neuronal differentiation in implanted fetal cortical tissue. *J Neurol Psychiatry* 1940;3:263.
4. Das GD, Altman J. Studies on the transplantation of developing neural tissue in the mammalian brain. I. Transplantation of cerebellar slabs into the cerebellum of neonate rats. *Brain Res.* 1972;38:233–249.
5. Das GD. Transplantation of embryonic neural tissue in the mammalian brain. I. Growth and differentiation of neuroblast from various regions of the embryonic brain in the cerebellum of neonatal rats. *J Life Sci.* 1974;4:93–124.
6. Seiger A, Olson L. Quantitation of fiber growth in transplanted central monoamine neurons. *Cell Tissue Res.* 1977;179:285–316.
7. Stenevi U, Bjorklund A, Svendgaard NA. Transplantation of central and peripheral monoamine neurons to the adult rat brain: Techniques and condition for survival. *Brain Res.* 1976;114:1–20.
8. Gash D, Sladek JR Jr. Vasopressin neurons grafted into Brattleboro rats: Viability and activity. *Peptides* 1980;1:11–14.
9. Lund RA, Hauschka SD. Transplanted neural tissue develops connections with host rat brain. *Science* 1976;193:582–584.
10. Stein DG, Mufson EJ. Morphological and behavioral characteristics of embryonic brain tissue transplants in adults. Brain damaged subjects, cell and tissue transplantation into the adult brain. *Ann NY Acad Sci.* 1987;495:444–464.
11. Sotelo C, Alvarado-Mallart RM. Cerebellar transplantations in adult mice with heredogenerative ataxia. I. Cell and tissue transplantation into the adult brain. *Ann NY Acad Sci* 1987;495:242–266.
12. Wyatt RJ, Freed WJ. Central nervous system grafting. In: Wilkins RH, Rengachary SS, eds. *Neurosurgery.* New York: McGraw-Hill; 1985.
13. Wallace RB, Das GD. *Neural Tissue Transplantation Research.* New York: Springer–Verlag; 1983.
14. Backlund EO, Granberg PO, Knutsson E, et al. Transplantation of adrenal medullary tissue to striatum in Parkinsonism. *J Neurosurg.* 1985;62:169–173.
15. Backlund EO, Olson L, Seiger A, Lindvall O. Toward a transplantation therapy in Parkinson's disease. A progress report from continuing clinical experiments. *Ann NY Acad Sci.* 1987;495:658–673.
16. Madrazo I, Leon V, Torres C, et al. Transplantation of fetal substantia nigra and adrenal medulla to the caudate nucleus in two patients with Parkinson's disease. *N Engl J Med.* 1987;318:51(letter).
17. Zhang Han-Qi, et al. The mitosis of Purkinje's cells of injured cerebellum in adult rats. *Acta Chinese Anat.* 1964;15(1):59–63.
18. Zhang Han-Qi, et al. An observation of the influence on the mitosis of Purkinje's cells by transplanting the cerebellum of neonatal rats into the injured cerebellum of Wistar rats. *Acta Shandong Medical University.* 1986;24(2):6–11.
19. Liu Yu-Mei, et al. A study of implantation of embryonic cerebellar tissue for a

type of injured cerebellar ataxia of Wistar rats. *Acta Shandong Medical University.* 1988;26(2):12–15.

20. Rosenberg RN, ed. *Neurology. The Science and Practice of Clinical Medicine*, Vol. 5. New York: Grune and Stratton Inc; 1980.

21. Vick NA. *Grinker's Neurology.* Springfield, Ill. Charles C Thomas; 1976.

22. Perlow MJ, Freed WJ, Hoffer BJ, Seiger A, et al. Brain grafts reduce motor abnormalities produced by destruction of nigrostriatal dopamine system. *Science.* 1979;204:641–643.

23. Seger M. Interactions between grafted serotonin neurons and adult host rat hippocampus. *Ann NY Acad Sci.* 1987;495:284–295.

24. Pezzoli G, Silani V, Motti E, et al. Human fetal adrenal medulla for transplantation in Parkinsonian patients. *Ann NY Acad Sci.* 1987;495:771–773.

25. Clarke DJ, Gage FH, Nilsson OG, Bjorklund A. Grafted septal neurons from synaptic connections in the dentate gyrus of behaviorally impaired aged rats. *J Comp Neurol.* 1986;252:483–492.

26. Clarke DJ, Gage FH, Dunnett SB, Nilsson OG, Bjorklund A. Synaptogenesis of grafted cholinergic neurons. *Ann NY Acad Sci.* 1987;495:268–283.

27. Gardette R, Alvarado-Mallart RM, Crepel F, Sotelo C. Electrophysiological demonstration of a synaptic integration of transplanted Purkinje cells into the cerebellum of the adult Purkinje cell degeneration mutant mouse. *Neuroscience.* (In press).

28. Oblinger MO, Das GD. Connectivity of transplants in the cerebellum: A model of developmental differences in neuroplasticity. In: Wallace RB, Gopan DD, eds. *Neural Tissue Transplantation Research.* New York: Springer–Verlag; 1983.

29. Bartus RT. Neural tissue transplantation: Comments on its role in general neuroscience and its potential as a therapeutic approach. *Ann NY Acad Sci.* 1987;495:355–361.

30. Sotelo C, Alvarado-Mallart RM. Embryonic and adult neurons interact to allow Purkinje cell replacements in mutant cerebellum. *Nature.* 1987;327:421–423.

31. Crain SM. CNS tissue culture analysis of trophic mechanisms in brain transplantation. *Ann NY Acad Sci.* 1987;495:103–107.

32. Crain SM. Trophic mechanism in transplantation: Summary (Part II). *Ann NY Acad Sci.* 1987;495:225–267.

33. Sabel B, Dunbar G, Stein DG. Gangliosides minimize behavioral deficits and enhance structural repair after brain injury. *J Neurosci Res.* 1984;12:429–443.

34. Hart T, Chaimas N, Moore RY, Stein DG. Effects of nerve growth factor on behavioral recovery following caudate nucleus lesion in rats. *Brain Res Bull.* 1978;3:245–250.

35. Nieto-Sampedro M, Kesslak JP, Gibbs R, Cotman CW. Effects of conditioning lesions on transplant survival, connectivity, and function: Role of neurotrophic factors. *Ann NY Acad Sci.* 1987;495:108–119.

36. Fishman PS. Neural transplantation: Scientific gains and clinical perspectives. *Neurology* 1986;36:389–392.

37. Clarke D, Gage FH, Dunnett SB, Nilsson OG, Bjorklund A. Synaptogenesis of grafted cholinergic neurons. *Ann NY Acad Sci.* 1986;495:268–283.

III. SURGICAL EXPERIENCE WITH THE SPINAL CORD INJURY

CHAPTER 10

Introduction to Intramedullary Tumors

Bennett M. Stein

Paul McCormick, M.D., chief resident, at The Neurological Institute, will review our experience in detail. We have a special interest in intramedullary tumors and arteriovenous malformations (AVMs). The intramedullary tumors are grouped according to histology and frequency in Table 10.1.

In light of what we have been discussing, intramedullary tumors offer a clinical correlate in which there is an unrelenting process within the interior of the spinal cord, gradually wasting away the spinal cord tissue by one means or another, sometimes producing dramatic clinical syndromes and at other times not so dramatic. Why is there such a difference in compliance of the spinal cord to the same size intramedullary mass?

The cavitation of the spinal cord that we see after removal of a lesion is often remarkable. For example, you can virtually see through the posterior column in some cases, and yet with the passage of time these white matter tracts begin to function in a reasonably normal fashion. The question that we were grappling with yesterday about regeneration or reorganization is paramount to the situation that we encounter in these cases.

A drawing (Fig. 10.1) shows the usual position of an intramedullary tumor, some larger than others with a varying degree of tissue compression. It would appear that there is equal compression of white matter tracts as there is of the gray matter. Notwithstanding, intramedullary tumors involving the cervical enlargement rarely produce atrophy of the intrinsic muscles of the hand, whereas function of the posterior and lateral white matter tracts may be severely impaired. It would appear that the gray matter function is more resistant to compression. These tumors tend to be oriented dorsal from the central canal, which must pertain to stress and resistance within the spinal cord that prevent tumors from growing in a concentric fashion from the central canal and going ventrally as far as they do dorsally. This eccentricity may be due to less tension in the posterior median raphae or perhaps related to the arterial supply of the spinal cord, which is prominent in the anterior raphae. These are purely speculations to which we cannot give specific justification.

Table 10.1. Intramedullary tumors incidence.

Astrocytoma	40%
Ependymoma	40%
Hemangioblastoma	10%
Miscellaneous	10%
Teratoma, Dermoid, Pigmented Neurofibroma, Cavernous Malformation	

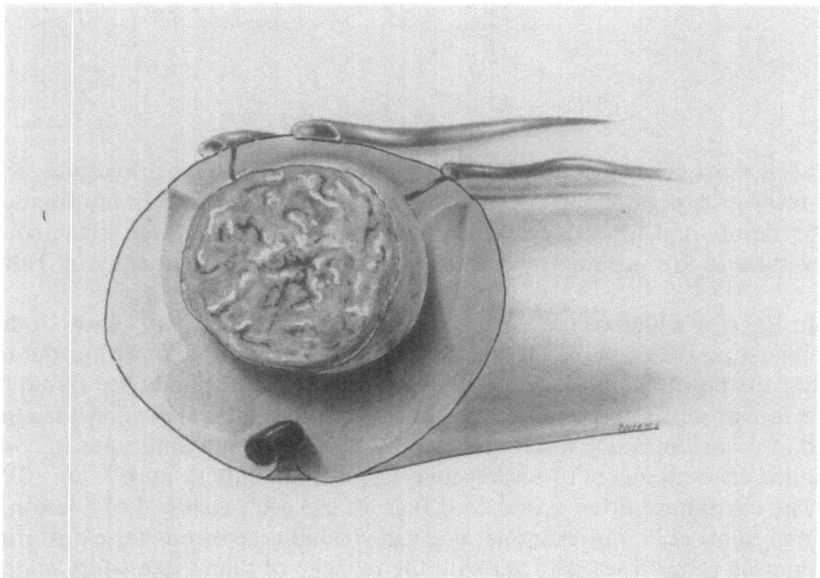

Figure 10.1. Drawing of intramedullary tumor expanding the interior of the cord. Note the dorsal direction of tumor growth and the fact that the dorsal element of the tumor lies deep to the pia.

A remarkable phenomenon is the enlargement that occurs in the cord adjacent and occasionally distal to an intramedullary tumor. This change was encountered in a number of hemangioblastomas, as illustrated in Fig. 10.2. Associated with the illustrated hemangioblastoma occurring at two levels was a multilevel widening of the caudal cord without cyst. In one patient there was a change on the magnetic resonance image (MRI) (presumed to be edema) that extended all the way into the medulla (Fig. 10.3). Therefore, the effects of these tumors may be not only local but extend well beyond. It would appear that local as well as distal changes are reversible after successful operation. In this example (Fig. 10.3), the tumor occupied a large part of the spinal cord and produced a syndrome of modest spasticity, mild loss of posterior column function, and weakness of the upper extremities that was not associated with atrophy. Surgery demon-

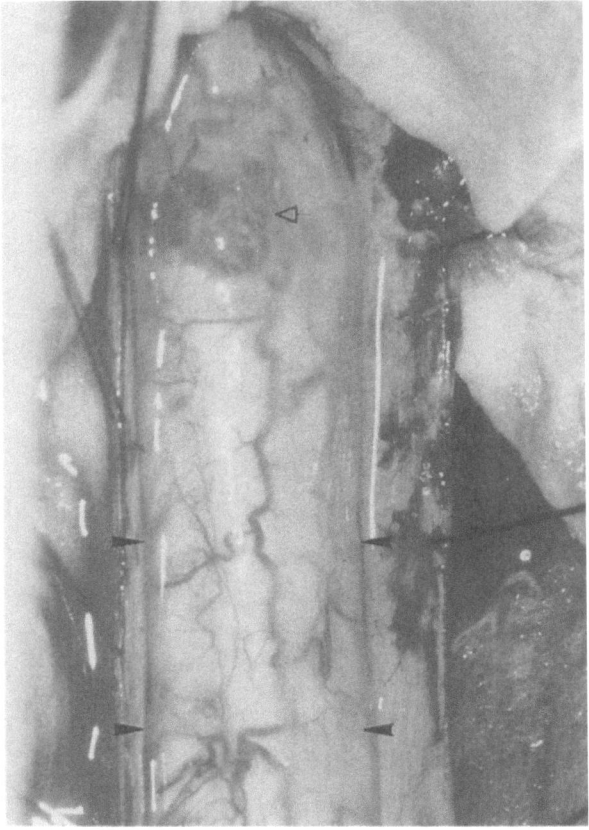

Figure 10.2. Operative photograph of hemangioblastoma located at the second cervical vertebral level (*arrow*) without caudal cyst but enlargement of the cervical spinal cord to the level of T-1, below the level of the lesion (*arrowheads*).

strated that the tumor was located more to the lateral side, but extended well into and thinned out the cord tremendously. After removal of such a tumor and passage of time the cord can become atrophic or develop small syrinxes. All of the cord widening in this patient that extended well up into the medulla and caudal to the tumor has remitted. With the loss of "mass effect" the cord became atrophic.

It is my impression that what is happening is an electrolyte shift, movement of extracellular fluid, or possibly demyelinization occurring in the compressed fiber tracts. Many of these changes are reversible. I think if it were cellular injury or axonal injury, then we would not see the reversibility after removal of the process, but this is purely speculation and we have little pathology to substantiate this contention.

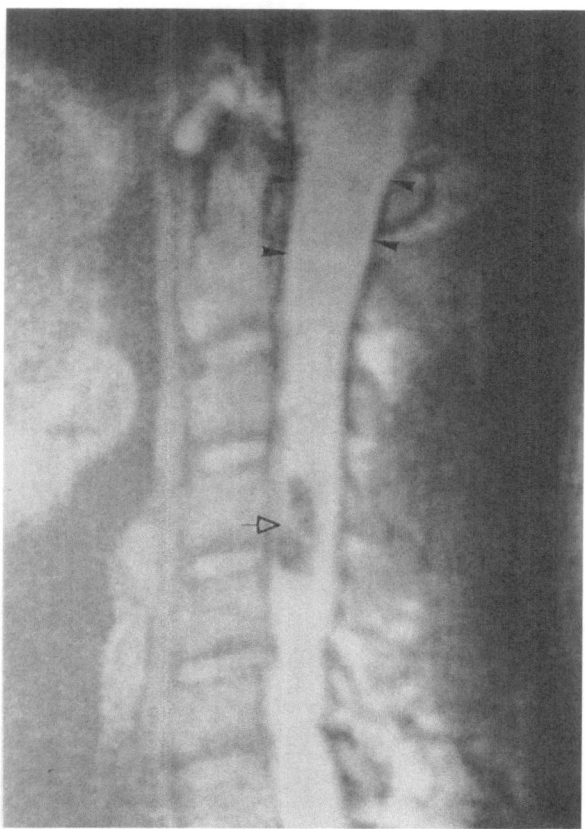

Figure 10.3. Sagittal MRI view showing focal hemangioblastoma *(arrow)* and spinal cord widening extending rostrally to the level of the medulla *(arrowheads)*.

We have recently had the opportunity, because of the MRI, to follow these patients postoperatively in detail. Much like the traumatized spinal cord that develops a syrinx at other levels, or the foramen magnum meningioma that develops a syrinx at the C-8 level, well removed from the tumor, we may be seeing syrinxes developing at future dates after an otherwise successful removal of a tumor. It remains to be seen if the formation of a syrinx is clinically important.

In another individual with an intramedullary ependymoma in the cervical region there was thinning of the dorsal columns, so that they were virtually translucent through the pia (Fig. 10.4). After the removal of the tumor, which had a good capsule, the anterior median raphe was seen (Fig. 10.5). The tumor extended farther dorsal or posterior than it did anterior. With a spinal cord so thin after tumor removal, you have to ask

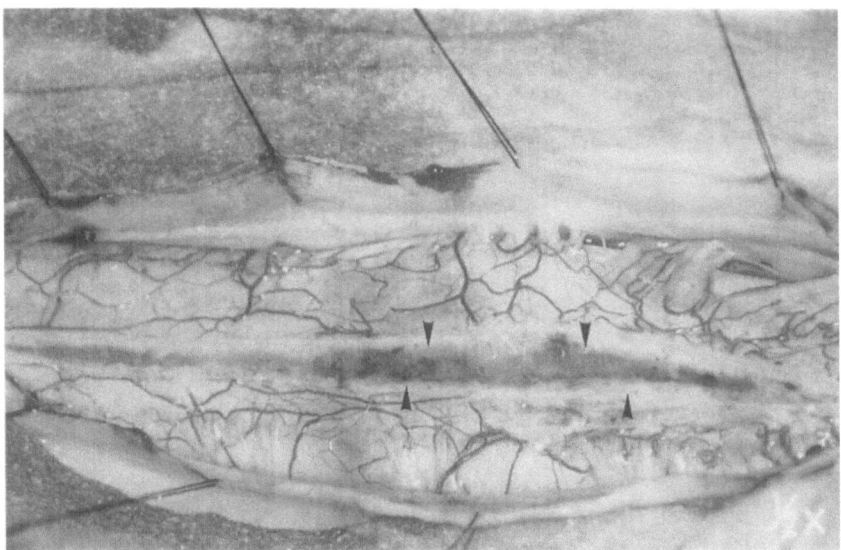

Figure 10.4. Operative photograph showing initial myelotomy and the presentation of tumor below the thinned out posterior columns (*arrowheads*).

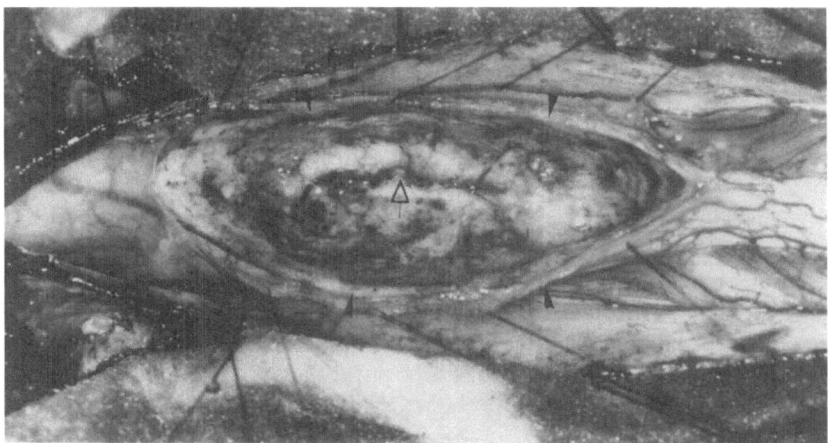

Figure 10.5. Operative photograph showing removal of large intramedullary ependymoma with anterior raphae (*arrow*) and thinned out posterior columns (*arrowheads*).

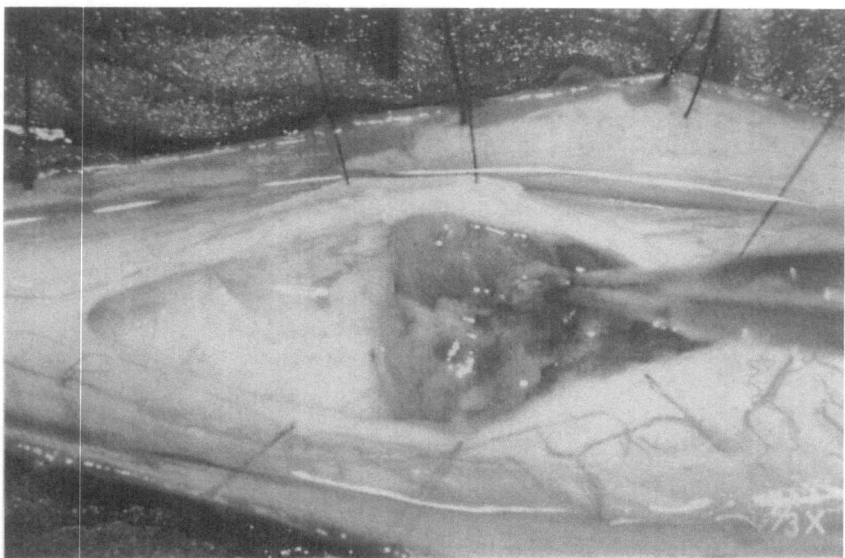

Figure 10.6. Operative photograph showing the removal of a large encapsulated astrocytoma from within the spinal cord. The large cavitation is due to both the solid and cystic nature of the tumor. The cord substance has been markedly thinned and cavitated by this long-standing tumor.

how an individual could possibly function, either immediately after the surgery or in the future. Improvement in the neurologic state may be seen almost immediately after operation, suggesting some shift in electrolytes or fluid, with maximum improvement occurring gradually, which makes me think that there is a remyelination process that takes over.

In another individual with a huge tumor (Fig. 10.6) solid and cystic, the patient had only a Babinski response and a little difficulty determining position of the great toe, modest pain in the shoulder, and no other abnormalities. This slow process of tumor growth produced compression of aspects of the spinal cord that were not essential for functional neurological activity. Despite the huge tumor and cavitation of the cervical spinal cord, the patient was little afflicted preoperatively and became normal postoperatively.

Another patient had a large epidermoid tumor located in the conus. After removal it was possible to see through the center of the cord (Fig. 10.7). This patient presented with a weak lower extremity, but he had normal bladder function before and after the surgery. You have to ask yourself the question, how can this conus, grossly distorted by the lesion and traumatized by surgery, be correlated with a normal functioning bladder?

Another patient who was operated 6 years previously, biopsied, and

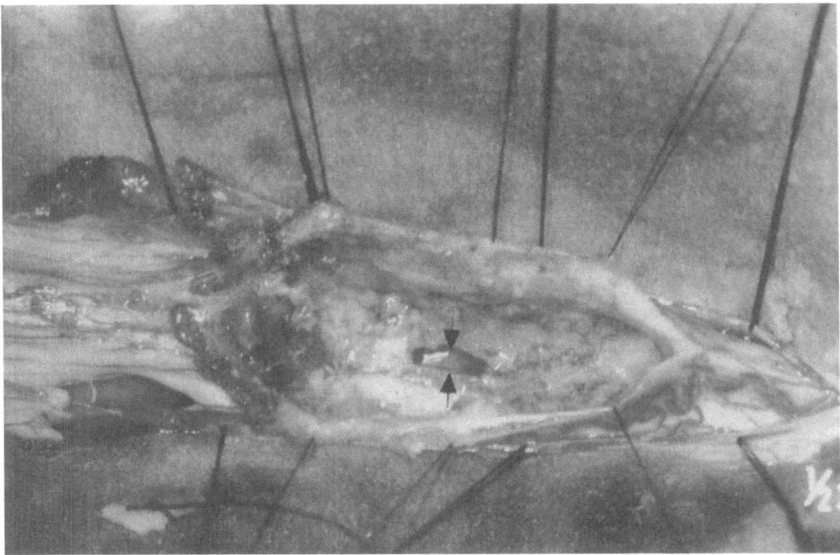

Figure 10.7. Operative photograph of the conus after removal of a large intramedullary epidermoid. The hole in the anterior cavitated conus is marked by arrows.

radiated for an intramedullary astrocytoma, came back with regrowth and was still ambulatory. Now we see a multicompartmental tumor. A subtotal removal was performed and her function improved!

Even with numerous insults to the spinal cord, growth of tumor, and radiation, the capacity for recovery of function is most remarkable. This attests to the resiliency of the neural (spinal cord) tissue.

I believe there are many unanswered questions. We do minimal physiological monitoring during the surgery, only monitoring posterior column function. You can see evoked potentials that turn on and off. You can see with traction or manipulation the potentials fall off in terms of amplitude and frequency, and see them come back after the manipulation is stopped, so that there is a flux situation during the surgery. Some people have been able to monitor motor function by stimulating the corticospinal tract above the area of the surgery and recording below, but that is much more difficult. Basically, we are looking at one primary sensory tract in terms of the monitoring.

It is interesting that although the recovery from surgery is remarkable in most cases, especially if the patient is not devastated before, one of the major problems has been pain, which appears to become worse as time goes by. This is not only pain related to the radicular elements in the area of the tumor resection, but it can be whole body pain. It can extend well below the actual level of the tumor and engulf the patient with painful paresthesias or dysesthesias; perhaps a posterior column phenomenon or a disturbance in the dorsal root entry zone.

This raises interesting speculation in terms of reorientation or regeneration in the spinal cord. It may be a double-edged sword that we are witnessing here; some form of aberrant regeneration, or cross-talk between the various nerve fibers that have now been injured at the dorsal root entry zone or the posterior columns, two areas that are exquisitely associated with sensation. When we talk about regeneration or reorganization of pathways then we may also be opening Pandora's box, in terms of function that we do not necessarily anticipate or want.

CHAPTER 11

Intramedullary Spinal Cord Ependymoma: Long-Term Clinical Evaluation after Complete Surgical Removal

Paul C. McCormick and Bennett M. Stein

Among the various intramedullary spinal cord neoplasms mentioned in the previous chapter by Dr. Stein, ependymomas present a number of intriguing clinical and biological characteristics that offer a rather unique opportunity to evaluate certain clinical aspects of spinal cord function and recovery. First, although ependymomas are glial derived, unencapsulated tumors, the vast majority of spinal ependymomas exist in a histologically benign form with little infiltrative potential and produce a progressive myelopathy by compression of the surrounding spinal cord rather than invading fiber tracts or gray matter. Second, biological growth of spinal ependymomas is extremely slow with prodromal symptom duration usually measured in years. This slow growth is further evidenced by the frequent finding of large intramedullary ependymomas producing a thin, translucent-appearing surrounding spinal cord in patients with rather mild neurological deficit. These findings indicate a rather remarkable ability of the spinal cord to tolerate mechanical deformation secondary to a slowly expanding mass. Finally, with advances in imaging and microsurgical techniques, it has become clear that total removal of intramedullary ependymomas with acceptable morbidity and a low incidence of recurrence is now possible.[1-11]

Thus, spinal ependymomas may be considered as a clinical model of a slowly progressive compressive myelopathy in which the course of the syndrome can be reversed or arrested by removal of the tumor. This chapter reviews in detail both the preoperative clinical presentation and long-term postoperative evaluation of a series of 23 patients with intramedullary spinal cord ependymoma treated by complete surgical removal. Although this information may be insufficient to address specific aspects of recovery, it is hoped that such a careful clinical evaluation may allow at least some insight into spinal cord function, response to injury, and capacity for recovery.

Table 11.1. Clinical/functional classification scheme.

Grade 1:	Neurologically normal; mild focal deficit not significantly affecting function of involved limb; mild spasticity or reflex abnormality; normal gait
Grade 2:	Presence of sensorimotor deficit affecting function of involved limb; mild to moderate gait difficulty; severe pain or dysesthetic syndrome impairing patient's quality of life; still functions and ambulates independently
Grade 3:	More severe neurological deficit; requires cane/brace for ambulation or significant bilateral upper extremity impairment; may or may not function independently
Grade 4:	Severe deficit; requires wheelchair or cane/brace with bilateral upper extremity impairment; usually not independent

Clinical Methods

A consecutive series of 23 patients underwent operative resection of an intramedullary spinal ependymoma between January, 1976 and September, 1988. Patients with filum terminale ependymomas were not included in this study. The location of the tumors was: cervical or cervicothoracic 17, thoracic 2, conus medullaris 4. Two conus tumors had both intramedullary and extramedullary components (cases 6 and 10). At operation, a grossly complete tumor removal was believed to be accomplished in each patient. No patient received postoperative radiation therapy but six patients had undergone previous operation and radiation therapy before clinical tumor recurrence and ultimate referral to this institution.

Preoperative clinical evaluation was performed carefully and each patient was assigned a clinical grade according to the clinical/functional classification scheme listed in Table 11.1. Neurological function was assessed during the immediate postoperative period and at approximately 3 months and 1 year postoperatively. Long-term follow-up, consisting of office visits and completion of a detailed questionnaire, has recently been performed (Table 11.2). Fourteen patients have had postoperative magnetic resonance imaging (MRI) performed at intervals ranging from 8 months to 10 years after operation. There have been no deaths and no patient has been lost to follow-up. The follow-up period ranged from 6 to 159 months (mean 62 months), with seven patients followed a minimum of 10 years after surgery.

Clinical Summary

The patient population consisted of 13 women and 10 men ranging in age from 19 to 70 years (mean 43 years) at the time of initial diagnosis (Table 11.2). Pain was the initial symptom in 15 (65%) patients and was present an average of 16 months before the onset of objective neurological complaints. The pain was localized to the back or neck in 12 patients and usually corresponded to the level of the tumor. Interscapular or shoulder pain was also common in patients with cervical or cervicothoracic tumors. Two patients had associated pain radiating to the arm or leg and one patient presented with isolated leg pain. Six patients described a sensory disturbance, consisting of numbness, paresthesiae, or dysesthesiae as the initial symptom. In four patients the sensory change began distally and later progressed to involve the proximal limb. Weakness was the initial complaint in two patients. The duration of symptoms preceding initial diagnosis ranged from 6 to 96 months (mean 34 months; median 26 months).

Objective neurological deficit was present in 22 patients at the time of initial diagnosis. The deficit was usually mild with 21 patients (91%), demonstrating independent ambulation, and 19 patients (83%) classified as clinical/functional grades 1 or 2. Eight patients had received previous treatment before tumor recurrence and referral.

The pattern and progression of neurological deficit was variable and related to tumor location. Cervical or cervicothoracic tumors (n = 17) tended initially to produce isolated deficit of the upper extremities of a predominant sensory (n = 8) or motor (n = 4) nature. Two patients complained of pain and noted no neurological deficit on admission interview. Five patients, with a mean symptom duration of 22 months, had neurological deficit confined to one or both arms. Five patients, with a mean symptom duration of 39 months, denied lower extremity symptoms but had mild leg deficit on admission exam. Seven patients complained of lower extremity weakness and/or numbness as the first noticeable deficit (one patient), concurrently with the onset of upper extremity deficit (one patient), or occurring on average 23 months after the onset of upper extremity deficits (five patients).

Atrophy of one or both hands was occasionally noted with tumors of the cervical spinal cord but was usually subtle and asymptomatic. Proximal muscle atrophy was present in two patients. Only one patient noted bowel/bladder difficulty.

Six patients had neurological deficit that was predominantly unilateral, with two patients demonstrating an incomplete Brown-Séquard syndrome.

Both patients with thoracic ependymomas (cases 20 and 22) presented with bilateral leg numbness. Minimal leg weakness or stiffness occurred 14 months and 2 years after the onset of numbness, respectively. One patient noted bowel/bladder difficulty. One patient (case 20), with a T3-4 ependymoma, had dissociated sensory loss in one arm secondary to a rostral cyst extending to the C-6 level.

All four patients with conus ependymomas presented with pain as the initial complaint. Neurological exam in one patient was normal. In two patients progressive weakness of one or both legs was the predominant neurological complaint. Unilateral leg numbness followed by leg weakness

Table 11.2. Clinical summary of 23 patients with intramedullary ependymoma[a].

Case no.	Age (yrs), sex[b]	Initial symptom	Duration of symptoms[a]	Cord enlargement (tumor level)	
1	50, M	Paresthesiae, hand	23 mos	C-1–T-1	(C-2–7)
2	19, M	Pain, back	16 mos	C-2–T-1	(C-3–T-1)
3	35, F	Pain, neck	86 mos	C-2–7	(C-3–7)
4	46, M	Pain, neck and arm	38 mos	C-2–7	(C-4–7)
5	48, F	Pain, leg	6 mos	T-12–L-1	(T-12–L-1)
6	24, M	Pain, back and leg	14 mos	T-8–L-2	(T-10–L-2)
7	41, F	Pain, neck	13 mos	C-2–T-2	(C-3–T-1)
8	36, M	Pain, neck	96 mos	C-1–T-3	(C-3–7)
9	43, F	Pain, neck	24 mos	C-2–T-3	(C-5–7)
10	33, F	Pain, back	92 mos	T-11–L-2	(T-11–L-2)
11	32, F	Pain, back	35 mos	C-4–T-1	(C7)
12	37, M	Pain, back	72 mos	C-4–L-2	(T-8–L-2)
13	32, M	Gait difficulty	7 mos	C-4–T-9	(C-5–T-2)
14	49, F	Pain, neck and back	17 mos	C-3–T-1	(C-5–7)
15	64, F	Numbness, hands	30 mos	C-2–5	(C-4–5)
16	70, F	Numbness, hands and feet	37 mos	C-3–7	(C-5–7)
17	52, F	Pain, neck	46 mos	C-4–T-1	(C-4–7)
18	42, M	Paresthesiae, arms	30 mos	C-3–T-1	(C-5–6)
19	48, M	Weakness, arm	14 mos	C-3–7	(C-4–7)
20	47, M	Paresthesiae, legs	17 mos	C-5–T-8	(T-3–4)
21	61, F	Pain, arm	26 mos	C-4–T-1	(C-5–7)
22	54, F	Dysesthesiae, feet	26 mos	C-7–T-3	(T-1–3)
23	35, F	Pain, back	10 mos	C-3–T-1	(C-4–7)

[a] C, cervical; T, thoracic; L, lumbar.
[b] Age at time of initial diagnosis.
[c] Duration of symptoms prior to initial diagnosis.

was noted by the remaining patient. One patient also complained of bilateral hand numbness and had dissociated sensory loss in the arms. A rostral cyst extending to the C-4 level was present. Three patients noted bowel/bladder difficulty.

The clinical course was slowly progressive in all patients. Several patients, however, noticed an accelerated progression in the 6 months to 1 year preceding diagnosis. Two patients had an acute worsening of neurological deficit from an intratumoral hemorrhage confirmed at surgery.

Radiological Investigation

Preoperative radiological evaluation consisted of plain films (12 patients), myelogram (7 patients), myelogram followed by computerized tomography (CT) (8 patients), and MRI (13 patients). Metrizamide or iohexol myelography followed by delayed CT was performed in five patients.

Initial preoperative (most recent preop.[e])	Immediate postop.	3 months postop.	1 year postop.	Recent follow-up (length[d])	Net grade change
1 (3)	4	3	3	3 (159 mos)	0
1 (3)	3	3	3	4 (159 mos)	−1
1 (3)	3	2	2	2 (156 mos)	+1
1	2	1	1	1 (146 mos)	0
1	1	1	1	1 (135 mos)	0
2 (4)	4	4	4	4 (125 mos)	0
1	2	2	2	1 (121 mos)	0
1 (4)	4	4	4	4 (89 mos)	0
3	3	2	1	1 (66 mos)	+2
1 (2)	3	3	2	2 (63 mos)	0
2	2	1	1	1 (59 mos)	+1
3	4	3	3	3 (54 mos)	0
3	3	3	2	2 (43 mos)	+1
2	2	2	1	1 (42 mos)	+1
1	2	2	2	2 (39 mos)	−1
2	3	2	2	2 (36 mos)	0
1	2	1	1	1 (33 mos)	0
1 (2)	2	2	2	1 (23 mos)	+1
1 (3)	4	2	2	2 (21 mos)	+2
1	2	1	1	1 (20 mos)	0
3	3	3	2	2 (14 mos)	+1
1	2	2	—	2 (8 mos)	−1
1	2	1	—	1 (6 mos)	0

[d]Length of follow-up following completion of most recent treatment.
[e]Cases 1, 2, 3, 6, 8, 10, 18, 19 had previous operation +/− radiation therapy. Clinical grade in parentheses indicates clinical status prior to most recent treatment.

Plain films revealed mild scoliosis of the upper or midthoracic spine in three patients. An enlarged spinal canal with vertebral body scalloping, medial pedicle erosion, and thinning of the laminae was noted in two patients.

Spinal cord enlargement was identified in all patients, ranging in length from 2 to 18 (mean 7) spinal segments. MRI was particularly useful in defining the level of the tumor and identifying associated spinal cord edema or cysts. Delayed CT scanning after water-soluble myelography did not reveal contrast uptake into the spinal cord in any patient.

Outcome

Neurological evaluation in the immediate postoperative period revealed either worsening of an existing deficit or onset of a new deficit, usually posterior column, in 20 patients. This resulted in a deterioration of the clinical grade in 12 patients. In general, however, significant recovery from the operative deficit was achieved by 3 months postoperatively. Only two patients (cases 15 and 22) have had a persistent net deterioration in clinical grade caused by surgery. Both of these patients were grade 1 preoperatively. One patient, neurologically unchanged after surgery, developed a severe dysesthetic pain syndrome. The other patient, currently grade 2 at 8 months postoperatively, continues to show slow improvement.

Recovery from a preoperative deficit resulting in an ultimate improvement in clinical grade was seen in eight patients. The timing of recovery was variable with relief of spasticity occurring early (< 6 months), whereas recovery of lower motor neuron and sensory deficit tended to appear later (> 6 months) with continued improvement noted up to 2 years postoperatively in two patients.

Bowel/bladder function improved in all patients with cervical, cervicothoracic, or thoracic tumors but in only one patient with a conus tumor. Two patients with conus tumors had permanent worsening of bowel/bladder function after surgery.

One patient (case 2), with severe neurological deficit before definitive tumor removal, experienced delayed neurological deterioration 10 years postoperatively. MRI demonstrated a huge cervical intramedullary cyst just above the level of previous resection. Operative exploration revealed a dense adhesive arachnoiditis in addition to the cyst but no gross tumor recurrence. No improvement in neurological function occurred after cyst drainage.

A frequent phenomenon after surgery was the appearance of a dysesthetic syndrome. Although subjective complaints of numbness, out of proportion to objective sensory deficit, were also common and usually of little functional consequence, dysesthetic complaints were perceived to be particularly annoying and often debilitating to the patient. The severity of the dysesthesiae, and the patient's emotional response, were quite variable, ranging from intermittent and clinically insignificant "pins and needles" sensations to persistent distressing, often causalgic-like, complaints of "itching," crawling," or "burning" dysesthesiae.

This syndrome generally appeared early in the postoperative period and frequently seemed to follow a posterior column or radicular distribution. Patients with preoperative dysesthesiae seemed particularly prone to develop this syndrome postoperatively but no other factors predicting occurrence could be identified.

The dysesthesiae were refractory to various forms of medical therapy but usually self-limited with resolution or amelioration of complaints several months after surgery. Only two patients had significant dysesthetic complaints at 1 year postoperatively.

The physiological basis of this syndrome is unclear but the anatomical distribution of the dysesthesiae suggests injury to the posterior columns or dorsal root entry zone.

With the exception of one patient (case 2), no patient has shown any clinical evidence of tumor recurrence at follow-up ranging from 6 to 159 months (mean 62 months). Comparison of most recent preoperative clinical grade and current follow-up evaluation revealed an improvement in clinical grade in 8 patients, no significant change in 12 patients, and deterioration in 3 patients.

Follow-up MRI has now been performed in 14 patients. Spinal cord atrophy, extending variable degrees above and below the level of tumor resection, dorsal tethering of the spinal cord to the posterior dura with a large ventral subarachnoid space, and diminution but persistence of cysts were the most common findings (Fig. 11.5). No patient showed definite evidence of tumor recurrence although, one patient had faint gadolinium uptake in the walls of the resection bed on MRI performed 6 months postoperatively. Repeated MRI over 3 years has shown no change. Although residual tumor cannot be ruled out, it seems more likely that this appearance represents a persistent postoperative change.

Discussion

Surgical pathology affecting the spinal cord generally involves either compressive lesions that may be extradural, intradural, or intramedullary in nature or vascular malformations. Preoperative considerations in these patients routinely include an assessment of operative risk, natural history of the disease process, and benefit of nonoperative therapy, but only to a limited degree is the potential for recovery adequately addressed. Clinical experience has shown that the timing, pattern, and extent of recovery are related to numerous variables including the type and location of pathology, duration and severity of the preoperative deficit, and the time course of neurological deterioration. Accumulated clinical data therefore allows statistical predictions for recovery but the estimation of recovery on an individual basis is difficult to ascertain preoperatively. This difficulty is related, in part, not only to an inhomogeneous patient population with respect to variable clinical effects produced by similar pathology but also by limitations in knowledge of spinal cord function, which allows examination of only a limited number of spinal cord tracts and cell groups. In addition, the pathophysiological mechanisms producing neurological deficit and the response of the spinal cord to this injury are poorly understood. Nevertheless, carefully performed clinical studies can provide information from which valuable insight into spinal cord function, plasticity, response to injury and possible mechanisms of recovery may be obtained.

In the present series, analysis of a detailed history and neurological examination and correlated with radiological studies and intraoperative findings indicate that the spinal cord displays an extraordinary tolerance to a slowly expanding mass. Despite an average symptom duration of just under 3 years and the frequent operative finding of a severely distorted spinal cord, most patients presented at initial diagnosis with only minor neurological deficit. The pattern of deficit was variable but ascending sensory and corticospinal tracts appeared clinically most susceptible to the expanding mass. Lower motor neuron and visceral function was least affected with cervical or cervicothoracic tumors. Unilateral deficits were common and usually correlated with an eccentric tumor location. A number of patients noted an accelerated progression of deficit before diagnosis, suggesting that there is a limit to spinal cord tolerance beyond which relatively rapid decompensation will occur.

In order to evaluate recovery it is important that the possible mechanisms responsible for the return of function be defined. Similarly, it is important to distinguish between true neurological recovery and functional recovery resulting from an adaptive response. Based on clinical experience and laboratory investigations, it is the authors' opinion that functional recovery may be explained by five mechanisms: resolution of focal physiological impairment, repair, plasticity, regeneration, and adaptation. Although it is difficult to define confidently the precise physiological phenomena underlying these mechanisms, particularly at the cellular or subcellular level, a careful analysis of the pattern and progression of deficit and the timing of postoperative recovery does allow reasonable postulations of the specific operative mechanisms effecting recovery.

Early recovery, which is often dramatic and may be witnessed in the first few hours to several days postoperatively, seems best explained by resolution of focal physiological impairment. This type of recovery is usually seen after removal of extramedullary compressive lesions in patients whose preoperative duration of deficit is relatively brief. It is occasionally witnessed in patients with a longer deficit duration, particularly, as Dr. Oldfield has shown, if the deficit is secondary to vascular insufficiency. Early recovery is rarely seen after removal of intramedullary tumors.

This type of recovery implies a reversible impairment to nerve impulse transmission, caused either by ischemia, membrane distortion, or edema, in neural tissue whose underlying functional and structural integrity is intact. It is, perhaps, similar to the effects seen with peripheral nerve compression.

We define intermediate recovery as occurring several weeks to several months after surgery. It tends to be less complete than early recovery and is commonly associated with more severe deficits of longer duration. It was frequently seen in the present series involving recovery from surgically induced deficits. Although the pathophysiological mechanisms may be similar to those seen in early recovery, the time course and quality of recovery suggests that the structural integrity of the neural tissue has been compromised. Thus, whereas surgery may restore the local physiological and anatomical environment, recovery is delayed until repair is effected. Intermediate recovery, therefore, may be viewed as both a physiological and reparative response of more severely injured but still functionally viable neural tissue. Whether the reparative process is due to remyelinization, membrane repair with ionic channel reorganization, or reestablishment of the correct metabolic milieu is not known.

Long-term recovery is somewhat arbitrarily defined as commencing about 6 months postoperatively or beyond. It is the most difficult aspect of recovery to evaluate for several reasons. First, functional recovery is frequently seen purely on the basis of an adaptive behavior rather than true neurological recovery. A frequent example in this series was the improved ambulation seen in patients with posterior column deficits compensated for through the increased reliance on visual input. Adaptation can been seen on many different levels and represents the cornerstone on which the field of rehabilitative medicine is based. Second, long-term true neurological recovery potentially involves the mechanisms of repair, plasticity, and regeneration, which are poorly understood, difficult to identify clinically, and may be present simultaneously. An example in this series was the eventual return of muscle bulk in atrophic hands or limbs. Whether this return was due to the adaptive response of enlargement of existing motor units, plasticity of the spinal cord with reinnervation through sprouting, or regeneration of anterior horn cells is unknown. It is hoped that detailed electrophysiological testing and further research in the area of regeneration and plasticity, similar to the important work of Dr. Kliot, may provide further insight into these poorly understood aspects of recovery.

References

1. Fisher G, Mansuy L. Total removal of intramedullary ependymomas: Follow-up study of 16 cases. *Surg Neurol.* 1980;14:243–249.
2. Garrido E, Stein BM. Microsurgical removal of intramedullary spinal cord tumors. *Surg Neurol.* 1977;7:215–219.
3. Greenwood J. Total removal of intramedullary tumors. *J Neurosurg.* 1954;11:616–624.
4. Greenwood J. Intramedullary tumors of the spinal cord. A follow-up study after total surgical removal. *J Neurosurg.* 1963;20:665–668.
5. Guidetti B. Intramedullary tumours of the spinal cord. *Acta Neurochir.* 1967;17:7–23.
6. Malis LI. Intramedullary spinal cord tumors. *Clin Neurosurg.* 1978;25:512–539.
7. Mork SJ, Loken AC. Ependymoma. A follow-up study of 101 cases. *Cancer.* 1977;40:907–915.
8. Post KD, Stein BM. Surgical management of spinal cord tumors and arteriovenous malformations. In: Schmidek HH, Sweet WH, eds. *Operative Neurosurgical Techniques.* vol 2. New York: Grune and Stratton; 1987:1487–1507.
9. Rawlings CE, Giangaspero F, Burger PC, et al. Ependymomas: A clinicopathologic study. *Surg Neurol.* 1988;29:271–281.
10. Sloof JL, Kernohan JW, MacCarthy CS. *Primary Intramedullary Tumors of the Spinal Cord and Filum Terminale.* New York: W B Saunders; 1964.
11. Stein BM. Surgery of intramedullary spinal cord tumors. *Clin Neurosurg.* 1979;26:529–542.

Discussion

Mechanisms of Spinal Cord Recovery

Dr. Kliot asked how is it possible to sort out the mechanisms causing spinal cord dysfunction and relate them to the potential for recovery of clinical neurological function. There is certainly no question about the size of the tumors compressing the neural tissues of the spinal cord and yet considerable function is preserved. Are there ways of determining what kind of reorganization has occurred preoperatively to maintain function and what has occurred postoperatively with the return of additional function? Are there ways we can assess how that is happening? Is it remyelination? There is experimental evidence showing that as the nerve fibers are compressed, conduction slows and as remyelination progresses conduction velocities change in very characteristic ways. Are there ways clinically or physiologically that we can get at these mechanisms?

Dr. McCormick responded that our ability to test the spinal cord still is limited to three tracts. We know little about the function of the remaining tracts. We have only scanty information about the interneurons. Based on what we do know and from what can be added by electrophysiologic transcranial magnetic stimulation of the motor pathways, it may be possible to quantify or to qualify to what extent function is preserved and the degree of recovery taking place. The same holds true for the somatosensory evoked potentials (SSEPs) that may be indicative of functional improvement, but cannot at present determine whether the phenomenon is reorganization, remyelination, or simply relief of neurogenic ischemia by relieving the compressive effect. Could it be both phenomena or all three working together?

Dr. Kliot responded that in the laboratory setting Steve Waxman and his group have shown beautifully that during compressive lesion you get demyelination with the redistribution of the sodium and calcium channels. When you remove the compressive forces, before you get remyelination axons fail at a certain rate. There are characteristic changes and then remyelination occurs, but the internodal lengths are not the same so I wonder if physiologists could tell us that if we study the three major spinal pathways over the timespan of demyelination and remyelination we might come to understand these mechanisms better.

Dr. Schlesinger added that when you look back at what is known taking a simpler model, such as the peripheral nerve, neurologists who had not had experience in the field would say shocking things when they saw a patient with an ulnar nerve injury decompressed with restoration of function within hours that the patient must have been hysterical. Anyone who has dealt with war injuries, which is where one sees the majority of peripheral nerve injuries, knows full well that there is a point at which there is sufficient pressure on a nerve to diminish its blood supply and suppress conduction, just as in Allen's experiments on the spinal cord. It does not necessarily entail remyelination or regeneration. The same is true for the patient who is paraparetic with a spinal meningioma and begins to move her legs in the next few days after surgery and regains control of her bladder and the ability to ambulate. Events occurring in that time frame, which all neurosurgeons have experienced, do not reflect remyelination. The biggest factor is restoration of blood supply permitting the return of nerve conduction.

Dr. Kliot asked what then about improvement over a 6-month period of time?

Dr. Schlesinger responded that now we are talking about a different phenomenon about which most of our discussion is speculative. As I emphasized before, the early recoveries from extramedullary spinal compressive lesions are more easily explained. Late recoveries are the subject of your speculation.

Factors Surrounding Patients with Repeat Surgery and Radiotherapy

Dr. Oldfield asked what about the experience with patients who have had repeat surgery or prior radiation therapy? Were they among the group of patients with incomplete excision of ependymomas? What were the outcomes in those seven patients who had had prior radiotherapy and then surgery?

Dr. McCormick responded: the literature points out that reoperations or operations after radiation therapy to the spinal cord or tumor bed are more difficult. Scarring and gliotic changes are present and the tumor planes are more difficult to establish. Our experience is that the risks of surgery are greater and the likelihood of reducing the patients' neurological deficits is less in those patients.

There were a number of patients who came to us who had been previously radiated. This does not imply that there was no effect from the radiotherapy. I clearly believe that radiation does have a positive effect on these tumors and the literature supports that. We are seeing a select group of patients who ultimately failed radiation therapy. I believe there were two such patients in whom we were unable to achieve a gross total removal. One, because the tumor had invaded the bones and we performed a conservative operation in view of the extensiveness of the tumor and she did not get worse postoperatively. The other patient had cephalad progression of the tumor within the spinal cord with worsening neurological status. We opened the spinal cord on more than one occasion and removed obvious tumor, but it continued to progress.

That left us with a number of other patients who had had previous radiation therapy. These patients had recurrences within a short period of time. Their surgery took more time than usual because of the scarring present. The tumor planes were obscured particularly on the ventral and inferior surfaces of the tumor.

We did not observe a specific increase in postoperative deficits in those patients of whom there were only four as compared to the rest of the group. Would we be surprised if 5 or 8 years from now one or two of those recurred because we were unable to clearly delineate the tumor plane? I think the answer is no. It could happen and we have observed in some series that there are recurrences after the surgeon has stated that the tumor was completely removed. There simply are times when it is difficult for a surgeon to be completely certain. One may say that there has been a gross total removal, but then you have to live with the possibility that 10 years later the tumor may recur.

I do not think that it increased our risk in this small group of patients with a short time to recurrence and we acknowledge that in some of the patients we did not attempt to achieve a gross total removal.

Spinal Cavernous Angiomas

Dr. Oldfield asked have you seen any cavernous angiomas of the spinal cord and did you perform angiography on them?

Dr. McCormick responded that they had seen two and, as we have experienced with those intracranially, the angiograms were normal.

Somatosensory Evoked Potentials and Use of Ultrasound

Dr. Oldfield asked if the feeling was that somatosensory evoked potentials (SSEPs) were useful. Dr. McCormick said he did not believe in their usefulness in terms of predicting the outcome after tumor removal. Dr. Oldfield said, I have come to the same conclusion.

Dr. Oldfield asked if the cord expansion seen in relation to hemangioblastomas was edema or syrinxes. We think those are syrinxes—you apparently believe that they represent edema. Have you examined any of these with ultrasound?

Dr. McCormick responded that ultrasound has not been used diagnostically by us, but we cannot exclude the possibility that they are multicompartmental cysts. However, we believe that these changes represent permeability changes. We have not proved it by testing for erythropoietin or other vascular permeability factors that Dr. Jeffrey Bruce has worked with. The MRI appearances have been more consistent with edema than with cysts. We did not open the spinal cord over these areas and they resolved postoperatively. We felt that they represented edema but could not completely exclude first stage cyst or syrinx formation.

Dr. Antunes added, I think in regard to the hemangioblastoma that that is correct. Some of them are clearly cysts. Some of them come to the surface and you can actually visualize the cysts.

Ependymomas of the Conus Medullaris versus the Filum Terminale

Dr. McCormick said that this study did not include filum terminale tumors that were wrapped in the roots of the cauda equina. Dr. Antunes stressed that the filum tumors are biologically different from those of the conus and that Dr. Schlesinger could attest to the fact that subtotal removal of a filum tumor was not infrequently associated with a 20- or 30-year functional survival, whereas you had recurrences in all within 16 months. Dr. McCormick said, yes they are different. Those of the filum are myxopapillary. We have no way of knowing how long they have existed before they become symptomatic by causing root compression. Dr. Antunes agreed and suggested that in part it may reflect the widening of the vertebral canal as a consequence of bony erosion because they have existed for so many years. Dr. McCormick continued that the problem must be viewed from another perspective. If you leaf through the radiologic literature from 1978 through 1986 there are at least a dozen studies that say do not aggressively resect these tumors because they are benign and radiosensitive and you can get long-term survivals.

That is not true because in our experience it is clearly better when you get a gross total resection of the tumor. There are reasons why a surgeon should not attempt gross total removal in certain cases and we have discussed those.

Dr. Antunes continued, the point I wished to make is that the filum terminale tumors usually do better and in many of them technical problems make it impossible to achieve a gross total removal. Since I returned to Portugal I have operated on at least three in which tumor was growing out of the neural foramina at several levels. Where you might be able to remove the tumor from within the vertebral canal working extraspinally or with nerve roots densely adherent to the tumor you may have to accept a subtotal resection. Despite this, the functional recoveries may be excellent.

Dr. Antunes added that another interesting point regarding the cysts associated with ependymomas is that they are mostly rostral to the tumor as if the tumor is plugging the central canal. In fact, you almost can see the central canal, which is quite wide and as you remove the tumor there is a funnel-shaped appearance of the canal. My concern is that in the tumor removals we are shedding cells into the central and yet as was indicated there are patients with no recurrence, which is very interesting.

Finally, concerning the subject of ectopic ependymomas, embryologically one can conceive of how they might occur. I recently had an instance of an ependymoma in the sacrum, extradurally located, and causing bony erosion. The tumor was posterior and the possibility exists that ependymal rest cells exist outside the dura.

Glial Proliferation and Remyelination

Dr. Friedman said, let me summarize some of the thoughts why loss of neurological function occurs with spinal cord tumors and mass lesions. To begin with, if you can envision the myelin sheath and its 40 lamellae surrounding an axon it must be stressed that that is not a static or dead structure such as keratin or hair. When myelin sheath proteins have been labeled there is a documented turnover in this membrane even in the 40th layer, which is tightly applied against the axon. There is a turnover of proteins and probably the paranodal loops of myelin, which are non-compacted, play some part in housing metabolic machinery whether it is mitochondria or ribosomes, which are responsible for churning out the new proteins that probably have a half-life of days and some of them weeks.

It has been estimated that in the adult, approximately 0.03% of our myelin is turned over every day. That is a phenomenal amount of work for the oligodendrocytes to perform. So, with pressure effects on the myelin sheaths such as occurs with tumors, one can imagine that a "preferential differential" may make it difficult for the normal myelin metabolism to function. Exactly how that "preferential differential" may interfere with the transport of new proteins along the myelin sheath is unclear.

In terms of the breakdown of the blood–brain barrier here we have looked at cavernous malformations of the spinal cord. There is evidence of hemorrhage, with hemosiderin deposits and proteases released from lysosomes. Myelin is 30% protein and the myelin basic protein is essential to the structure of myelin sheaths. The proteases released by a small hemorrhage can locally cause an extreme degree of demyelination. Once that occurs one can see not only conduction delay, but conduction block. We all are aware of the effect on neurological function that patchy and incomplete areas of demyelination in multiple sclerosis can have.

Calcium metabolism is thought to be intimately involved with the disruption of function and demyelination as a consequence of axonal injury. If it were just pressure, any impairment in fast transport in the axon will result in the release of calcium from the axon. This causes extensive destruction to the myelin, which is extremely sensitive to calcium.

Another point worth mentioning is the role of Schwann cells in remyelination. For instance, local damage to the spinal cord has been shown in animal models of CSF barbotage or injury due to dropping weights on the exposed spinal cord to bring about disruption of myelin. One observation is that Schwann cells run in from the dorsal roots and locally remyelinate. Now, admittedly they do not migrate very far and they cannot accomplish much myelination, but they do accomplish local remyelination in the region of the dorsal root entry zone and their myelin is different from normal myelin. It is possible that there may be Schwann cell remyelination after pressure injury from a tumor to a greater extent than has been previously realized. Schwann cells create a peripheral basal lamina when they remyelinate that is totally different from that occurring in the central nervous system. In fact, their lamina production has been shown to have different effects than the lamina production of the central nervous system. Perhaps this is playing a role in some of the pathological processes that occur in the CNS.

Last, I think we have to look at animal models. These problems will not be solved by our subjective appreciation of who improves and who walks better, but by return to the laboratory setting in which we carefully create models of spinal cord trauma, vascular injury, and tumors and then look at the actual effects of the axons. This work is going to be done by physiologists and biochemists and has to go hand-in-hand with our clinical assessments.

Questions Regarding the Topographic Classification of Intramedullary Tumors

Dr. Lazorthes mentioned that the speaker proposed a terminology for the topographic classification of intramedullary tumors based on the spine and not on the spinal cord. I think this classification is not good because there is tumor inside the spinal cord, which includes lumbar and sacral segments as well as cervical and cervicothoracic. I know that the spinal cord ends at D-12–L-1 level and thereafter there is cauda equina. I do not believe this is an accurate classification for intramedullary tumors.

Dr. McCormick responded: I understand what you are suggesting Dr. Lazorthes. I did not classify the tumors according to any variable that I was going to look at. It was purely an anatomical reference point choosing the spinal vertebrae rather than the spinal segments. I do not think there is any difference in terms of tumor growth potential or recovery whether the tumors occur in the cervical or cervicothoracic regions. Clearly there are different clinical syndromes. I think it helps the surgeons to think about the location when referring to the vertebral segments. To reiterate, we had 10 cervical and 7 cervicothoracic tumors and the classification was created purely for anatomical reference. I do not think it makes sense to classify tumors within the spinal cord according to spinal segments other than to say intramedullary versus extramedullary.

Dr. Holtzman added: perhaps Dr. Lazorthes is thinking about the blood supply to a given tumor in a given segment of the spinal cord and the importance of that blood supply either to tumor growth or in the surgical management of these lesions.

Dr. Lazorthes concurred.

CHAPTER 12

Electrical Stimulation and Microsurgery of the Spinal Cord

Arcady V. Livshits

All-Union Center of Spinal Cord Neurosurgery and Electrostimulation of Organs

Spinal shock is one of the most demonstrative functional disturbances in the activity of the spinal cord in an acute period. Accurate electrophysiological diagnosis made it possible not only to control the development of spinal shock, but the dynamics of withdrawal from it as well, although pathophysiological mechanisms of this complex process remain obscure.

To accelerate the reversal of spinal shock, we have suggested the technique of radiofrequency electrical stimulation of the spinal cord in an acute period of trauma, as the pulse current exerts trigger and trophic effects on the nerve tissue.

With this purpose in view we open the vertebral canal and dura mater in the injured area of the spinal cord and stitch two to four platinum plate electrodes, connected to a radiofrequency receiver, implanted under the skin or thoracic muscles, to the internal surface of the dura mater above or below the injured zone (on the anterior and posterior surfaces of the spinal cord). The radiofrequency generator, tuned to resonate with the receiver, emits signals received by an implanted receiver, which are detected at 20 Hz, 0.5 msec, and subthreshold force, and are transmitted to the cord structures (Fig. 12.1).

The appearance of the formerly absent reflex activity of the spinal cord, registered many times during the whole period of the spinal shock by analyzing H-reflex, coupled stimuli, evoked potentials (EP), and audio-spinal effect, was the criterion for the withdrawal from spinal shock (Fig. 12.2).

It has been established that an early subthreshold electrostimulation of the spinal cord is able to activate functionally inhibited spinal structures as a result of an injury and located close to the injured zone, by withdrawing them from the state of inhibition. This in turn reduced the duration of the spinal shock, caused by major trauma, to 7 to 14 days (Fig. 12.3, 12.4).

Experimental morphological studies of the spinal cord in dogs with hemisection of the spinal cord and its electrostimulation, conducted for 3 years, revealed the hypertrophy of intact motoneurons and spinal conduction tract in the zone of electrostimulation, the formation of a sprouting

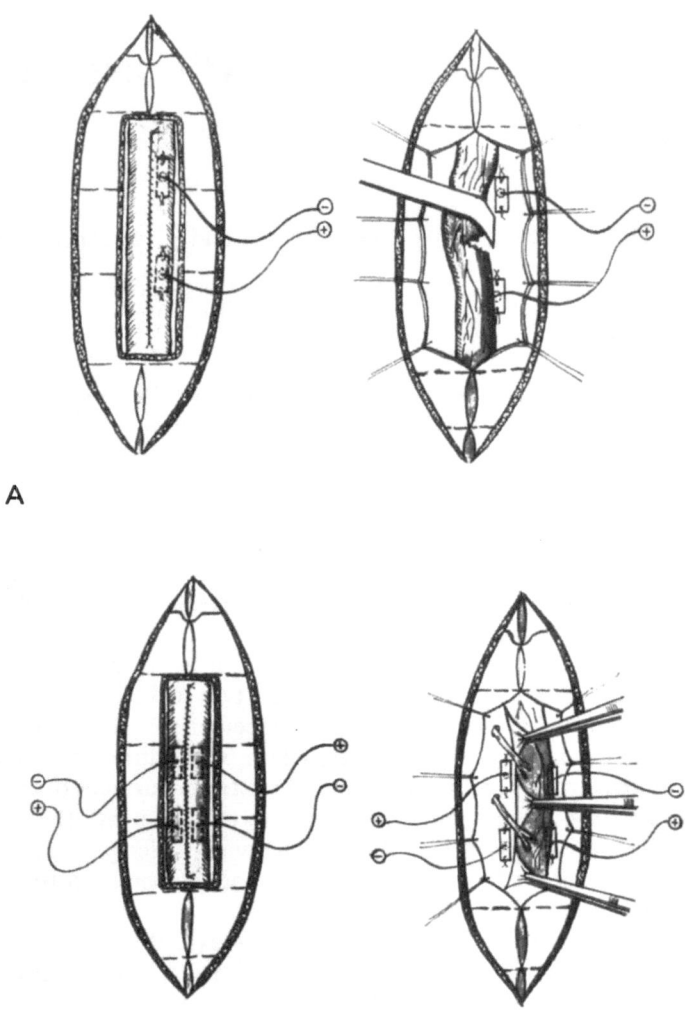

A

B

Figure 12.1. The scheme of electrostimulation of the spinal cord in an acute period of trauma. **A**, Two electrodes. **B**, Four electrodes.

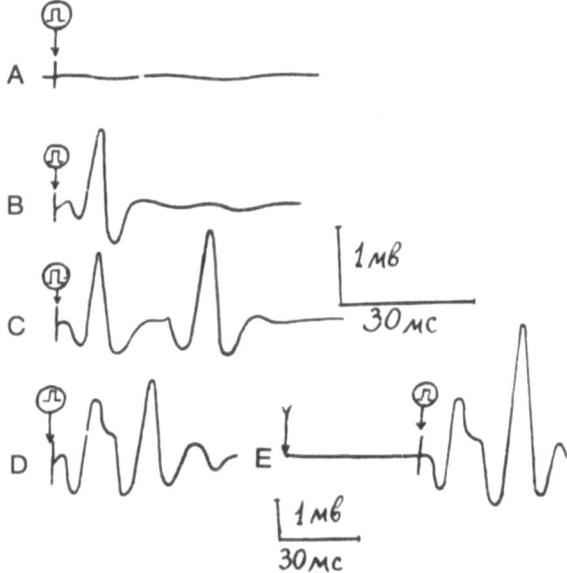

Figure 12.2. Audiospinal reflex in patients. **A–D**, The appearance of response, which was absent before. **E**, One year after electrostimulation.

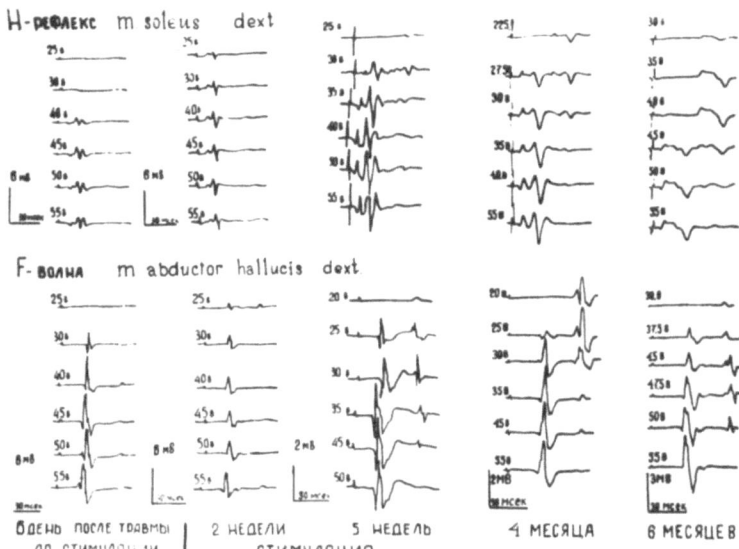

Figure 12.3. Electrophysiological investigations in the early period of trauma before and after electrostimulation.

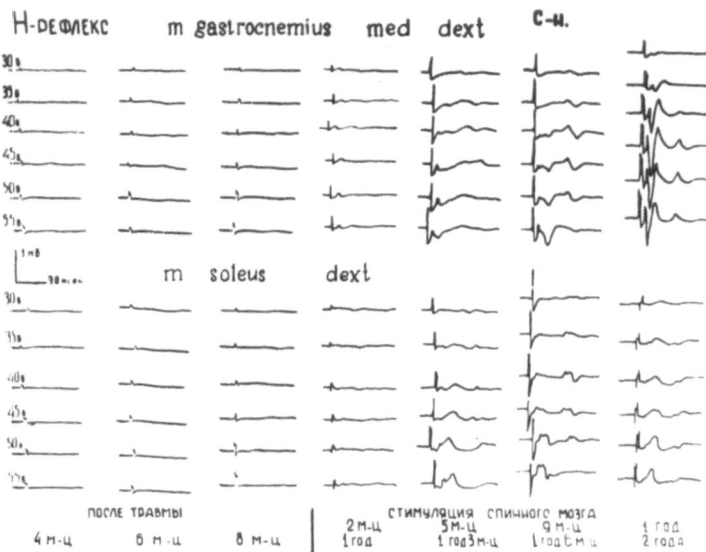

Figure 12.4. Electrophysiological investigations in the late period of trauma before and after electrostimulation.

effect, which was manifested clinically in the activation of motor visceral functions (Fig. 12.5).

A peculiarity of the late period of spinal trauma is the emergence of a number of pathologic syndromes that require functional neurosurgical interference to correct the impaired functions. Among them are algesic, spastic, and adhesive syndromes and dysfunctions of pelvic organs.

The problem of eliminating the algesic syndrome is extremely difficult; apparently it cannot be solved by one or two methods as it is dependent on many factors; among them are ethiopathogenetic, morphofunctional, psychological, and so forth.

The difficulties of this problem spring from the absence of objective criteria in diagnosing pain. Until now we attempt an objective diagnosis of pain by registering EPs (evoked potentials) in response to nociceptive stimulation.[1]

We have described similar EPs with electrical stimulation of the forearm skin and registered the inhibition of these EPs under effective percu-

Figure 12.5. Experimental morphological investigations. **A,** Hemisection of the spinal cord without electrostimulation. **B,** Hemisection of the spinal cord after electrostimulation. **C,** Hypertrophy of motoneuron with electrostimulation. **D,** Atrophy of the spinal cord in the zone of trauma. **E,** Sprouting effect in the zone near the trauma with electrostimulation.

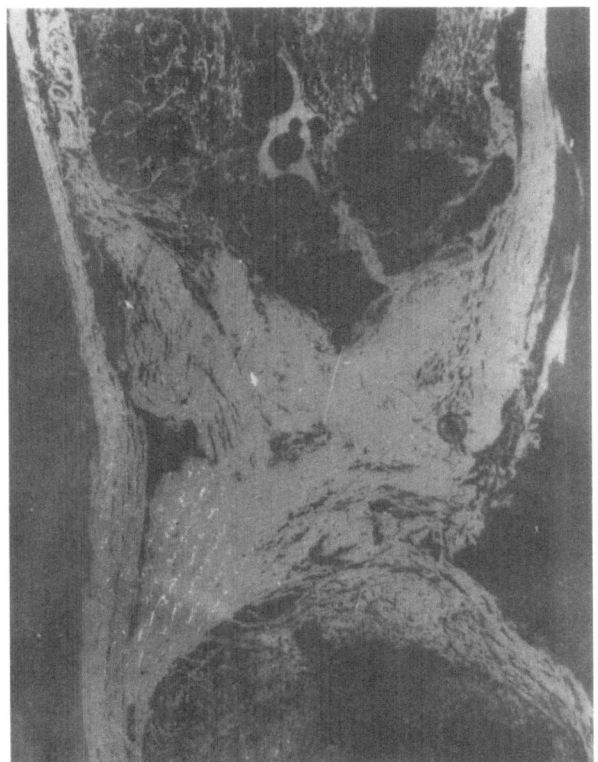

A

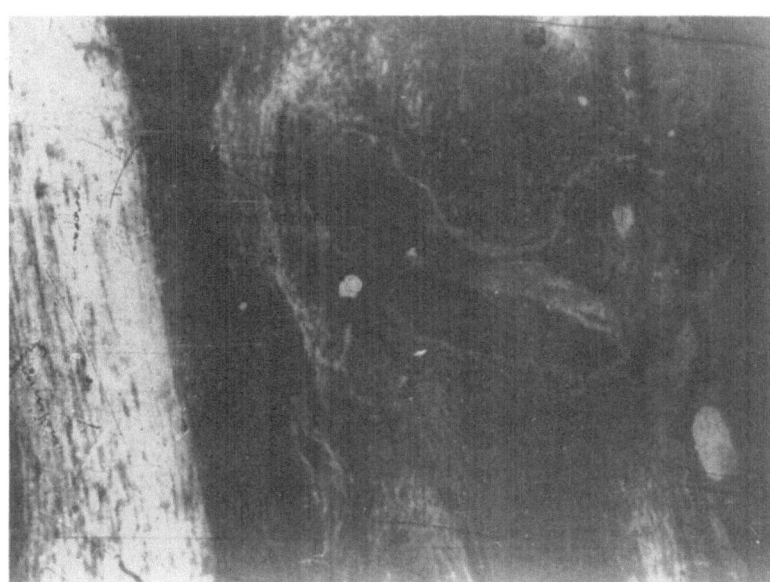

B

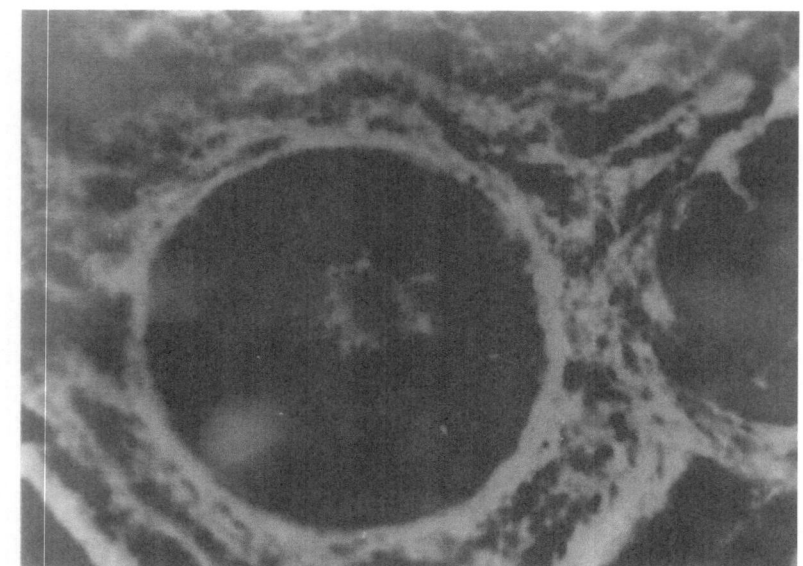

C

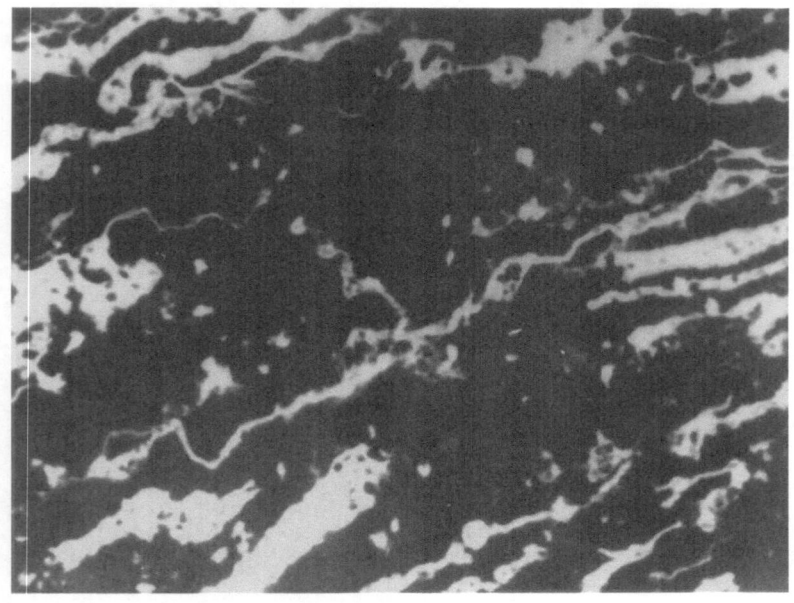

D

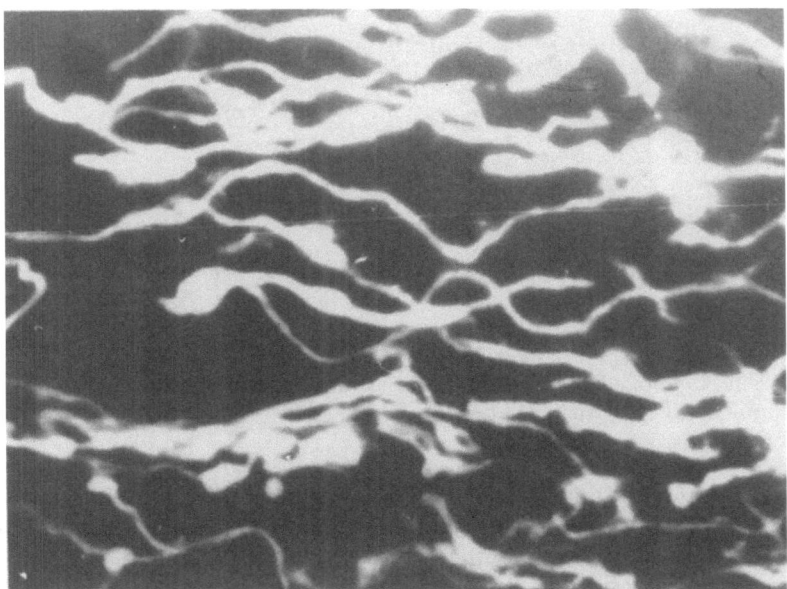

E

taneous analgesic electrical stimulation. We made an attempt to use EPs to evaluate not only acute algesic attacks, but to evaluate prolonged algesic syndromes and the effect of analgesic electrical stimulation on the posterior spinal columns. Before the employment of analgesic electrical stimulation of posterior columns with a pronounced algesic syndrome, the somatosensory cortex, in response to electrical skin stimulation, revealed high amplitude (15 μv) slow positive oscillation with a latent peak period of 220 msec mainly in point C-0, whereas it was virtually absent in point C-3 (Fig. 12.6).

A sharp reduction of this potential (to 5 μv) has been registered after analgesic electrical stimulation when pain virtually disappeared. Pain appeared after a temporary termination of the analgesic electrical stimulation and, at the same time, positive oscillation in point C-0 with a peak latent period of 220 msec and the amplitude of 14 μv appeared with the registration of somatosensory EPs.

A clearly pronounced high amplitude (12–15 μv) positive oscillation with a latent period peak of 240 msec preserved in case of ineffective analgesic electrical stimulation of posterior columns.

In our series a slow potential, related to algesic afferentation, reached its maximum values not in the somatosensory zone of the cortex (which corresponds to point C-3) but in point C-0, which corresponds to the vertex zone, and which, according to modern concepts, is the projection zone to the cortex of big hemispheres of nonspecific structures.

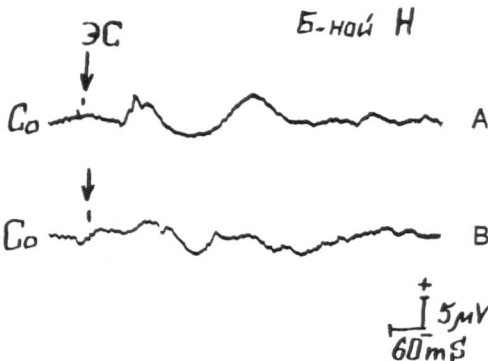

Figure 12.6. Evoked potentials by pain syndrome. Registration of P_{240} by pain syndrome (**A**) before and (**B**) after.

We assume that this potential is not a component of the somatosensory EP but is related to the projection to the cortex of the cerebral hemispheres of nonspecific structures.

We may now assume that the inhibition of the somatosensory EP P_{240} component by analgesic electrical stimulation may point to the relation of this component to the algesic syndrome.

The anteroposterior commissurotomy developed by Greenfeld and performed for the first time by Donald Armur in 1926 is known to be the most effective operation against an algesic syndrome.

This operation, performed on 28 patients in cervical and thoracic areas, was effective in 88.6% of cases. Neurological "losses" are insignificant.

Histology of the spinal cord of the patient subjected to commissurotomy has revealed that it leads to a bilateral ascending degeneration of the spinothalamic tract. Posterior spinal columns are sometimes damaged during commissurotomy. The possibility of injuring the pyramidal path of the lateral column is almost impossible. Histopathologic changes in the spinal cord are not fully reflected in the clinical picture, which points to a high level of plasticity of the nervous system.

The spastic syndrome is another rather frequent complication of the spinal trauma. The treatment of spastic phenomena in patients with a spinal injury represents a difficult problem that has not yet been completely solved. The literature devoted to this problem highlights the search for the most effective techniques of surgery and conservative treatment of spasticity.

Lateral longitudinal frontal myelotomy in L-1–S-1 segments worked out by Bischoff in 1951 was the first attempt to implement selective interference for interrupting reflex arcs of segmental reflexes within the spinal cord. Later this operation has been modified by Pourpre et al. The effectiveness of antispastic operations, performed by national neurosurgeons, was studied in 93 patients. Good results in our series were obtained in 57.7%, satisfactory in 23.1%, and unsatisfactory in 19.2% of patients.

The use of lateral accesses resulted in complete areflexia and atony. We consider that lateral accesses should be performed only in patients with a complete transection of the spinal cord verified during previous operations and subsequent functional studies. The dorsal access alone should be used in cases of spastic paraparesis with intact motor function, as it allows preservation of lateral corticospinal tracts and residual motor function.

The commissural process leading to subarachnoid space block often forms in the late period of the spinal trauma, after operations in an acute period. We have chosen an active tactic by performing a repeated operation—meningomyeloradiculolysis, irrespective of the period that elapsed since the first operation. The employment of microsurgery to prevent the spinal cord, spinal roots, and membranes from adhesions and the reestablishment of circulation with the subsequent plasty of the dural sac to enlarge the subdural space promote the improvement of segmental and conduction functions of the spinal cord in 72% of cases. This conclusion was drawn from 115 operations, performed in patients with various injuries of the spinal cord, 1 to 10 years after the first operation. A contraindication for this operation is the finding of the complete transection of the spinal cord in combination with old age of the patient and cardiovascular and hepatorenal decompensation.

Complete transection of the spinal cord in young people with a formed block of the subarachnoid space is not a contraindication for an operation, as the liberation of distal and proximal spinal sections from adhesions and cicatrices promotes the improvement of segmental spinal functions, which is important for initiating restorative processes.

Another important problem of spinal trauma consequences is the dysfunction of pelvic organs and mostly of the urinary bladder.

The development of microneurosurgery and radioelectronics enabled us to promote a coordinated voluntary controlled act of urination, although the reduction of resistance of the cervical–sphincter system of the urinary bladder and the enhancement of the influence of the ways of voluntary innervation of the urinary bladder still pose a big problem (Fig. 12.7A).

A study of the effect of radiofrequency electrical stimulation in 50 patients and 15 years of observations showed the possibility of the complete evacuation of the urinary bladder with flaccid lower paraplegia and intact electrical excitability of the detrusor (Fig. 12.7B). In other cases we had a problem with the resistance of the urinary bladder sphincter system, its cervix, and musculus perinei. This problem has been solved by blocking n.n. pudendi or their resection and transurethral electroresection of the urinary bladder, cervix, or its sphincters. Electrostimulation of the detrusor promoted, as an additional effect, the enhancement of the motor function of the intestine and also activated the spinal memory, which faded in the process of evolution, and this boosted the development of urination

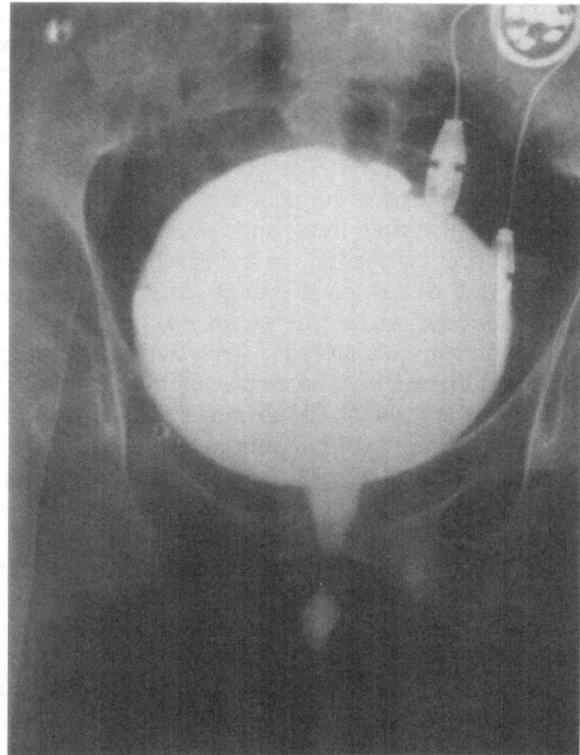

Figure 12.7. A, The cystogram before the bladder electrostimulation.

reflex in an appropriate time. This ability of spinal neurons to preserve, for a definite period, the traces of stimulations in the spinal memory promoted the development of temporary parameters of urination suitable for life. Ileocystoplasty is used with an injury of the thoracolumbar section of the spinal cord and secondary sclerosis of the urinary bladder, caused by a prolonged use of the drain. We have performed 25 operations with a follow-up period of up to 18 years (Fig. 12.8).

A section of the small intestine, innervated above the spinal injury zone, on the vascular–nervous limb, is transferred to the small pelvis and is anastomosed with the residual tissue of the urinary bladder or with the urethra, providing there is no tissue, and ureters are stitched to it. Wire electrodes are implanted for a direct electrostimulation of the transplant, preventing its dilation. A marked urge to urinate as well as the feeling that the bladder is full, are formed 2 to 3 months after the functioning of the artificial urinary bladder, although baroreception is not envisaged by nature for the small intestine. However, this operation has no future as the proper

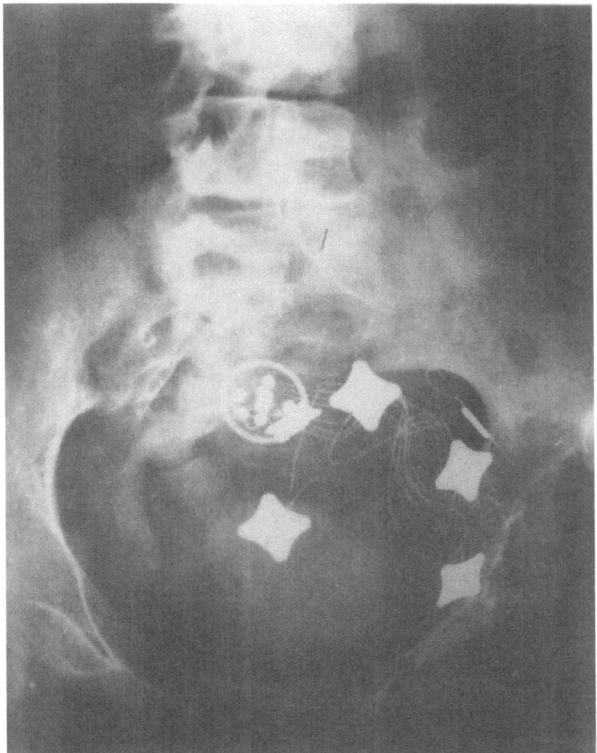

Figure 12.7. B, The cystogram 5 minutes after the bladder electrostimulation.

organization of treatment may prevent the development of the secondary sclerosis of the urinary bladder. The task of the comprehensive innervation of the urinary bladder has not been fully solved in creating a coordinated act of urination. Back in 1908 N.N. Burdenko pioneered and began to study experimentally the possibility of paving a new innervation path for the urinary bladder by surgery, creating anastomoses between spinal roots above and below the injury zone.

Carlsson and Sundin (1967) suggested the creation of anastomoses with an injury of the spinal cord at L-1 level between the abovelying T-12 roots and S-2–S-3 to pave a new innervation path for the urinary bladder.

During the last 2 years we also studied the problem of reinnervation of the urinary bladder by creating anastomoses between T-11–12 and S-2–4, by employing microneurosurgery and a surgical microscope.

We have performed 26 operations of laminectomy, meningomyelora-diculolysis, neurolysis of T-11 and T-12 intercostal nerves, and created anastomosis between them and S-2 and S-4 roots, identified by a urological

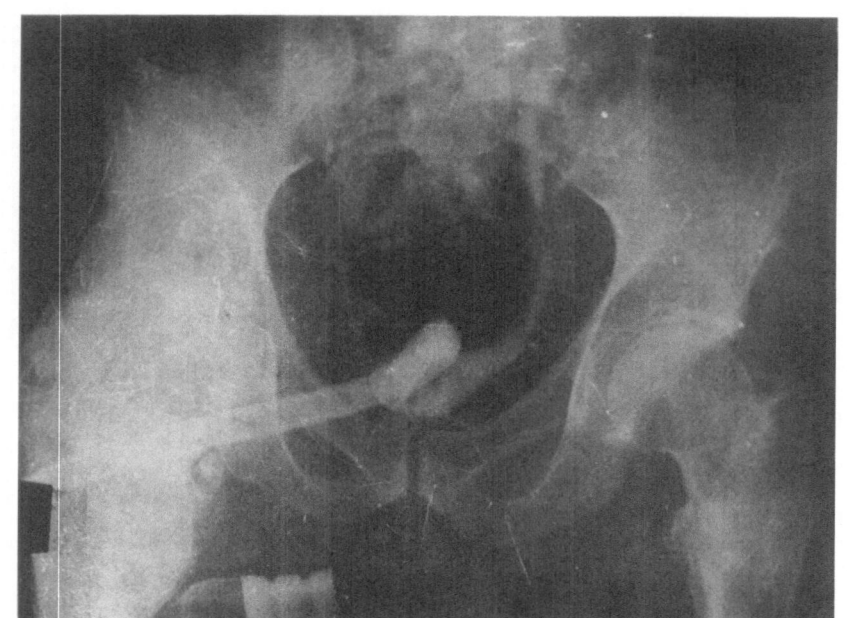

A

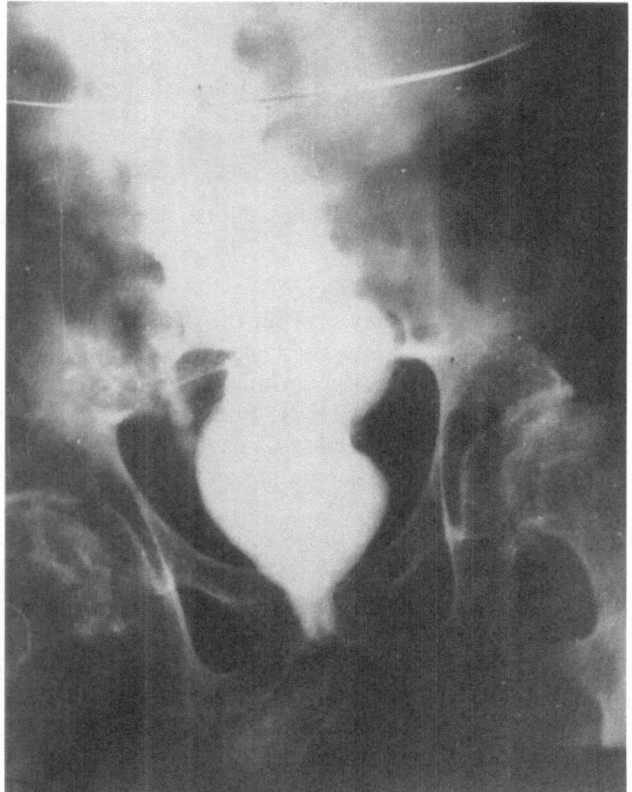

B

272

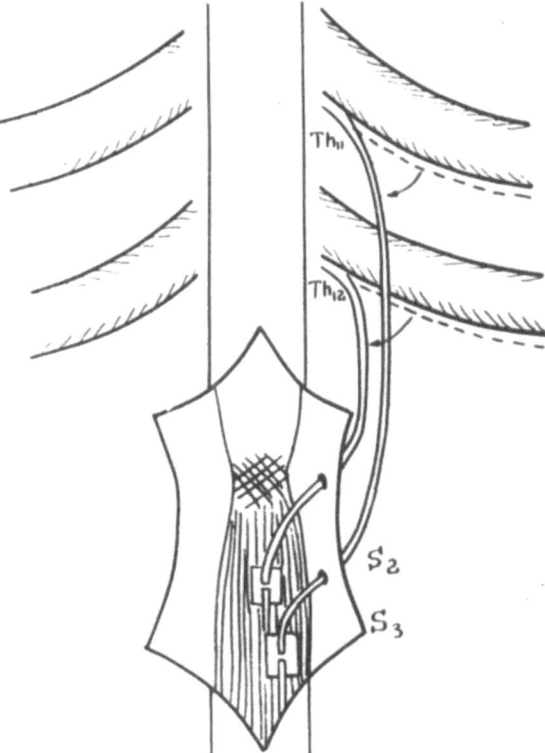

Figure 12.9. The bladder reinnervation: anastomosis between the intercostal nerve and S-2 root.

computer. (Fig. 12.9) There is a certain improvement in the function of the urinary bladder; however, the complexity of innervation mechanisms in regulating urination does not allow one to draw conclusions. The best results were received in groups with areflexic and hyporeflexic bladders. The effect is good in 75% to 80% of cases.

It should be underlined in conclusion that modern achievements in microsurgery, electronics, and operative optics allowed for the development of active surgery in acute and late periods of spinal trauma, for the improvement of the techniques of functional neurosurgery which, in its turn, promoted progress in the recovery of the impaired functions of the spinal cord.

◁—————————————————————————

Figure 12.8. A, The cystogram (microcysticus). **B**, X ray of artificial bladder (enterocystoplasty).

Reference

Carlsson CA, Sundin T. Reconstruction of efferent pathways to the urinary bladder in a paraplegic child. *Rev Surg.* 1967;34:73–76.

Discussion

Aspects of Technique

Dr. Hecht-Nielsen asked if the patient activates the switch or is the switch activated by a nurse or physician. Dr. Livshitz responded that the urine output is registered on a computer and regulates the impulses.

Intercostal nerves are transposed into the spinal canal connecting motor roots by microsurgical technique to sacral motor roots and then stimulation takes place by transcutaneous stimulation. Platinum plates are utilized. One of the big problems that we face is the antagonism, due to reciprocal innervation, between the detrussor and the urethral sphincters. Initially we may perform a nerve block for the pudendal nerve and may ultimately transect the pudendal nerve, which may lead to impotence in the male. If that is not successful we perform a transurethral resection of the neck of the bladder.

Timing of the Operation in Relation to Spinal Transection and Spinal Shock

Dr. Friedman asked how soon after transection are you performing these operations?

Dr. Livshitz said ideally the procedure should be done as soon as possible. Placing electrodes on the roots may lead to hypertrophy of the motor neurons and sprouting in the regions of myelopathy. In cases of total spinal transection surgical decompression is undertaken to prevent scar formation and to improve the environment as regards spinal vascular supply.

In some senses then success in the management of bladder dysfunction is attributed to the management of spinal shock with cold water irrigation and hyperbaric oxygenation. The earlier subthreshold electrical stimulation of the spinal centers begins, the better the outcome in our experience.

Dr. Kliot asked if the electrical stimulation was inducing growth of fibers, as is evidenced by sprouting, or is it improving recovery on a functional basis. Dr. Tator in Toronto has been performing electrical stimulation in spinal cord injury. His animals recover better when an alternating current of DC battery current is applied to the site of spinal injury in cases of incomplete injuries. They do not know whether this represents regeneration or reduction in the impact of the injury on surviving neurons. They just call it recovery.

Dr. Livshitz answered, I think that the mechanism of influence of electrical stimulation of the spinal cord in incomplete transections is compensative because of hypertrophy in the adjacent nontraumatized zones. In other words, there might be more utilization of surviving neurons in the areas surrounding the injury, which would not be the case if it were not for the electrical stimulation.

Dr. Hecht-Nielsen added there is certainly no question that one of the truisms of the nervous system is that you either use them or you lose them; neurons either work or they are not there any more.

Dr. Livshitz indicated that there was no evidence of neural atrophy in the region of stimulating electrodes when subthreshold stimuli are given. This was not the case with suprathreshold stimuli. We use 210 mamp with a frequency of 20 Hz and a duration of 0.5 msec.

Dr. Holtzman inquired about the dog who underwent hemisection of the spinal cord. Dr. Livshitz responded that electrical stimulation was begun the next day and the dog was able to stand within 1 month of the trauma. He pointed out that there was function in both lower extremities, and that the dog could stand and ambulate to a degree and was not spastic.

CHAPTER 13

Venous Congestion of the Spinal Cord: A Reversible Mechanism of Myelopathy

Edward H. Oldfield

Recent observations in patients with myelopathy associated with spinal dural arteriovenous (AV) fistulas, which drain intrathecally into the veins of the spinal cord, indicate that venous hypertension can produce myelopathy.[1-8] This clinical circumstance proves not only that venous congestion alone can produce myelopathy, but also indicates the type of clinical syndrome and the type of pathological injury that occurs to the cord with venous stagnation. It also calls for reevaluation of venous congestion as a more common mechanism of early and reversible cord injury in other conditions than has been generally recognized.

Venous congestion previously has been implicated as a mechanism of spinal cord injury in several neurological diseases affecting the spinal cord, including some of the more common ones. Brain in 1948, in an early discussion on the myelopathy of gradual cord compression by protruded discs and cervical spondylosis, suggested that venous congestion might be more important as the etiology of myelopathy than arterial insufficiency or mechanical distortion.[9] He wrote "No doubt the earliest changes produced by a protruding intervertebral disc are circulatory, and these must be important at all stages. The veins with their thin walls and pressure would naturally be compressed first and since the flow in them is upward, edema of the anterior and anterolateral region of the cord at the subsegments below the site of compression would cause symptoms related to these segments."

Evidence produced by John Doppman and his colleagues in the early 1970s, in experiments in subhuman primates designed to reproduce acute bony or tumorous impaction of the spinal cord, suggested that acute mass compression from the anterior aspect of the spinal canal produced loss of venous flow before arterial flow was compromised and before mechanical deformation occurred sufficient to account for the neurological deficits.[10-14]

For many years the Foix-Alajouanine syndrome was considered a syndrome of venous thrombosis of the spinal veins, and as such cord injury in this syndrome was considered irreversible. However, our recent experience indicates that, at least in the early phases of this clinical syndrome, myelopathy is produced by impairment of venous drainage, and not by venous thrombosis.[15] Therefore, in these patients recognition of venous congestion as a form of reversible myelopathy and implementation of early treatment to eliminate it can reverse cord dysfunction and prevent paraplegia.

However, venous hypertension generally has not been accepted as a mechanism of cord injury, as there has been no disease that clearly produced venous congestion of the spinal cord in which cord dysfunction could not also be attributed to arterial ischemia, hemorrhage, or mechanical deformation. Thus, explanations other than venous congestion were always possible, as no problem clearly was caused by venous congestion alone. In the past decade it has become apparent that the most common form of spinal arteriovenous malformation, the spinal dural AV fistula, elicits cord injury by draining arterial blood into the veins of the spinal cord and producing venous hypertension. Thus, dural AV fistulas with spinal venous drainage provide a clinical model of venous congestion and secondary cord injury.

Spinal Dural AV Fistulas

It is now generally recognized that there are two main types of arteriovenous malformations of the spine, dural arteriovenous fistulas, in which the nidus of the AV fistula is imbedded in the dural covering of the nerve root and the adjacent spinal dura, and intradural arteriovenous malformations (AVMs) of the spinal cord, AVMs in which the nidus of the AVM is either within the tissue of the spinal cord or is imbedded in the pia.[1–8] The intradural AVMs are further subclassified into juvenile and glomus lesions and direct AV fistulas (Table 13.1). However, this is a recent classification. For many years all spinal AVMs were considered to be intradural and to be comprised of an arteriovenous nidus in the spinal cord or the pia. Paradoxically, the initial concept of spinal AVMs was that most of them were venous in origin.

The first successful operation for a spinal AVM was performed in 1914 by Dr. Charles Elsberg. The clinical description of his patient and the operative findings are described in his text of 1916, *Surgical Diseases of the Spinal Cord*.[5] The patient suffered severe paraparesis and sensory loss to T-9. At surgery Elsberg interrupted a dilated posterior spinal vein as it entered the dura adjacent to the eighth thoracic nerve root and removed a 2-cm segment. The patient enjoyed complete neurological recovery within 3 months of the procedure.

The initial classifications of vascular lesions of the spinal cord were based on the pathology. In 1925, as a result of his review of the previously reported 19 patients and 2 patients of his own, Sargent concluded that most

Table 13.1. Spinal arteriovenous malformations.

Dural arteriovenous fistulas
Intradural arteriovenous malformations
  Juvenile AVMs
  Glomus AVMs
  Arteriovenous fistulas

spinal AVMs were comprised of abnormal veins.[16] In 1943 Wyburn-Mason, after reviewing 110 patients with spinal AVMs, concluded that there were two main types of spinal AVMs.[17] The most common type he described as a mass of turgid, blue, thin-walled veins on the cord surface. He designated this type "angioma racemosum venosum" in keeping with Virchow's original nomeclature of central nervous system (CNS) vascular anomalies.

With the introduction of spinal arteriography in the 1960s the vascular anatomy of these lesions could be seen for the first time in vivo. As a result, the classification of spinal AVMs changed from being based on pathology to being based on the vascular anatomy and pattern of blood flow as interpreted from arteriography. The result was a classification into three types of spinal AVMs: juvenile, glomus, and single-coiled vessel types. In the juvenile and glomus AVMs, which comprised only 15% to 20% of all spinal AVMs, the site of the AV fistula, the transition from arterial to venous elements, was obvious. The feeding vessel was always an enlarged medullary artery, which had the potential of also supplying the spinal cord. Since most of these were AVMs with rapid blood flow and as the arterial supply was from medullary arteries that also supplied the spinal cord, spinal ischemia as a result of vascular steal, hemorrhage by the AVM, and cord compression by the vessels of the AVM were the postulated mechanisms of cord injury.

In the most common type of spinal AVM, the single coiled vessel type, which comprised 80% to 85% of spinal AVMs, arteriography demonstrated a single, tightly coiled, continuous vessel on the cord surface with very slow flow, often requiring 16 to 20 seconds for clearance of the contrast. These were supplied by one, occasionally two, feeding vessels, which themselves did not provide blood supply to the spinal cord. The arterial to venous transition, the nidus of the AV fistula, was not clearly identified; many small communicating vessels between the dorsolateral arterial plexus and the single coiled vessel on the cord surface were considered likely shunting sites and the mechanism of cord injury was considered to be similar to that which produced myelopathy in the other types of spinal AVMs: that is, by vascular steal and ischemia or by cord compression. It was not until 1977 that Brian Kendall and Valentine Logue described nine patients in whom the site of the AV fistula was identified as the dura.[3] The patients were treated by excision of the dural AV fistula and most enjoyed considerable improvement.

Spinal dural AV fistulas injure the cord by passing arterial blood from a fistula in the dural covering of the nerve root and adjacent spinal dura into the venous system of the spinal cord. The dual AV fistula is supplied by a dural artery, an artery that does not also provide blood supply to the spinal cord, and the fistula is drained by a medullary vein, which carries blood from the dural AV fistula into the coronal venous plexus on the cord surface.[4,5] Since the only potential mechanism of cord injury in these patients is venous congestion, spinal dural AV fistulas provide a model of cord injury that is purely by increased venous pressure. The evidence for venous congestion as a mechanism of cord injury is reviewed below.

Spinal Vascular Anatomy

Evidence that the mechanism of cord injury with dural AV fistulas is venous congestion is based on the vascular anatomy of the spinal cord. Two markedly different systems supply blood to the spinal cord, an anterior and a posterior arterial network (Fig. 13.1). The anterior arterial chain, the anterior spinal artery, which supplies the anterior two thirds of the cord, including the corticospinal tracts, extends without interruption along the entire anterior surface of the spinal cord. The posterior spinal arteries are two plexiform interconnecting channels running along the posterior and lateral surfaces of the spinal cord. They perfuse the posterior one third of the spinal cord.

In the developing fetus medullary arteries supply the spinal cord at each segmental level. However, most of these regress before the sixth month of gestation, and only a limited number of the medullary arteries, which supply the anterior and posterior spinal arteries, remain. Persisting at each segmental level in the adult, however, are radicular arteries, which supply the nerve roots, and dural arteries, which supply the proximal nerve root sleeve and the adjacent spinal dura. Medullary arteries, radicular arteries, and dural arteries are all derived from the intervertebral segment of the spinal ramus of the posterior segmental arteries (Fig. 13.1), which, in turn, arise from the aorta and from the vertebral, subclavian, and iliac arteries at irregular intervals.[18] Spinal rami from the vertebral, subclavian, and aortic intercostals supply 6 to 10 anterior medullary arteries that inoscultate with the anterior spinal artery. Particularly important is the artery of Adam-

---

Figure 13.1. Normal arterial supply and venous drainage of the spinal cord. At each segmental level the spinal ramus of each intercostal artery divides, after entering the intervertebral foramen and penetrating the outer surface of the dura, into dural arteries, which provide arterial blood supply to the root sleeve and spinal

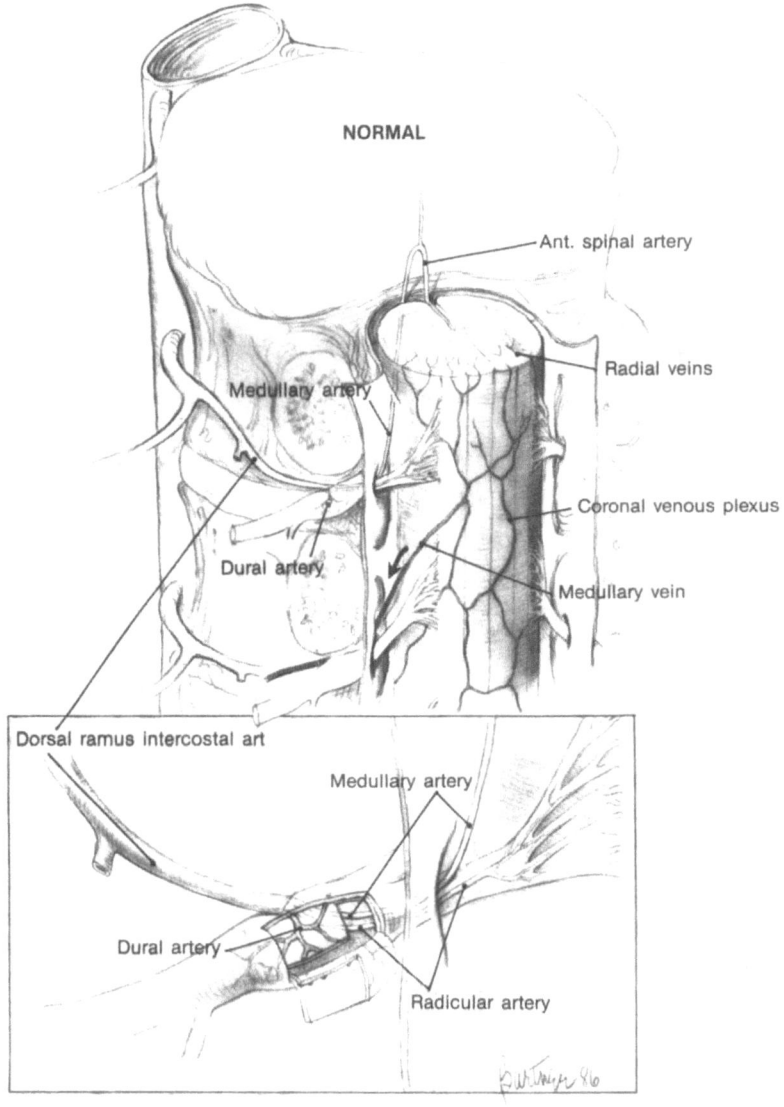

dura, and radicular arteries, which supply the anterior and posterior nerve roots. In addition, at some levels and in a sporadic manner, the spinal ramus of the intercostal artery also is the origin of a medullary artery, which enters the dura adjacent to the nerve root ganglion, ascends, and joins an anterior or posterolateral spinal artery to supply the spinal cord. The cord is drained by radial veins, which carry blood to the coronal venous plexus or longitudinal veins. These veins are drained by medullary veins which pierce the dura adjacent to the dural penetration of the nerve roots. (From Oldfield EH, Doppman JL. Spinal arteriovenous malformations. *Clin Neurosurg.* 1986;34:161–183. Reprinted with permission.)

kiewicz, a medullary artery that provides the anterior spinal artery with blood below the midportion of the spinal cord. This artery arises from an aortic intercostal between T-8 and L-4.

In the adult, therefore, at each segmental level the spinal ramus of each intercostal artery divides, after entering the intervertebral foramen and penetrating the outer leaflet of the dura, into dural arteries, which provide arterial blood to the root sleeve and spinal dura, and radicular arteries, which supply the anterior and posterior nerve roots. In addition, at some levels, and in a sporadic manner, the spinal ramus of an intercostal artery also is the origin of a medullary artery, which enters the dura adjacent to the nerve root ganglion, ascends, and joins the anterior or posterior spinal artery to supply the spinal cord (Fig. 13.1).

The spinal cord is initially drained by radial veins, which drain the blood centrifugally from the cord parenchyma to the surface where they empty into the coronal venous plexus, a plexiform venous network in the pia on the cord surface.[19] The venous blood passes from the intradural to the epidural veins via medullary veins. These traverse the subarachnoid space from the coronal venous plexus to the dura where they penetrate the dura adjacent to the dural entry of the nerve roots and join the intervertebral veins of the epidural venous plexus (Fig. 13.1). The medullary veins, like the medullary arteries, are not present at every segmental level but have an inconstant occurrence along the longitudinal axis of the spine. There are functional valves at the level of the dura, as substances within the epidural venous system do not reach the intradural venous system or the spinal cord. However, there are no valves in the intrathecal or intraparenchymal veins.

Selected Examples of Myelopathy by Venous Congestion: Spinal Dural AV Fistulas

Analysis of the following two patients demonstrates that venous congestion alone can produce myelopathy and that the myelopathy from venous stagnation is reversible if venous hypertension is eliminated. The first patient is typical of patients with spinal dural AV fistulas. He has been reported previously.[4,15]

Patient 1. A 56-year-old man developed urinary hesitancy and left leg weakness 5 months before admission. His condition was then stable until 2 weeks before admission when he developed progressive weakness in both legs. He could walk only a few feet with the aid of a cane; his perineum became numb and he developed urinary retention. He entered the hospital in a wheelchair with an indwelling bladder catheter.

Myelography revealed a long coiled filling defect in the subarachnoid space that extended from midthoracic to midlumbar levels. Selective spinal

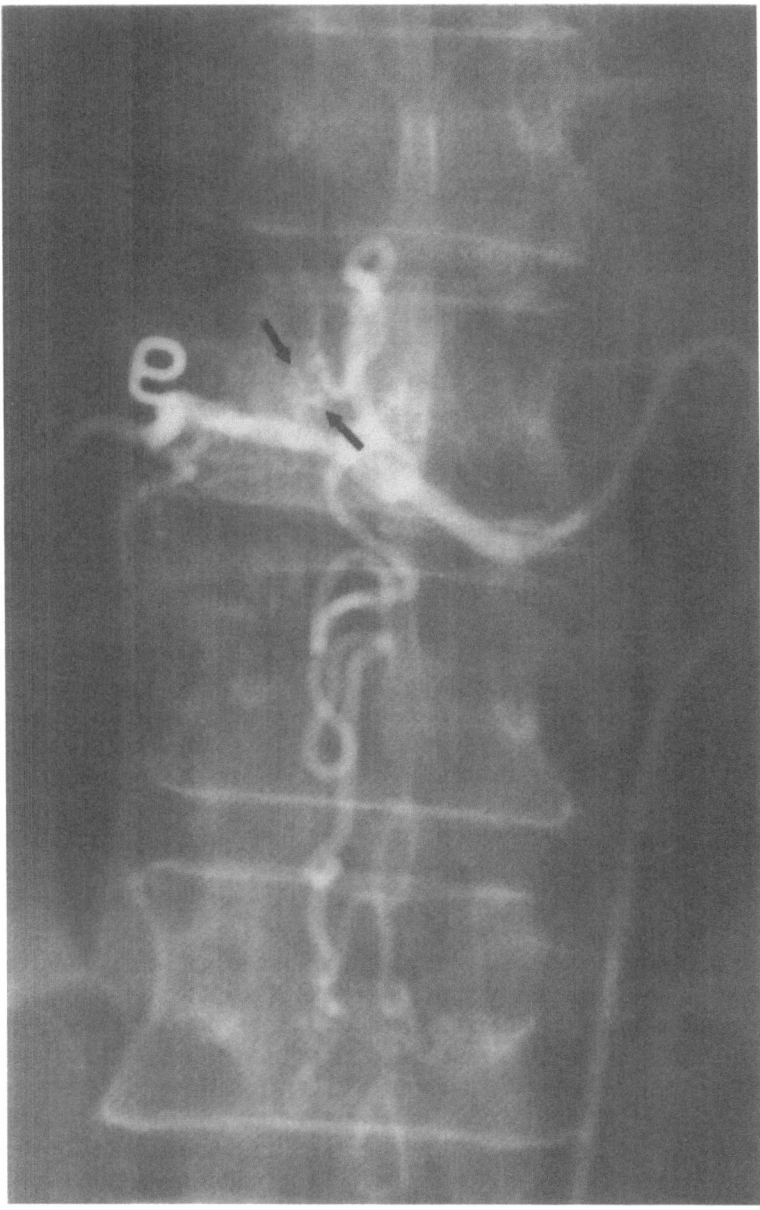

Figure 13.2. Selective spinal arteriogram of spinal dural AV fistula imbedded in the root sleeve of the ninth thoracic nerve root and the adjacent spinal dura. The nidus of spinal dural AV fistula is typically in the intervertebral foramen and the lateral aspect of the spinal canal and drains into the dilated, tortuous intradural veins on the cord surface. The artery of Adamkiewicz was supplied from the left ninth thoracic intercostal, which arose from a separate orifice of the aorta.

arteriography demonstrated a collection of fine vessels in the intervertebral foramen and the lateral aspect of the spinal canal at T9-10, the nidus of
a dural AV fistula, which was supplied by a single feeding vessel from the
right ninth thoracic intercostal (Fig. 13.2). Contrast flowed through the
fistula and intradurally, into a tightly coiled, continuous vessel on the cord
surface. The artery of Adamkiewicz arose from the left thoracic intercostal
at the same level. At surgery after removing the lamina of T-9 and T-10
and unroofing intervertebral foramen on the right at T9-10, the AV nidus
of abnormal-appearing small vessels was exposed imbedded in the dura of
the nerve root sleeve and the adjacent spinal dura. After opening the dura
a thin-walled arterialized vessel was found overlying the dorsal aspect of
the spinal cord. It entered the dura adjacent to, but slightly separate from,
the dural penetration of the right T-9 nerve root (as illustrated in Fig.
13.3). The dural nidus was obliterated with bipolar coagulation and the
vessel draining the dural AV fistula intradurally into the coronal venous
plexus was divided intradurally between ligatures.

After surgery the patient's neurological function improved daily. His
strength returned to normal within 2 weeks, the numbness resolved almost
completely, and he developed normal bladder function. Postoperative
selective spinal arteriography demonstrated no residual filling of the spinal
dural AV fistula.

Fig. 13.3 schematically shows the anatomy of spinal dural AV fistulas
and demonstrates the route of transmission of arterial blood to the spinal
venous system via retrograde flow in the medullary vein that occurs in
these patients. The dural branch of the intervertebral artery supplies the
dural AV fistula. Blood flowing through the dural AV fistula is carried
through the medullary vein, the solitary venous outflow of the dural AV
fistula, in a retrograde direction to the coronal venous plexus, which becomes dilated, tortuous, and elongated by the reception of arterial blood,
which is under higher flow and pressure than would normally occur in the
spinal venous system. Since there are no valves between the coronal
venous plexus and the radial veins that drain the spinal cord, the increased
venous pressure is transmitted directly to the cord and myelopathy results.
By interrupting the vessel that carries blood from the dural AV fistula to
the coronal venous plexus, venous hypertension is eliminated and the cord
recovers.

That the blood draining the AV fistula can cause an acquired transfigura-
tion of the coronal venous plexus by elongation, dilatation, and tortuosity
of its component vessels is demonstrated by a similar alteration in appearance by lesions that we know are acquired, such as spinal cord hemangioblastomas. Fig. 13.4 shows the spinal arteriogram of a patient with a hemangioblastoma in the midthoracic portion of the spinal cord. The rapid and
excessive blood flow through this tumor has caused the normal coronal
venous plexus to become transfigured so that its appearance is similar to
that which occurs with dural AV fistulas, which demonstrates that the tor-

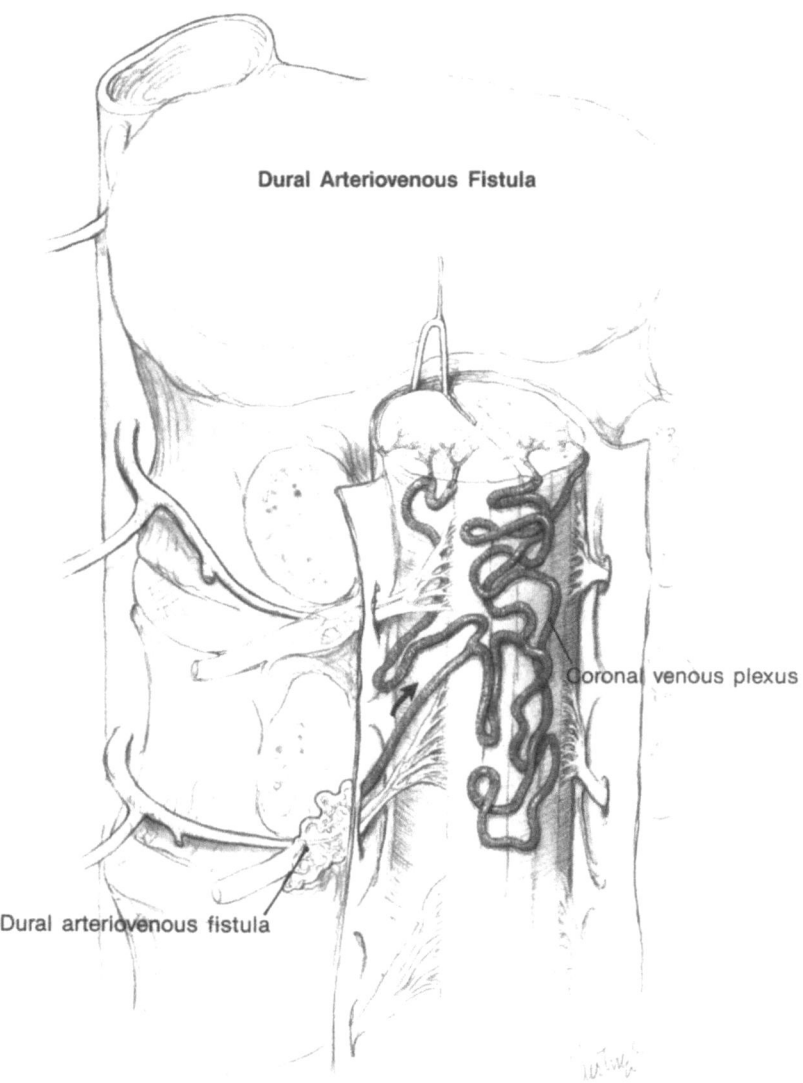

Figure 13.3. Dural AV fistula is supplied by a dural artery and is drained by a medullary vein, which carries blood retrograde to the normal direction of venous drainage to the coronal venous plexus, which becomes elongated, tortuous, and dilated by the reception of arterial blood. Increased venous pressure is transmitted to the cord tissue and causes myelopathy. (From Oldfield EH, Doppman JL. Spinal arteriovenous malformations. *Clin Neurosurg.* 1986;34:161–183. Reprinted with permission.)

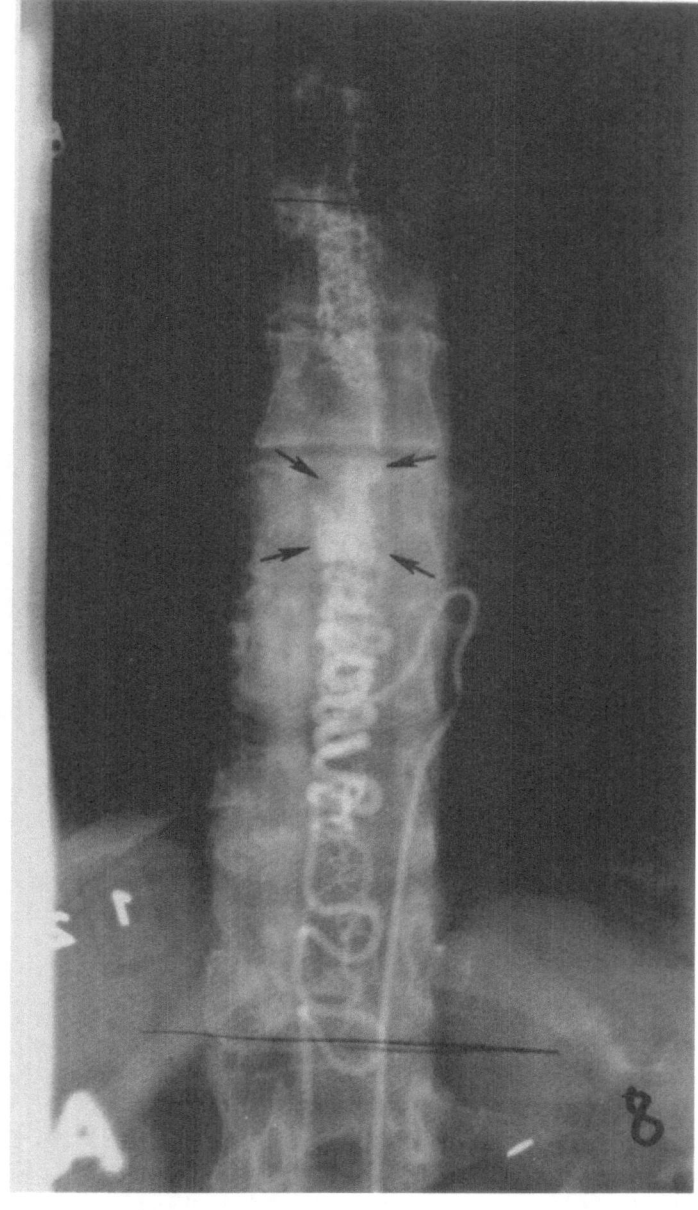

Figure 13.4. Selective spinal arteriogram demonstrating hemangioblastoma of the thoracic segment of the spinal cord and the venous drainage of the excess blood flowing through the vascular tumor. The hemangioblastoma is confined to the area bordered by arrows. The abnormal appearance with tortuosity, elongation, and dilation of the veins of the coronal venous plexus is an acquired alteration in these

tuous vessels on the surface of the cord can evolve from normal veins that receive arterial blood from an AV shunt of any type.

Several years ago it was considered that vascular steal of blood away from the spinal cord accounted for ischemic cord injury in patients with this type of spinal AVM. However, the patient discussed above, with the dural AV fistula on the right at T9-10, has only one vessel supplying the dural AV fistula, the right ninth thoracic intercostal. A separate injection of contrast, with the catheter in the left ninth thoracic intercostal, which arises from a separate orifice of the aorta, fills the artery of Adamkiewicz, the only supply to his spinal cord at this level (Fig. 13.2B). For this AV fistula to cause cord injury by vascular steal, it would have to have such high flow to reduce the intraaortic pressure significantly, which is unlikely, since the flow of contrast through this malformation was so slow that it took more than 20 seconds to disappear. In fact, only 4 of our 27 patients with spinal dural AV fistulas have had common arterial supply to the dural AV fistula and the spinal cord from the same intercostal artery.[6]

In other examples of dural AV fistulas, patients with cranial AV fistulas, the argument for venous congestion as a mechanism of producing cord injury, without contribution from any other potential mechanism, is even clearer.

Patient 2. A 43-year-old man noticed numbness in the left lower quadrant and left leg incoordination early in 1983 (this description is taken directly from a previous report of this patient by Wrobel et al.[20]). Over several months these symptoms became more prominent and left hand numbness developed. A myelogram revealed a coiled filling defect extending from cervical to midthoracic levels (Fig. 13.5). Extensive spinal arteriography failed to opacify any abnormal vessels. His symptoms progressed and bladder dysfunction developed. In 1985 he had sudden onset of quadraparesis that resolved over several hours and another myelogram revealed changes consistent with a spinal AVM, but spinal arteriography was again negative. Carotid arteriography revealed a cranial dural AV fistula of the tentorium with intradural venous drainage into the petrosal vein and then inferiorly into the spinal veins. Frontotemporal craniotomy and interruption of feeding vessels was attempted, but was unsuccessful because of excessive bleeding. After surgery he was able to ambulate with a walker until September 1986, when abrupt lower extremity deterioration occurred. He was admitted to our care 8 weeks after becoming wheelchair-bound.

Examination disclosed normal cranial nerves, moderate weakness of the

◁———————————————————————————————

normal vessels, which results from the reception of arterialized blood with high flow and pressure. A similar alteration in appearance of the normal veins of the coronal venous plexus occurs in patients with spinal dural AV fistulas. (From Oldfield EH, Doppman JL. Spinal arteriovenous malformations. *Clin Neurosurg.* 1986;34:161–183. Reprinted with permission.)

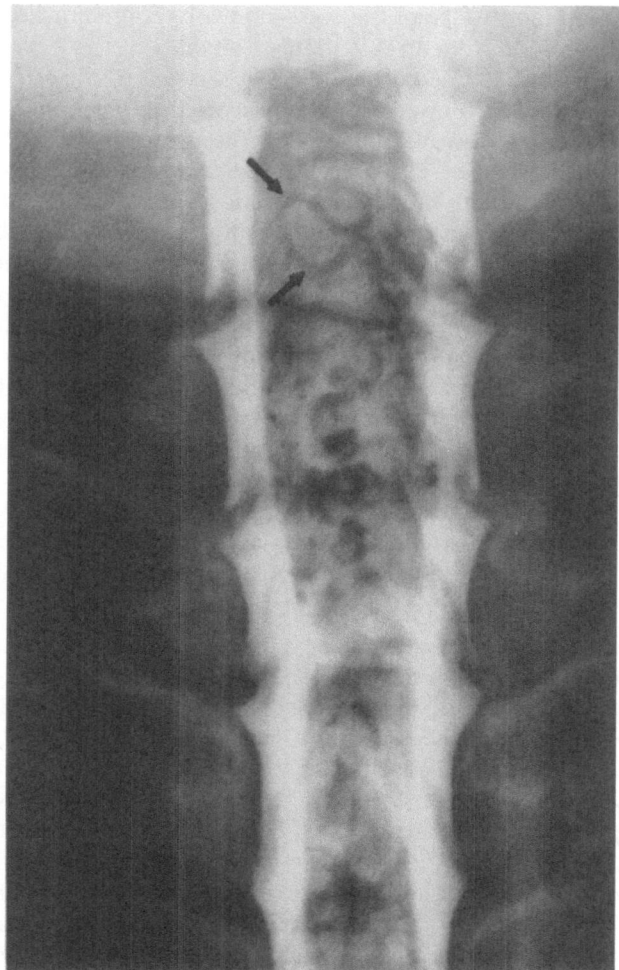

Figure 13.5. Myelogram showing local expansion of the spinal cord and a serpentine subarachnoid filling defect at the lower cervical levels. (From Wrobel, et al. Myelopathy due to intracranial dural arteriovenous fistulas draining intrathecally into spinal medullary veins. *J Neurosurg.* 1988;69:934–939. Reprinted with permission.)

left upper extremity, and mild right hand weakness. Marked weakness and spasticity affected the lower extremities. All stretch reflexes were hyperactive. Position sense was diminished in the lower extremities and pinprick sensation was diminished below T1-2. A spinal MRI indicated swelling and increased signal of the cervical segments of the spinal cord (Fig. 13.6A). Cerebral arteriography defined a right petrous apex dural AV fistula supplied by the occipital branch of the external carotid artery and the mening-

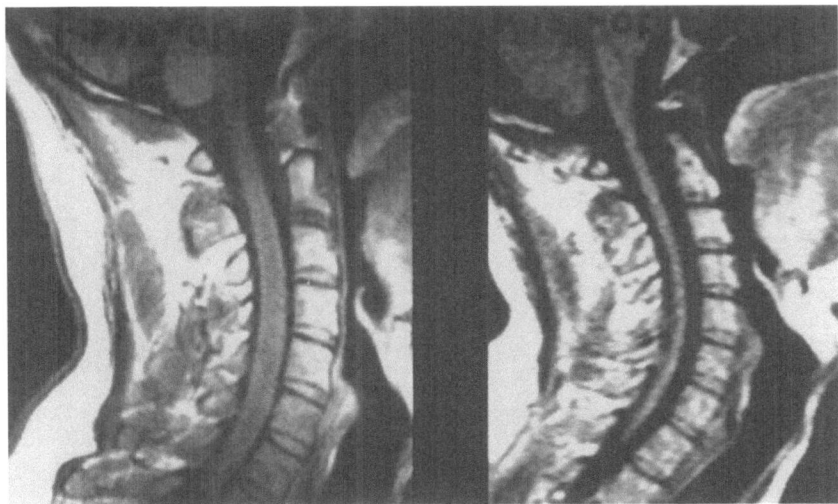

A   B

Figure 13.6. T1-weighted magnetic resonance imaging of the cervical portion of the spinal cord in Patient 2 before (**A**) and after (**B**) interruption of cranial dural AV fistula of the tentorium with venous drainage into the spinal veins. **A,** Preoperative study reveals swelling and edema of the spinal cord resulting from venous congestion of the spinal cord. **B,** After interruption of the dural AV fistula the patient had clinical improvement and the cord edema resolved.

ohypophyseal trunk of the intracavernous segment of the internal carotid artery (Fig. 13.7A). Venous drainage of the fistula was via the anterior pontomesencephalic vein and anterior medullary vein into the intradural veins on the anterior and posterior surfaces of the spinal cord to the mid-thoracic level (Fig. 13.7B).

At surgery, after a suboccipital craniectomy and exposure of the cerebellopontine angle, the petrosal vein was interrupted as it entered the dura. Postoperative arteriography was normal. Three weeks after surgery his spasticity had lessened and within 3 months he could ambulate with a walker and had regained the ability to initiate voiding. MRI of the spinal cord revealed resolution of the preexisting cervical cord swelling (Fig. 13.6B). Nine months after surgery his upper extremity strength was normal and he could ambulate short distances unaided. Repeat postoperative arteriography again revealed no reestablishment of flow in the dural AV fistula.

This patient and the three similar patients that previously have been described[20] establish that cranial dural AV fistulas, fed by arteries unrelated to the spinal cord blood supply, may drain into intrathecal spinal veins and cause myelopathy at a distant level.

These findings establish: (a) that patients with myelography indicating a

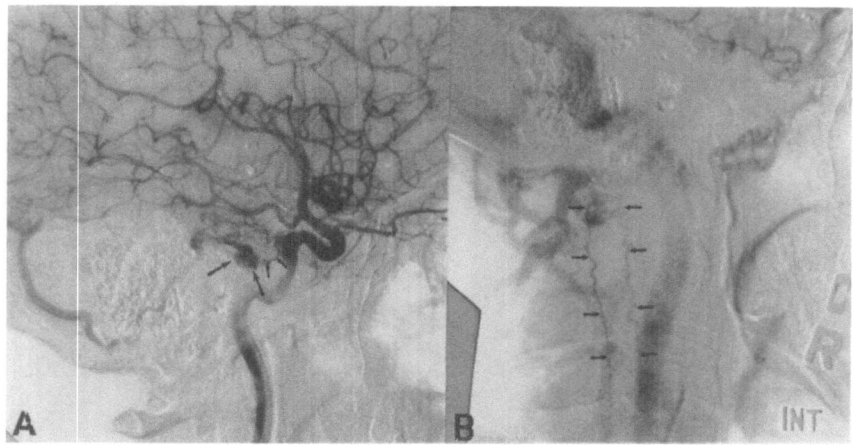

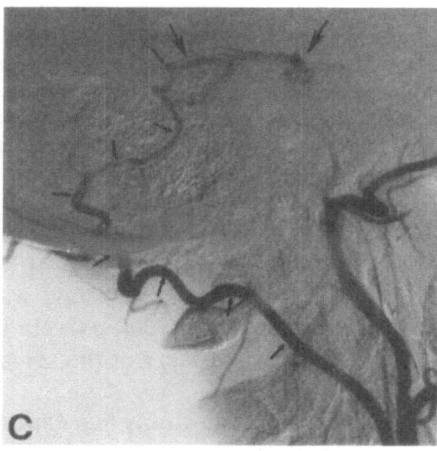

Figure 13.7. Carotid arteriography demonstrating an intracranial dural arteriovenous fistula (**A** and **C**, *large arrows*) supplied by the tentorial branch of the internal carotid artery (**A**, *small arrows*) and by the occipital branch of the right external carotid artery (**C**, *small arrows*). The venous phase demonstrates drainage of the fistula via the petrosal vein into the anterior and posterior spinal veins after internal carotid artery (**B**) and external carotid artery (**D** and **E**) injection (*arrows*). Panels **D** and **E** show prolonged spinal venous drainage. (From Wrobel et al. Myelopathy due to intracranial arteriovenous fistulas draining intrathecally into spinal medullary veins. *J Neurosurg.* 1988;69:934–939. Reprinted with permission.)

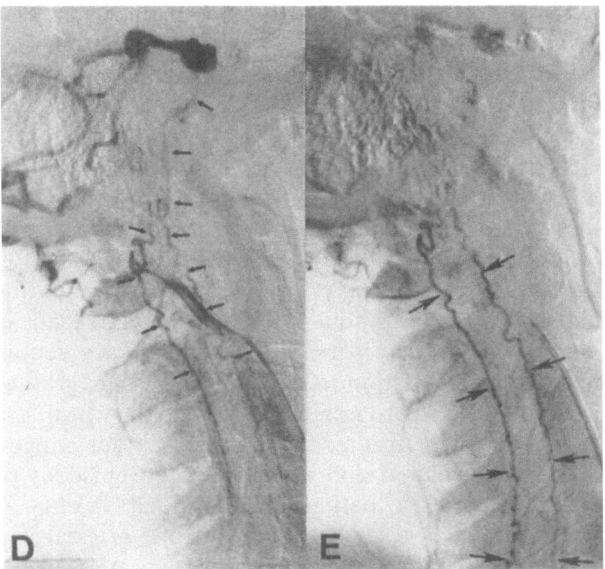

"spinal AVM" and negative spinal arteriography may have cranial dural AV fistulas, (b) venous hypertension as a pathophysiologic mechanism of myelopathy, and (c) that interruption of a dural fistula draining into the spinal veins permits recovery of myelopathy caused by venous congestion.

Therefore, dural AV fistulas with medullary venous drainage serve as a model of venous congestion in which no other potential source of tissue injury is present. What happens to the parenchyma and microvasculature of the cord with excess venous pressure? How are patients with venous hypertension of the spinal cord affected clinically?

Histological Alterations Produced by Venous Congestion of the Spinal Cord

A previous report by Aminoff, Barnard, and Logue from an autopsy of a patient with paraparesis due to a spinal AVM demonstrates the effect on the spinal cord of chronic venous congestion.[21] Despite that this description was made before it had been discovered that most spinal AVMs are dural AV fistulas and not true AVMs of the spinal cord, the authors attributed cord injury to venous hypertension and cogently argue for venous congestion as the pathophysiological basis of spinal cord injury in these patients. They described the spinal cord of a 49-year-old man with a spinal AVM in whom there was no nidus of an AVM in the spinal cord. The cord was examined at autopsy 8 years after complete paraplegia below T-8.

There was extensive dilatation and tortuosity of the veins within the leptomeninges over the entire length of the spinal cord. Within the spinal cord there were abnormal dilated venous channels with thickened, hyalinized walls. Thrombosis was not present in the abnormal extramedullary or intramedullary venous channels. In the posterior and lateral portions of the lower thoracic segments of the cord there was extensive proliferaton of the intrinsic capillary-sized vessels with concentric hyalinization of the walls.

On the basis of the pathological findings in this patient and an extensive clinical review of 60 patients with spinal AVMs by Aminoff and Logue,[22,23] they postulated, and convincingly argued, that the shunting of blood through spinal AVMs to the venous system of the cord leads to increased pressure in the coronal veins, increased intramedullary venous pressure, venous congestion and stagnation, reduced AV pressure gradient, lowered intramedullary blood flow, cord ischemia, and capillary proliferation. They also hypothesized transient further increases in venous congestion as the mechanism of posture-related and activity-related episodes of increased neurological impairment in patients with spinal AVMs (neurogenic claudication).[21] Moreover, their argument against arterial ischemia by a vascular steal phenomenon was based on the separate vascular supply of the AVM and the spinal cord in most patients, and they discounted cord compression by the enlarged draining veins based on observations of no evident compression of the cord at surgery, absence of myelographic block in most patients, and the failure of decompressive laminectomy to halt clinical progression in their patients. Today, their observations and hypotheses appear particularly foresighted, as they made them before it was recognized that most spinal AVMs are actually dural AV fistulas.

Clinical Presentation and Natural History of Venous Congestion of the Spinal Cord

We recently reviewed the clinical syndrome, diagnostic features, and outcome after treatment of 81 patients with spinal AVMs.[6] The clinical course of the 27 patients with spinal dural AV fistulas represent the clinical effects of venous congestion. Twenty three of the 27 (85%) patients with dural AV fistulas presented with a gradual onset and progressive loss of neurological function. Bending, standing, or activity elicited exacerbation of symptoms in 75% of these patients. The natural history of these patients was that of stepwise increases in neurological deficit against a background of progressive loss of cord function, as had been previously noted in patients with spinal AVMs in general.[22,23] In most patients neurological deficits were at least partially reversible with treatment.[5,6] Seventy two percent of the 27 patients improved postoperatively (85% were able to walk, although about half of them required aid with a cane or crutches).[5,6]

The progression of untreated venous congestion of the cord is illustrated by patients who ultimately develop sufficient stasis of flow that venous thrombosis occurs or in whom venous hypertension occurs to a degree that low perfusion pressure of the cord causes cord ischemia. Our experience with several patients with Foix-Alajouanine syndrome, one of whom is described below, demonstrates that venous hypertension ultimately leads to stagnant venous flow and to venous thrombosis and infarction if untreated, but that in many of these patients at clinical presentation the problem is venous congestion, and not venous thrombosis, as was previously thought, in the early phases of acute deterioration of cord function.[15,24]

·Patient 3. A 61-year-old man developed progressive weakness and sensory loss in his lower extremities, urinary incontinence, and constipation over an interval of 4 weeks (the following description of this patient is from a prior report by Criscuolo et al.[15]). On the day of admission complete paralysis of his lower extremities and a progressive, ascending sensory deficit developed over several hours. Neurological examination revealed flaccid paraplegia, complete sensory loss below the T-10 dermatome, and diminished rectal sphincter tone. At spinal arteriography, selective injection of the right lumbar artery at L-2 showed a dural AV fistula at L-2 with a characteristic vein draining the blood from the fistula into dilated tortuous subarachnoid veins. The dural AV fistula was occluded by embolization with particles of polyvinyl alcohol (Ivalon). Within 24 hours of the embolization motor and sensory function began to recover. The patient was discharged after regaining antigravity strength and with improving sensory function, but without voluntary control of bowel or bladder function.

As his recovery progressed he was able to walk using parallel bars, but could not ambulate independently. He regained normal lower extremity sensation, but still required self-catheterization. On the day before admission, he rapidly became paraplegic and was given intravenous dexamethasone. He regained antigravity function that evening. Early the next morning he again lost all lower extremity function and had been in that condition for approximately 12 hours at admission. He had flaccid paraplegia with total loss of sensation below T-10. There was no response to plantar stimulation, and deep tendon, abdominal, and cremasteric reflexes were absent. Repeat selective spinal arteriography revealed reestablishment of flow through the spinal dural arteriovenous fistula. The feeding vessels were again occluded by embolization with Ivalon. Motor and sensory function began to recover within hours after embolization. Within 48 hours, he regained some antigravity function and no longer had a detectable sensory level. Four days after embolization the patient underwent surgery. Laminectomy exposed the cluster of tortuous arteries surrounding and embedded in the L-2 nerve root sleeve and the adjacent spinal dura. The AV fistula was drained by a single intrathecal vessel that traversed the subarachnoid space to join the coronal venous plexus on the ventral surface of the spinal cord. There were several small areas of thrombosis in radicular veins at isolated nerve roots. The feeding vessels and nidus of the AV fistula were coagulated as they entered the dura, and the vessel draining the fistula was interrupted as it pierced the inner layer of dura. Lower extremity strength gradually improved after surgery. Two weeks later, the patient had regained bilateral proximal antigravity strength and had only minimally impaired position sense in the left leg with normal position sense in the right leg. At 14 months after surgery, slow but progressive improvement continued. He was able to walk unaided approximately 150 yards, the previous impairment of position sense fully resolved, and he was voiding voluntarily without urinary retention.

We have treated five patients with dural AV fistulas who experienced acute or subacute onset of myelopathy without hemorrhage, and who improved substantially after interruption of the dural AV fistula.[15] The outcome of these patients indicates that acute and subacute progression of myelopathy with spinal dural AV fistulas may be caused by venous congestion, and not thrombosis. Therefore, in patients with spinal dural AV fistulas and rapidly progressive myelopathy (Foix-Alajouanine syndrome), myelopathy is probably caused by deterioration of the compensatory capacity of the spinal cord to accommodate venous congestion and, in the early stages, is not a result of venous thrombosis, which occurs at a later stage in the evolution of lesions that impart increased venous pressure and venous stagnation on the cord tissue. Early diagnosis and proper management of venous congestion can result in a successful outcome, whereas progression to thrombosis causes irreversible cord injury.

Venous Congestion as a Mechanism of Cord Injury in Other Conditions

The discussion above indicates venous congestion as a mechanism of cord injury that alone can produce reversible cord injury in patients with spinal dural AV fistulas, in patients with cranial dural AV fistulas with venous drainage into the venous system of the spinal cord, and in patients with Foix-Alajouanine syndrome. If we accept venous congestion as a mechanism of cord injury in these circumstances, particularly early and reversible injury, might it not be present and play a significant role in other types of cord injury?

About half of the patients with intradural AVMs of the spinal cord (juvenile and glomus AVMs and direct AV fistulas of the cord or the pia) also present initally with gradual and progressive loss of neurological function.[6] Although they almost always have blood supply from a vessel that also supplies the spinal cord, and therefore could have cord injury from arterial ischemia by an arterial steal mechanism, the extensive blood flow into the venous system could also produce increased venous pressure and cord injury by venous stagnation in many of these patients.

Cord compression, acutely or chronically, from degenerative disc, tumor, or trauma may also produce cord injury, at least initially, by venous congestion. In the mid-1970s John Doppman and his coworkers at NIH performed a series of experiments that support consideration of venous congestion as a mechanism of cord dysfunction when the cord is compressed by a mass in the spinal canal.[10-14] They placed a balloon in the spinal canal of rhesus monkeys and acutely expanded it to varying sizes, over 1 to 2 minutes, and observed the effect on neurological function and on spinal cord blood flow, as determined by spinal arteriography and by in vivo perfusion studies with radio-opaque barium-containing solutions. When an anteriorly placed balloon first reached a size that consistently produced neurological deficit it compromised flow in the spinal veins as seen arteriographically, but flow in the anterior spinal artery, which was immediately dorsal to the balloon, remained unaffected. Furthermore, the perfusion studies indicated that at this stage of expansion of the balloon that flow in the sulcal arteries, terminal small vessels in the anterior median fissure, was impaired. A similar result was obtained when the balloon was placed posteriorly in the spinal canal. In animals in which a balloon was placed anteriorly and a laminectomy was performed, and in which flow was re-established through the spinal veins by the laminectomy, there was no disturbance in filling of the sulcal arteries in the perfusion studies and no neurological deficit occurred.

These results are consistent with an initial neurological deficit after acute cord compression from impaired venous flow which, in turn, produced reduced perfusion pressure and cord ischemia. It is therefore reasonable to consider that successful decompression with recovery of neurological function under similar circumstances of acute or chronic cord compression in the clinic may occur by eliminating impaired venous flow and by doing so secondarily permitting recovery of arterial perfusion of the spinal cord.

Summary

Venous congestion is a relatively unstudied mechanism of spinal cord injury. Venous congestion of the spinal cord may be produced by any cranial or dural AV fistula that gains access to the venous system of the spinal cord and produces elevated pressure in the coronal venous plexus or the medullary veins. As the intradural spinal venous system is valveless, with increased pressure in the medullary veins or the coronal venous plexus pressure in the radially oriented intramedullary veins increases. Our observations and the work of others, some of which has been reviewed here, support venous hypertension as a pathophysiological mechanism of myelopathy, and indicate that certain neurological disorders that traditionally have been considered to cause spinal cord injury primarily by mechanical distortion of the cord or by compromising arterial flow may impair cord function initially by producing venous congestion. Further experimental investigation of the physiological events of venous congestion of the spinal cord, of venous congestion as an etiology of spinal cord dysfunction in myelopathy caused by diseases in addition to spinal dural AV fistulas, and as a potentially reversible mechanism of cord dysfunction is needed.

References

1. Doppman JL, Di Chiro G, Oldfield EH. Origin of spinal arteriovenous malformation and normal cord vasculature from a common segmental artery: Angiographic and therapeutic considerations. *Radiology*. 1985;154:687–689.
2. Doppman JL, Dwyer AJ, Frank JL, Di Chiro G, Oldfield EH. Magnetic resonance imaging of spinal arteriovenous malformations. *J Neurosurg*. 1987; 66:830–834.
3. Kendall BE, Logue V. Spinal epidural angiomatous malformations draining into intrathecal veins. *Neuroradiology*. 1977;3:181–189.
4. Oldfield EH, Di Chiro G, Quindlen EA, Reith KG, Doppman JL. Successful treatment of a group of spinal cord arteriovenous malformations by interruption of dural fistula. *J Neurosurg* 1983;59:1019–1030.
5. Oldfield EH, and Doppman JL. Spinal arteriovenous malformations. *Clin Neurosurg*. 1986;34:161–183.
6. Rosenblum B, Oldfield EH, Doppman JL, Di Chiro G. Spinal arteriovenous malformations: A comparison of dural arteriovenous fistulas and intradural AVM's in 81 patients. *J Neurosurg*. 1987;67:795–802.
7. Symon L, Kuyama H, Kendall B. Dural arteriovenous malformations of the spine: Clinical features and surgical results in 55 cases. *J Neurosurg*. 1984;60:238–247.
8. Yasargil MG, Symon L, Teddy PJ. Arteriovenous malformations of the spinal cord. In: Symon L, ed. *Advances and Technical Standards in Neurosurgery*. vol 11. Wien: Springer–Verlag;1984:61–102.
9. Brain WR, Knight GC, Bull JWD. Discussion of rupture of the intervertebral disc in the cervical region. *Proc R Soc Med*. 1948;41:509–516.
10. Doppman JL. The mechanism of ischemia in anteroposterior compression of the spinal cord. *Invest Radiol*. 1975;10:543–551.
11. Doppman JL. Angiographic changes following acute spinal cord compression: an experimental study in monkeys. *Br J Radiology*. 1976;49:398–406.
12. Doppman JL, Girton M. Angiographic study of the effect of laminectomy in the presence of acute anterior epidural masses. *J Neurosurg*. 1976;45:195–202.
13. Doppman JL, Girton M, Popovsky MA. Acute occlusion of the posterior spinal vein: experimental study in monkeys. *J Neurosurg*. 1979;51:201–205.
14. Ramsey R, Doppman JL. The effects of epidural masses on spinal cord blood flow. *Radiology*. 1973;107:99–103.
15. Criscuolo GR, Oldfield EH, Doppman JL. Reversible acute and subacute myelopathy in patients with dural arteriovenous fistulas: Foix-Alajouanine syndrome reconsidered. *J Neurosurg*. 1989;70:354–359.
16. Sargent P. Hemangioma of the pia mater causing compression paraplegia. *Brain*. 1925;48:259–267.
17. Wyburn-Mason R. *The Vascular Abnormalities and Tumours of the Spinal Cord and its Membranes*. London: H. Klimpton; 1943.
18. Gillilan LA. The arterial blood supply to the human spinal cord. *J Comp Neurol*. 1958;110:75–100.
19. Gillilan LA. Veins of the spinal cord. Anatomic details; suggested clinical applications. *Neurology*. 1970;20:860–868.
20. Wrobel C, Oldfield EH, Di Chiro G, Tarlov EC, Baker RA, Doppman JL.

Myelopathy due to intracranial dural arteriovenous fistulas draining intrathecally into spinal medullary veins. *J Neurosurg.* 1988;69:934–939.

21. Aminoff MF, Barnard RO, Logue V. The pathophysiology of spinal vascular malformations. *J Neurol Sci.* 1974;23:255–263.

22. Aminoff MJ, Logue V. The prognosis of patients with spinal vascular malformations. *Brain.* 1974;97:211–218.

23. Aminoff MJ, Logue V. Clinical features of spinal vascular malformations. *Brain.* 1974;97:197–210.

24. Hall WA, Oldfield EH, Doppman JL. Recanalization of spinal arteriovenous malformations following obliteration by embolization. *J Neurosurg.* 1989; 70:714–720.

Note. Portions of this chapter discussing spinal dural AV fistulas and the anatomy of the spinal vasculature are modified from Oldfield EH, Doppman JL. Spinal arteriovenous malformations. *Clin Neurosurg.* 1986;34:161–183 and from Oldfield EH: An update on spinal arteriovenous malformations. In: Wilkins RH, Rengachary SS, eds. *Neurosurgery Update.* New York: McGraw-Hill Book Co; 1989.

Discussion

Dr. Kliot: "How long is the follow-up in the patients who have had either surgical or endovascular obliteration of the fistula, but leaving the nidus. Is there a chance of curing the lesion for a while and then having another fistula open and the process recur?"

Dr. Oldfield: "I usually ablate the fistula. I accepted interruption of the vein draining the fistula intradurally in the spine, in 4 of 27 patients with dural arteriovenous fistulas in which the artery of Adamkiewicz was at the same level as the dural AVM and the artery was so intertwined with the AV fistula that it could not be separated from it. In the two patients who were treated with simple interruption of the vein, both were followed for a year with repeat angiography without evidence of recanalization of the dural AV fistula and for 4 years without either of them developing a recurrent neurological deficit.

I have treated three patients now with cranial dural AV fistulas in which the only venous drainage was intrathecal. I think that is the key to being able to treat those patients successfully. If the vein is interrupted there is no evidence of reflow through the fistula and no evidence of clinical recurrence. We have two patients that we have followed for 6 months and 10 months and we know of two others. In fact, there is a French patient who was reported with a cranial dural AV fistula of a similar nature who was cured of quadriplegia by embolic interruption of a posterior fossa dural AV fistula."

Dr. Lazorthes: "Concerning the normal anatomical and physiologic point of view there is a system of protection of the brain's and spinal cord's venous circulation. With Valsalva maneuvers we see increased pressure transmitted to the epidural venous plexus but not to the venous system of the spinal cord. The same is true with venous angiography. The veins of the spine pass through the dura obliquely so the dura acts as a valve to protect the circulation of the spinal cord."

Dr. Oldfield: "I agree. There is certainly a protective mechanism, otherwise everybody with advanced cirrhosis of the liver and increased venous pressure would potentially be developing a myelopathy that rarely occurs. Spinal metastases would not only occur principally in the epidural space, but would also occur with reasonable frequency in the intrathecal space of the spine. The problem with the venous anatomy at that level is that nobody has been able to anatomically show a valve.

As you know, Dr. Michael Sisti and I were trying to create a model of this venous congestion of the spinal cord so that we could study it. Dr. John Doppman put balloons in above and below the atrium to occlude the azygous vein and then we swung the internal carotid artery down on one side in rhesus monkeys and did an end-to-side anastomosis into the azygous vein and ligated the entrance of the azygous vein into the right atrium where it meets the cava.

Thus, we had an isolated segment of the azygous vein into which we were putting aortic-pressure type arterial blood. We followed those animals for 3 years with arteriography, initially monthly, later, every 3 months, and then every 6 months. They ended up dying of complications of the AV shunts, which were tremendous, but neither of them ever developed drainage of the fistula into the intrathecal venous system.

These recent three patients with dural AV fistulas in the head that drain into the spinal venous system and produced myelopathy have demonstrated to us a way of now producing a model of venous congestion in animals. All we need to do is isolate a segment of the transverse or sigmoid sinus that also includes the petrosal vein and make an AV shunt there."

Dr. Holtzman: "I am curious what you think the mechanism is of neural dysfunction in venous congestion? Is it hypercarbia? Is it toxic? Is it fluid congestion and edema?"

Dr. Oldfield: "It seems that there are two potential mechanisms. One is venous stagnation that reaches the point where thrombosis occurs. Under those circumstances I would not expect complete or major neurological recovery and the other is that the perfusion pressure has dropped to the point that the blood flow is being compromised."

CHAPTER 14

Surgical Treatment of Arteriovenous Malformations of the Spinal Cord

Y.M. Filatov, T.P. Tissen, and S.S. Eliava

Despite recent progress, current vascular neurosurgical diagnostic techniques and the treatment of arteriovenous malformations (AVMs) remain complicated problems due to the anatomicotopographical peculiarities of blood supply to the spinal cord. Thanks to the introduction and development of selective spinal angiography (SSA), vascular pathology of the spinal cord received a new interpretation, which broadened our conception of the anatomy and physiology of blood supply.[1] Application of SSA opened new possibilities for the exposure of spinal cord AVMs and allowed for the simultaneous introduction of new methods for their treatment.

Considering the complexity of treating patients with spinal cord AVMs, at the Burdenko Institute, varying methods of approach must be applied. Along with traditional, direct surgical operations, where the afferent arteries of the malformation are clipped, and occlusion and resection of the pathological vessels of AVMs occur, a nonstandard method of treatment—endovascular, artificial thrombosis of AVM vessels—has been used. This method of artificial thrombosis of spinal cord AVMs through the afferent vessels was first used in 1968.[2-4] Surgeons used solidifying compounds in combination with plastic spheres as material. However, substances and methods used in the embolization of spinal cord AVMs have been constantly updated. Parts of muscle and dura mater, gel foam, and silicon substances, as well as Ivalon and isobutylcyanacrylate have been used as thrombogenic materials.[5-7]

The first direct surgical operations on large spinal cord AVMs were performed at the Burdenko Institute in 1971. Beginning in 1974, the institute initiated the development of a method of embolization of spinal cord AVMs and vascular tumors at various levels of the spinal cord.[8] In the beginning of endovascular treatment of the above-stated diseases of the spinal cord, fragments of hemostatic sponge were used as material. Later, only small polyvinylacetate (PVA) emboli (from 0.2 to 0.5 mm), and detachable balloons were used, according to the Serbinenko method.[9]

Materials and Method

At the Burdenko Institute, experiments involving surgical treatment of patients with spinal cord AVMs were based on 44 observed cases. Surgery was performed on 14 of these: three patients had AVMs in the cervical area of the spinal cord, eight in the thoracic area, and three in the lumbar area. Selective embolization of AVMs through the afferent vessels was performed on 30 patients. Patients' ages ranged from 6 to 58 years.

In this report, greater emphasis has been placed on nonstandard methods of treating spinal cord AVMs, i.e., endovascular embolization of malformations, which, along with direct operations, succeeded in significantly increasing the proportion of patients who are receptive to surgery.

In all, embolization was performed on 48 afferent arteries of AVMs. In 11 of these cases, thrombogenic material was injected through the Adamkiewicz artery of the spinal cord. In 4 cases, AVMs were distributed in the cervical area, in 20 cases, in the thoracic area, and in 6 cases, in the lumbar area of the spinal cord. In two patients, both children, occlusion of the AVM in the cervical area proceeded in two steps: (a) injection of the embolus, and (b) placement of the occluding balloon. In 18 cases the disease was manifested by subarachnoid and parenchymatous hemorrhages. Ten patients experienced recurring hemorrhages, accompanied by severe neurological deterioration. Paraparesis of the lower extremities with periodic disturbances in functions of the genitourinary system (GUS) occurred in 15 patients, paraplegia with persistent disturbances in the GUS in 12 patients, tetraplegia in 2 patients, and tetraparesis in 2 patients, accompanied by disturbances in GUS. All patients experienced sensory disturbances, and pain syndromes were noted in 23 cases. Repeated embolization was carried out on five patients, 5 to 8 years after the first treatment of the AVM.

During embolization, a catheter, used in SSA, was placed in the opening of the intercostal, lumbar, thyrocervical arteries, and radicular branches of the vertebral artery, from which the afferent vessels of spinal cord AVMs emerge. After placing a catheter in the opening of the necessary artery, a corresponding catheter was introduced and a hydrodynamic probe was performed using a physiological solution or a contrasting medium. During this procedure, the distal end of the catheter should remain in the prescribed lumen of the artery. However, the contrasting medium, with a volume of 3 to 5 ml, which is introduced quickly and under pressure, should not escape from the prescribed vessel. The emboli used to occlude the distal section of the afferent vessel and AVM were selected after analysis of the angiogram. PVA particles, together with the physiological solution, slowly passed along the catheter to the afferent vessel of the AVM. At this point, an identification of the vessel was possible on the television screen due to the injection (3 ml) of the contrasting medium. In addition to identification on the television screen, in some cases, post-injection angiography was performed. (Angiography is important in the evaluation of the restructuring of blood circulation within the spinal cord AVM, as well as in identifying changes in its size.)

Results and Discussion

Clinical syndromes in patients with spinal cord AVMs develop as a result of ischemic processes and as a consequence of compression due to the dilated and constantly pulsating vessels of the AVM. In the case of a sharp increase in blood flow within the AVM itself, the veins, unaccustomed to high blood pressure, burst and bleeding occurs. In these cases patients experience subarachnoid and parenchymatous hemorrhages with accompanying neurological deterioration in both the immediate and delayed postictal periods. Surgery of AVMs removes, on the whole, pathophysiological manifestations, which cause ischemic changes and compression of the spinal cord. We also used this method after hemorrhagic strokes with the goal of excluding repeated hemorrhage and improving blood supply to undamaged cells of the spinal cord, in an attempt to eliminate the symptoms of a steal syndrome and compression of the spinal cord by vessels of the AVM. In order to study changes in the pathological vessels, occurring in the AVM as a result of embolization, we performed a control angiogram and myelogram with a water-soluble contrasting medium, several days after the embolization. In almost all cases, in the absence of accompanying arachnoiditis, the subarachnoid space was clearly visible on the myelogram, whereas before the embolization the blockage of the contrast medium at the level of the AVM was visible. On the basis of information received from the dynamic myelographic investigation, we came to the conclusion that, as a result of occlusion of the afferent vessels of the AVM, collapse of the dilated venous collectors occurs, the result of which is the restoration of patency of the subarachnoid space (Fig. 14.1). However, in the presence of accompanying fibrotic, adhesive processes, which are characteristic of spinal AVMs, the blockage continued to be visible on the myelogram after the embolization of the AVM.

Direct surgery of AVMs in the cervical area of the spinal cord was carried out on three patients. In all three cases, the afferent arteries of the malformation were clipped and occlusion of the pathological vessels of the AVM occurred. Endovascular intervention was implemented in four patients, and six vessels were occluded in the cervical area. In one patient embolization was repeated three times at time intervals of a year. The first two embolizations were performed with spongostan; the third time PVA particles were used as emboli. Each time a patient was discharged with improvement, the marked tetraparesis regressed. After the last embolization the patient returned to work. The AVM in the given case was supplied simultaneously by three vessels: the inominate artery, which comes

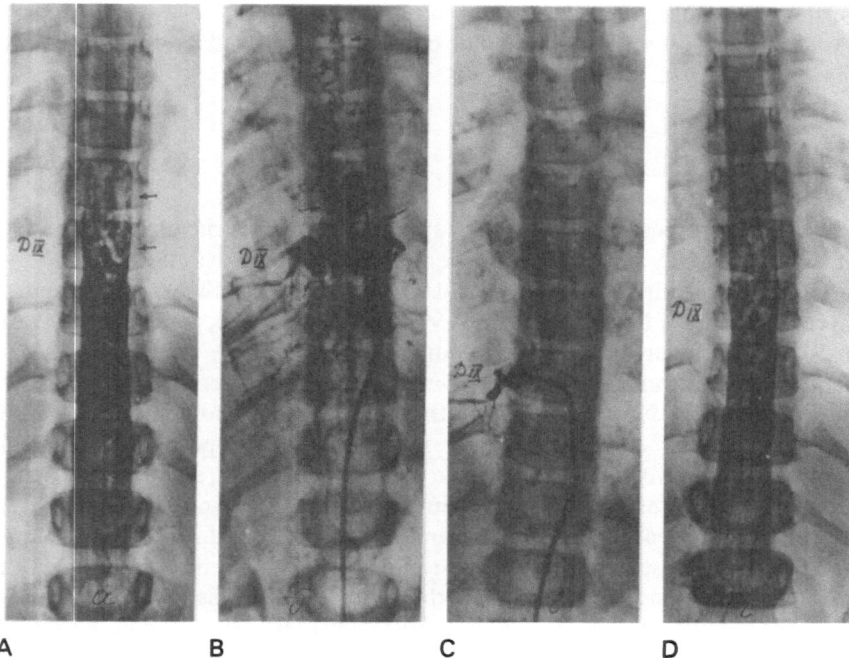

A   B   C   D

Figure 14.1. Arteriovenous malformation (AVM) of the thoracic spinal cord. **A,** Myelogram depicting the vascular pattern of the malformation (as shown by the *arrows*) and the partial block of contrast material at the D_8 vertebral level. **B,** AVM being fed by a short radicular artery at the D_9 vertebral level. The outflow of blood from the malformation is directed both cephalad and caudad by a draining vein along the spinal cord. **C,** Selective angiography of the afferent vessel after embolization demonstrates obliteration of the malformation. **D,** Repeat contrast study of the subarachnoid space after embolization of the malformation demonstrates its patency.

from the aorta; the radicular artery, a branch of the thyrocervical trunk; and the third vessel originated from the vertebral artery. The AVM was localized on the posterior and lateral surfaces of the spinal cord. The control angiogram, performed after embolization, revealed the total occlusion of the AVM (Fig. 14.2). In a second patient, who had tetraplegia for 9 years, a single vessel was occluded by two balloons (Fig. 14.3). Tetraplegia

————————————————————————————▷

Figure 14.2. AVM of the cervical portion of the spinal cord. **A,** The blood supply is derived from a hypertrophied ascending branch of the intercostal artery at the D_3 vertebral level on the left. A second nutrient source is a radicular artery coming off the thyrocervical trunk. **B, C, D,** Selective angiography following embolization of the malformation depicts the complete exclusion of the malformation, extending from C_4 to D_1 vertebral levels, from the circulation.

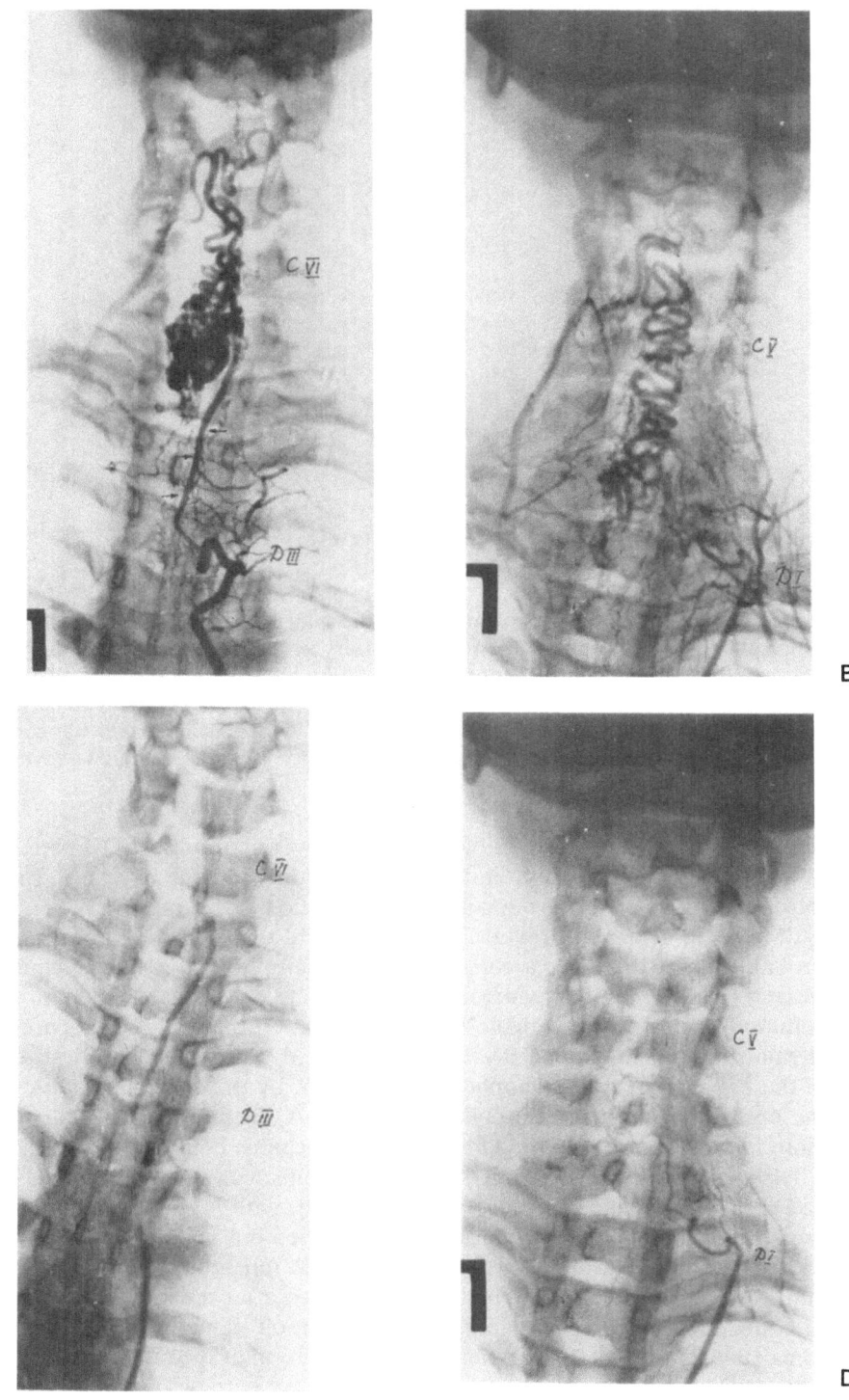

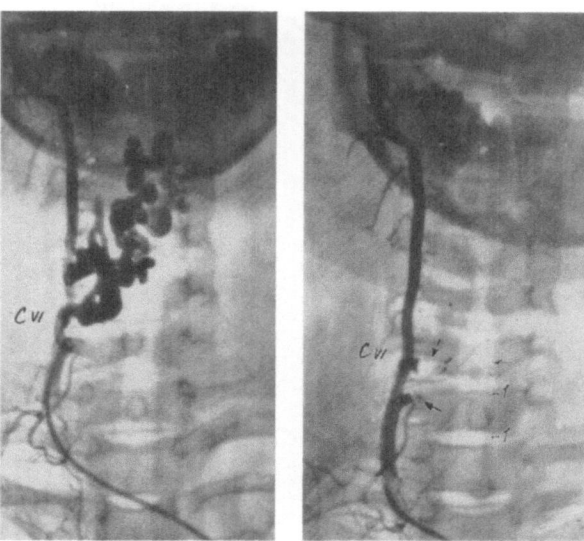

Figure 14.3. AVM of the cervical portion of the spinal cord in a 9-year-old girl. **A,** Blood supply is derived from the radicular artery at the C_6 vertebral level on the right. **B,** Selective angiography of the spinal artery after occlusion of the afferent vessel by two balloons with markers (as shown by the *arrows*) demonstrated the exclusion of the malformation from the circulation. The radicular artery was compared and contrasted in selective angiograms after occlusion (as indicated above).

regressed and turned into paraparesis of the lower extremities. The patient (a girl) can now move about independently and is studying in school. In a third patient from the group, after embolization, total occlusion of the AVM was in evidence. Reversal of neurological symptoms did not occur. Probably this patient, as a consequence of multiple hemorrhages, which were verified by lumbar puncture (on 5 separate occasions), experienced hematomyelia with irreversible ischemic change in the spinal cord parenchyma. In a fourth patient, 8 years old, a large AVM, which was localized in the cervical area, was supplied, in the main, by the radicular artery of the costocervical trunk. Embolization of the AVM and occlusion of the afferent vessel were performed by using a detachable balloon.

Direct surgery was performed on eight patients with AVMs in the thoracic area of the spinal cord, and on three patients with AVMs in the lumbar area of the spinal cord. Embolization was carried out in 26 patients in the thoracic and lumbar areas of the spinal cord. A repeated occlusion of the AVM was performed on five patients 5 to 8 years after the initial operation in connection with the appearance and evolution of neurological symptoms, and signs on the angiograms of recanalization of the afferent vessels. The earlier embolizations were performed on all patients using spongos-

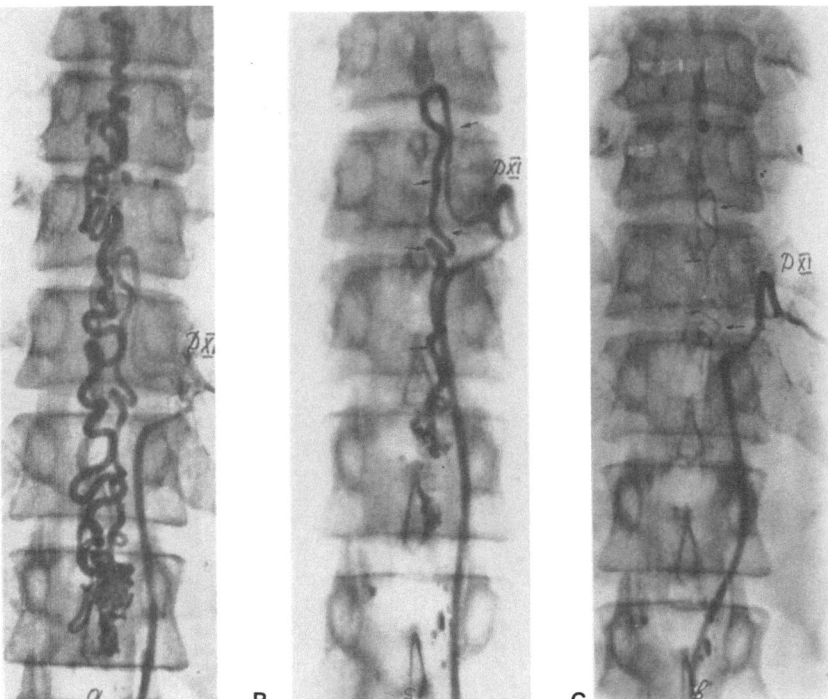

Figure 14.4. **A,** AVM of the thoracic portion of the spinal cord extending from the D_6 to L_1 vertebral levels is fed from the artery of Adamkiewicz. **B,** After embolization of the malformation the hypertrophied artery of Adamkiewicz is more clearly defined (*arrows*). The nidus is excluded from the circulation. **C,** Selective angiography of that vessel 6 days later demonstrates a marked reduction in its diameter.

tan. PVA particles were used in the second operations with good results. In some cases blood was supplied to the AVM from three sources at various segmental levels. Consequently, embolization was carried out with preservation of blood supply routes to the AVM and spinal cord. Preservation of the trunk of the afferent vessel before it enters the venous system is important; it is necessary especially when the AVM is supplied from the anterior spinal artery and Adamkiewicz artery of the spinal cord (Fig. 14.4). Intermediate control angiograms must be made during embolization in order to detect normal spinal vessels, which simultaneously supply the spinal cord. Occlusion of these vessels carries serious consequences.

Direct surgical treatment is based on the following: accurate identification of the afferent arteries of the spinal cord malformation, and application of microsurgical methods and operational optics, which allow for the preservation of normal arterial stems that participate in supplying blood to

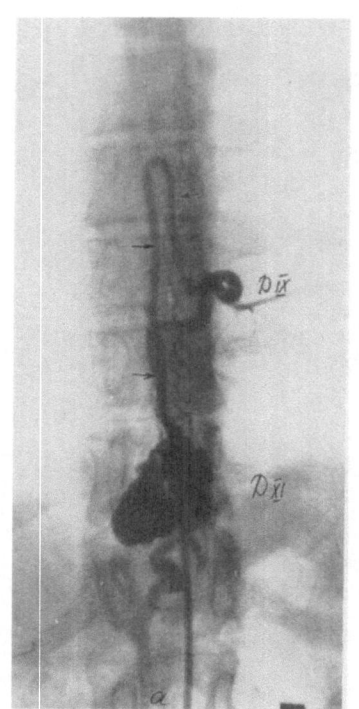
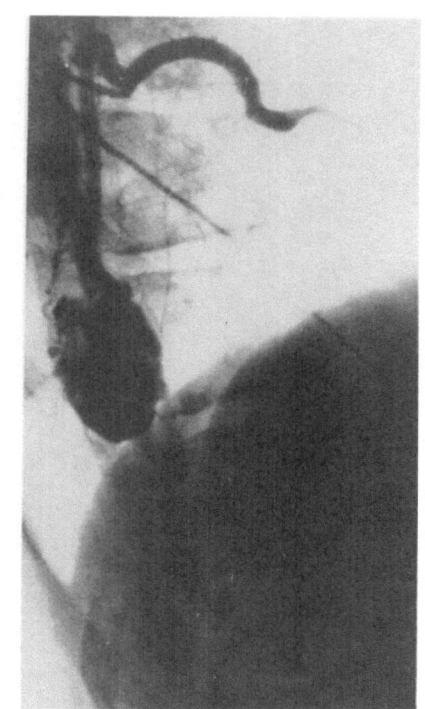

A

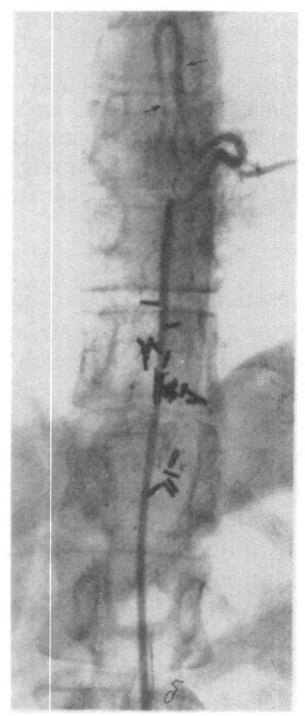
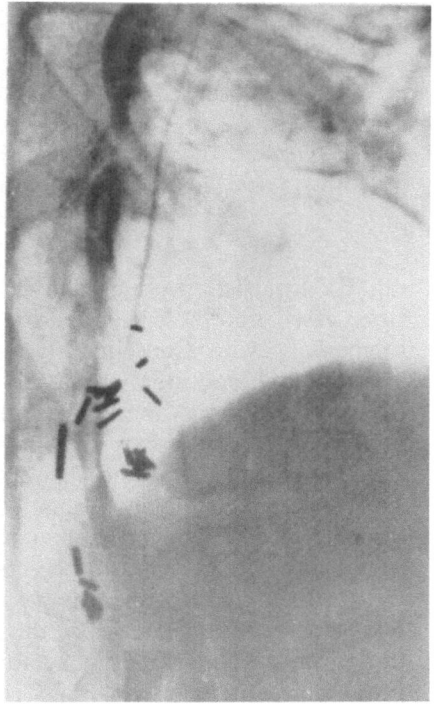

B

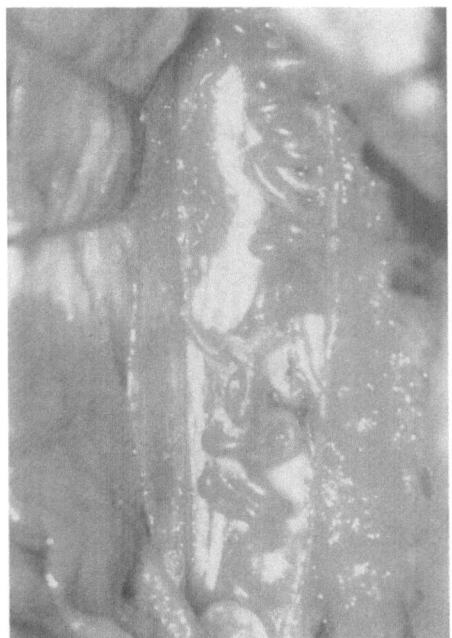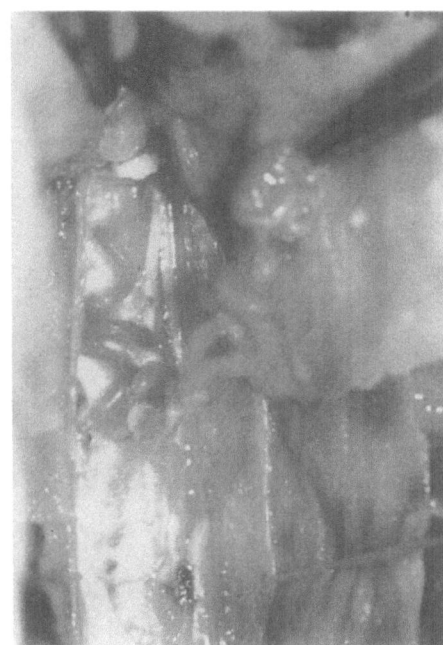

A   B

Figure 14.6. Intraoperative stages in the removal of an AVM.

adjacent areas of the spinal cord. There is a greater possibility for preservation when a subpial localization of the malformation is in evidence. This localization also allows for identification of the feeding arteries and draining veins of the AVM without severe damage to the spinal cord. A special attempt should be made to preserve the Adamkiewicz artery.

Figure 14.5 shows an AVM in the thoracic area of the spinal cord before the operation and after clipping of the afferent artery and transection of the pathological vessels of the AVM. The AVM was supplied by the Adamkiewicz artery, the stem of which, as the control angiogram confirmed, was kept intact. The malformation did not appear on the control angiogram. Figure 14.6 shows the stages of removal of a spinal cord AVM.

◁——————————————————————————————————————

Figure 14.5. AVM of the spinal cord (A-P and lateral projections) deriving its vascular supply from a hypertrophied artery of Adamkiewicz (as shown by *arrows*). **A,** A conglomerate of vessels located at the D_{11} vertebral level. **B,** Selective spinal angiography after clipping and coagulation of the malformation demonstrates its exclusion from the circulation (artery of Adamkiewicz is indicated by *arrows*) and its location on the ventral surface of the spinal cord.

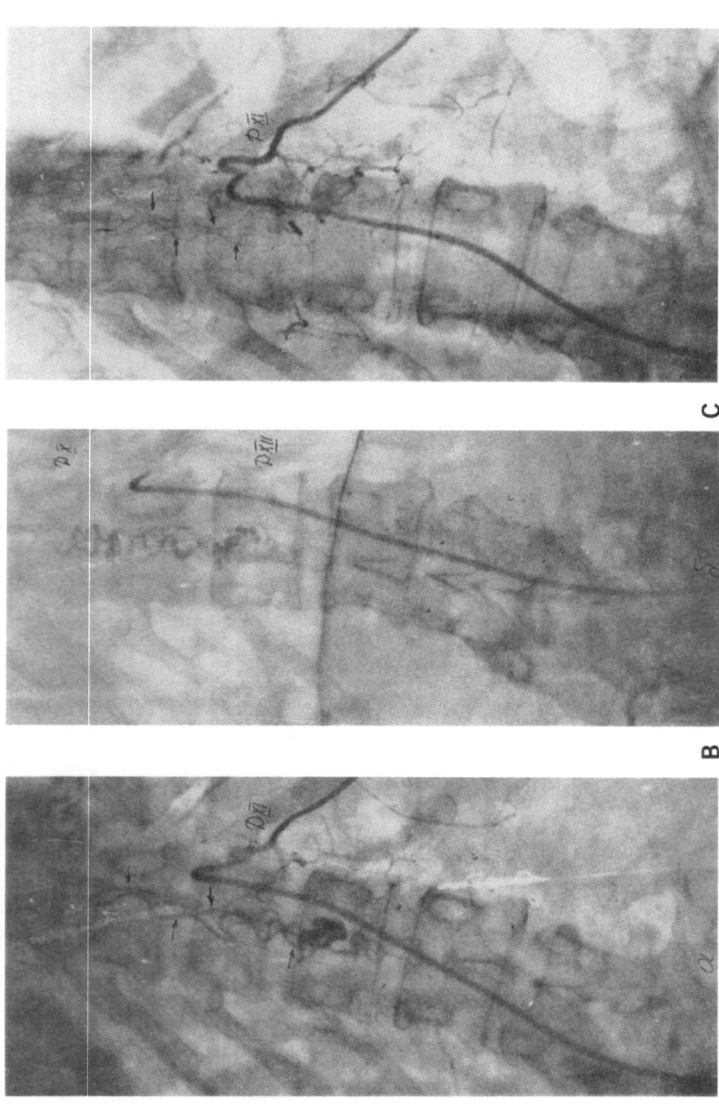

Figure 14.7. A, AVM of the thoracic portion of the spinal cord at the D_{10} to D_{12} vertebral levels (anterior projection). The malformation derives its vascular supply from a large radicular artery (indicated by *arrows*) and the D_{11} vertebral level. **B**, Venous phase. **C**, Selective angiography after coagulation of the malformation discloses the absence of contrast in the malformation. The afferent artery is smaller in diameter (as indicated by *arrows*).

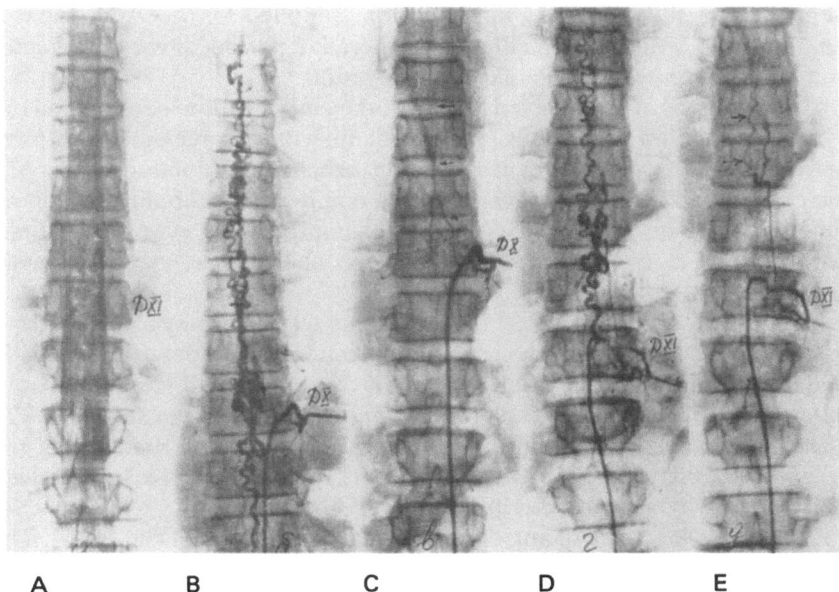

A   B   C   D   E

Figure 14.8. AVM of the thoracic portion of the spinal cord in an 11-year-old girl extending from the D_4 to D_{10} vertebral levels, which derives its blood supply from 2 radicular arteries at the D_{10} to D_{11} levels on the left. **A,** Myelogram. **B,** An extensive AVM lying on the ventrolateral surface of the spinal cord. **C,** Selective angiography after embolization demonstrates the complete occlusion of the malformation from the circulation with preservation of the anterior spinal artery (as shown by *arrows*). **D,** The second source of blood supply to the malformation is at the D_{11} vertebral level. **E,** A selective angiographic study disclosed the exclusion of the basic portion (nidus) of the malformation with preservation of the draining vein (*arrows*).

Figure 14.7 shows a second observed case of AVM in the thoracic area of the spinal cord pre- and postoperation, where the afferent arteries of the AVM were clipped and occlusion of the pathological vessels of the AVM occurred. The control angiogram showed the absence of contrast in the AVM. The vascular system of the spinal cord was preserved. The above-mentioned manipulations, performed on the afferent arteries of the malformation and on the adjacent normal stems, are impossible without microsurgical techniques and operational optics.

As has been mentioned earlier, in 11 patients AVMs were supplied by the Adamkiewicz artery. The embolization of this artery must be carried out taking care not to occlude it in the proximal area or at the level where the ascending branch arises (in our material this occurred in six cases) (Fig. 14.8), otherwise the patient may experience threatening neurological complications, analogous to the occlusion of the anterior spinal artery. Evalua-

312 Y.M. Filatov, T.P. Tissen, and S.S. Eliava

tion of the results of AVM embolization, supplied by the Adamkiewicz artery during both the immediate postoperative period, several days later and after several years, brought positive results.

Examinations of the delayed results of the embolization were carried out 1 to 12 years after operations. In 12 patients with paraplegia of the lower extremities, sensory disturbances, and disturbances of functions in the pelvic organs, significant improvement was noted, after embolization, in all functions in four patients. No significant improvement was noted in six patients, and in two patients no changes in neurological symptoms were noted.

The second group consisted of 14 patients with paraplegia of the lower extremities, sensory disturbances, and functional disorders of the GUS. Significant improvement of all functions was noted in 13 cases; functions deteriorated in one patient. Deterioration arose during the second AVM embolization and resulted in thrombosis of the ascending branches of the Adamkiewicz artery (Fig. 14.9a, b). Later, the patient experienced deep spastic paraparesis with deterioration of GUS functions.

In 7 to 10 days, control angiograms revealed occlusion of the AVM. The result was a decrease in diameter of the afferent vessel and neurological symptoms quickly regressed.

Classification of spinal cord AVMs is based upon angiographic indicators and a developing clinical picture. Malformations, which are supplied by the system of anterior spinal arteries are, as a rule, intramedullary. In these cases the radicular artery usually participates in supplying blood to the AVM. Blood can flow from the AVM in two possible directions: anterograde or retrograde, along the anterior spinal vein or along the radicular vein. Transection of the afferent vessel should be made carefully in order to avoid blocking the anterior spinal artery in the proximal area. In some cases during embolization the draining vein should be fully preserved, whereas the anterior and posterior spinal veins can be occluded together with the nidus of the AVM.

According to localization, in 21 cases AVMs were distributed on the anterior surface of the spinal cord (eight of these were intramedullary), in nine cases on the posterior surface. In all 14 cases where the direct surgical approach was used, AVMs were distributed on the posterior or posterior lateral surfaces of the spinal cord.

AVMs located on the posterior surface of the spinal cord, supplied by the radicular arteries (usually a single one), clinically at first show sensory disturbances that progress to motor deterioration. AVMs of the aforementioned localization can have extremely serious consequences if left untreated. All patients with AVMs in the dorsal area had total occlusion from the blood supply to the spinal cord and continuing regression of neurological symptoms as well as improvement of sociological rehabilitation.

It is interesting to note that pain syndromes were evident in 23 cases, including five patients who did not suffer subarachnoid hemorrhages. Disappearance of pain syndrome was noted in all cases after embolization.

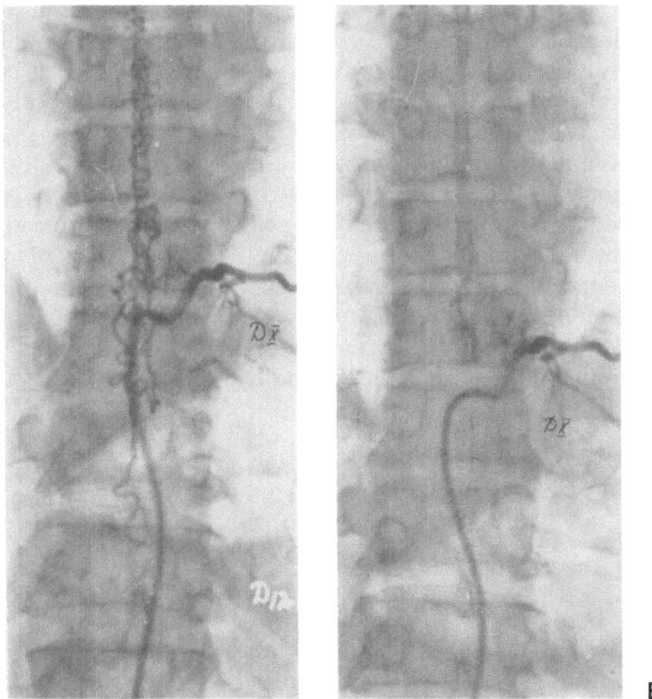

A   B

Figure 14.9. AVM located on the posterior surface of the thoracic portion of the spinal cord. **A**, Angiogram of the AVM at the D_6 to D_{10} vertebral levels deriving its blood supply from a short posterior radicular artery of the intercostal trunk at the D_9 vertebral level on the left. **B**, A selective study of the afferent vessel during embolization demonstrates the exclusion of the malformation from the circulation and the preservation of the patency of the spinal artery (9).

After analysis of neurological changes that occurred as a result of embolization of spinal cord AVMs at various levels, we can state with assurance that the endovascular aberrant vessels have been occluded with positive clinical results, even in patients with paraplegia and tetraplegia. Neurological improvement after embolization allowed a larger group of patients, formerly without hope, to resume their professional and social lives.

Summary

Greater emphasis has been placed on endovascular methods in the treatment of AVMs. Embolization of spinal cord AVMs was performed at various levels of the spinal cord in 30 patients, ages 6 to 58 years. Fragments of hemostatic sponge "spongostan" and PVA particles (0.2 to 0.5 mm)

were used as thrombogenic substances. Afferent vessels were occluded using detachable balloons, according to the Serbinenko method, in two patients, children, with AVMs. AVMs were distributed in the cervical area of the spinal cord in 4 patients, in the thoracic area in 20 patients, and in the lumbar area in 6 patients. Twenty patients experienced significant improvement in neurological status after embolization and occlusion, by balloon, of the AVM; the spinal cord was affected to varying degrees including paraplegia and tetraplegia. Social activity resumed after endovascular surgery; several patients returned to their previous work. No significant improvement was observed in six patients; no changes in neurological status were noted in three (Table 14.1). Deterioration, in connection with increasing thrombosis of the ascending branch of the Adamkiewicz artery, occurred in one patient after the second embolism.

References

1. Tissen TP. Selective spinal angiography. In: Konovalov AN, Romodanov AP, Filatov UM, Lyass FM, Vassin HYA, eds. *Neurosurgical Pathology of Cerebral Vessels.* Moscow, 1974:173–183.
2. Newton TH, Adams JE. Angiographic demonstration and nonsurgical embolization of spinal cord angiomas. *Radiology.* 1968;91:873–876.
3. Djindjian R, Houdart R, Cophignon J, Hurth M, Comoy J. Premiers essais d'embolisation par voie fémorale de fragments de muscle dans un cas d'angiome médullaire et dans un cas d'angiome alimenté par la carotide externe. *Rev Neurol.* 1971;125/2:119–130.
4. Doppman JL, Di Chiro G, Ommaya AK. Percutaneous embolization of spinal cord arteriovenous malformations. 1971;34:48.
5. Voigt K. Interventionale Neuroradiologie. II. Vertebro-spinale embolisationen. *Der Radiologe.* 1981;21:227–236.
6. Scialta G, Scotti G, Biondi A, De Grandi C. Embolization of vascular malformations of the spinal cord. *J Neurosurg Sci.* 1985;29:I,I–9.
7. Rosenblum BR, Oldfield EH, Doppman JL, Di Chiro G. Spinal arteriovenous malformations: a comparison of dural arteriovenous fistulas and intradural AVM's in 81 patients. *J Neurosurg.* 1987;67:795.
8. Tissen TP. In: *Endovascular (Catheterization) Therapy.* Moscow, 1979:25–26.
9. Serbinenko FA. The possibilities of a method to catheterize and occlude cerebral blood vessels. In: Konovalov AN, Romodanov AP, Filatov UM, Lyass FM, Vassin HYA, eds. *Neurosurgical Pathology of Cerebral Vessels.* Moscow, 1974:221–233.

CHAPTER 15

Syringomyelia

J. Lobo Antunes

The choice of syringomyelia as one of the topics in a seminar dedicated to spinal cord pathology is, in my view, quite fitting. This is not a new disorder. In fact, cavitation of the spinal cord was already recognized by Estienne in 1546,[1] and the term "syringomyelia," meaning literally "cavity within the spinal cord" was coined by Olivier d'Angers in 1827.[2] One other important landmark in the history of this condition is the distinction between hydromyelia, in which the cavity results from the dilatation of the central canal, and syringomyelia, in which the two are independent, made by Simon.[3]

Yet the diagnosis still often eludes us, we still argue about the correct method of treating it, and the mechanisms of its development are, to this day, controversial.

Two other contributions to our understanding of the disease should be mentioned. First, the description by Chiari of the various congenital anomalies of the posterior fossa, and the recognition of their association with syringomyelia.[4] Second, the seminal work by Gardner, who proposed a rational therapeutic approach based on a pathophysiological interpretation of this condition.[5,6]

The introduction of magnetic resonance imaging (MRI) represents a major step in the early diagnosis of syringomyelia and may help in clarifying how it develops.

The pathological changes in the spinal cord in cases of syringomyelia are not limited to a dilated central canal with a perserved ependymal lining, or a simple cyst with a glial wall. In fact, there are many secondary changes including neuronal loss, demyelination, not only of the decussating tracts, but also of the long ascending and descending pathways, and, to a variable degree, edema and gliosis. These alterations may actually extend quite far below the level of the cavity, and certainly explain why a number of these patients do not respond to any therapeutic maneuver (Fig. 15.1).

Furthermore, there are also vascular changes, such as thickening of the wall, and hyalinization and endothelial hyperplasia. These may lead to hemorrhage within the syrinx, which may be the cause of the sudden

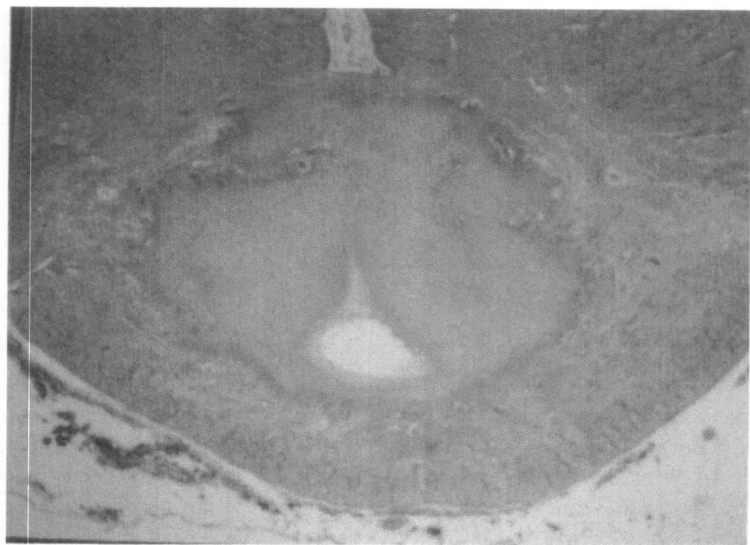

Figure 15.1. Syringomyelia, thoracic cord. Note the marked gliosis surrounding the dilated central canal.

deterioration of a previously stable clinical picture. This was actually described by Gowers many years ago.[7]

Rarely, the disease extends to the medulla (syringobulbia). In this location, there is usually not a well formed cavity but a slit that comes deeply from the floor of the fourth ventricle. The association of syringomyelia and syringobulbia is, however, exceedingly rare.

The classification of the various types of syringomyelia that is usually accepted is the one suggested by Barnett,[8] which we have simplified as Table 15.1.

For practical purposes, there are in fact three types of syringomyelia. The first, and more common one, is the *communicating* form of the disorder or

Table 15.1. Classification of syringomyelia.

Communicating syringomyelia (hydromyelia)
  Secondary to congenital abnormalities, e.g. Chiari type I and type II malformations
  Secondary to acquired lesions, e.g., basal arachnoiditis, posterior fossa tumors, hydrocephalus, etc.

Noncommunicating syringomyelia
  Posttraumatic, arachnoiditis, spinal cord tumors, etc.

Idiopathic syringomyelia

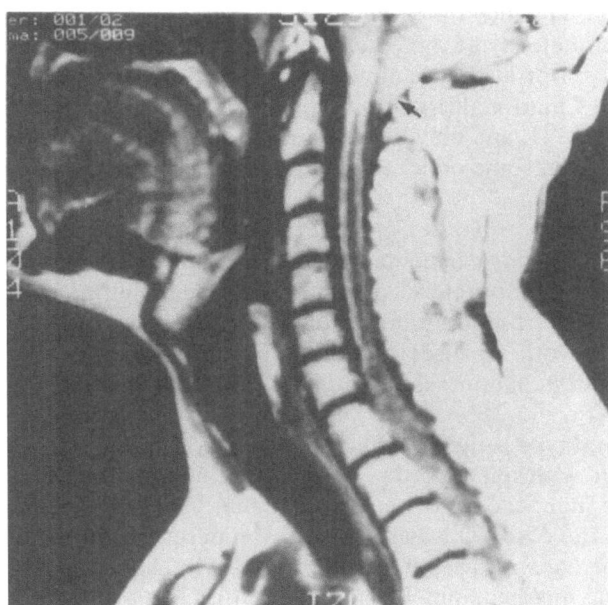

Figure 15.2A. MRI of a syringomyelia secondary to a Chiari I malformation. Note the descended tonsil (*arrow*). (TR = 600 msec; TE = 30 msec).

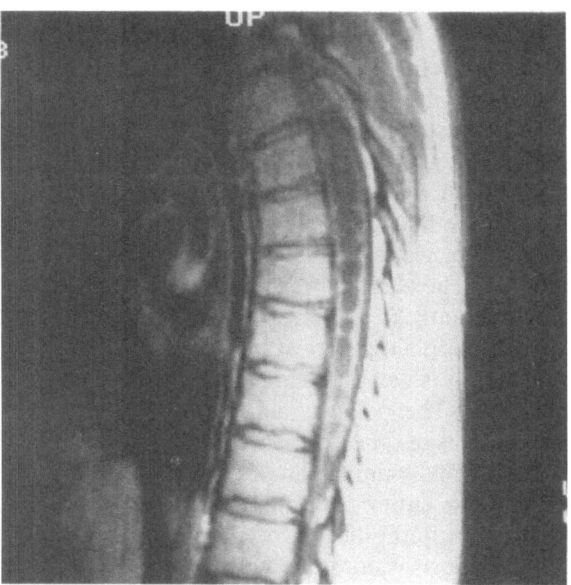

Figure 15.2B. Same case; thoracic spinal cord. Segmentation of the syrinx is quite obvious (TR = 500 msec; TE = 220 msec).

hydromyelia, in which the pathological substrate is a dilated central canal. In the great majority of the cases it is due to pathological processes in the posterior fossa or at the craniovertebral junction. Probably the most frequent is the Chiari malformation type I (Fig. 15.2). It may also be due to the Chiari type II, and may be the cause of the late neurological deterioration observed in some children who have been operated on for meningomyeloceles.

In recent years a number of rather interesting cases of acquired Chiari I malformations have been reported. These have developed in patients who received lumboureteral or lumboperitoneal shunts for treatment of hydrocephalus or pseudotumor cerebri.[9]

Among the other causes of communicating syringomyelia, we should mention brain stem or cerebellar tumors, basal arachnoiditis, and posterior fossa cysts (Fig. 15.3).

The second type is the *noncommunicating syringomyelia*, which is usually associated with spinal cord pathology. In this situation, the syrinx cavity may not be independent of the central canal, and may be due to ischemic necrosis of the cord. This variety has been described in patients who suffered spinal cord injuries,[10] or associated with intrinsic tumors such as astrocytomas and hemangioblastomas.[11] Other less common causes are extradural compressive lesions such as metastatic tumors or Pott's disease.

The third type includes the *idiopathic* cases. In these patients we are unable to define a causal lesion. I believe, however, that the use of MRI will reduce substantially the number of patients that have to be fitted into this category.

This classification is quite useful because it has pathogenetic, and, as we will see, therapeutic implications.

As far as the clinical manifestations of the disease I will focus mainly on the communicating type. The age spectrum is quite wide, but the disease affects mostly people in the third and fourth decades of life.

It is important to emphasize that if we are waiting for the typical syringomyelia syndrome to develop, we will miss the correct diagnosis in a substantial number of patients. The clinical presentation is deceptive, and the symptoms may actually fluctuate, to a point that the diagnosis of multiple sclerosis has been entertained in a number of our cases. Probably the most common form of presentation is weakness and sensory changes in a distal segment of one upper limb. The patients complain of loss of dexterity, atrophy of the intrinsic muscles of the hand, and numbness with an "ulnar" distribution. The picture is usually unilateral or at least asymmetrical in its intensity. Quite often patients suffer from pain, which may be of several different types—nuchal or occipital discomfort, or with a radicular or interscapular distribution. Scoliosis is not uncommon in the younger patients (Fig. 15.3). Syncope, lower cranial nerve dysfunction, and numbness in the trigeminal region have all been reported.

We have previously analyzed a series of 60 patients and have found mul-

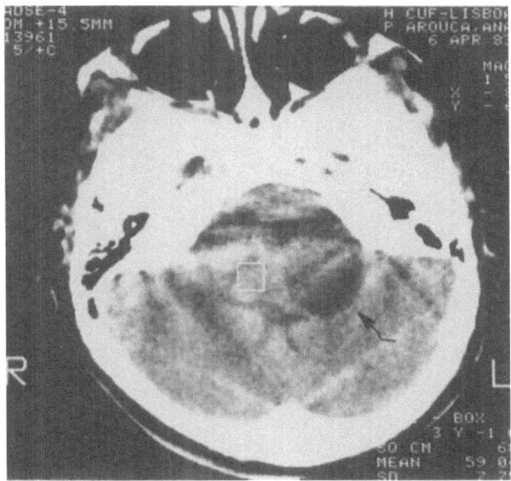

Figure 15.3A. CT scan of a patient with a syringomyelia demonstrating the presence of a posterior fossa cyst (*arrow*).

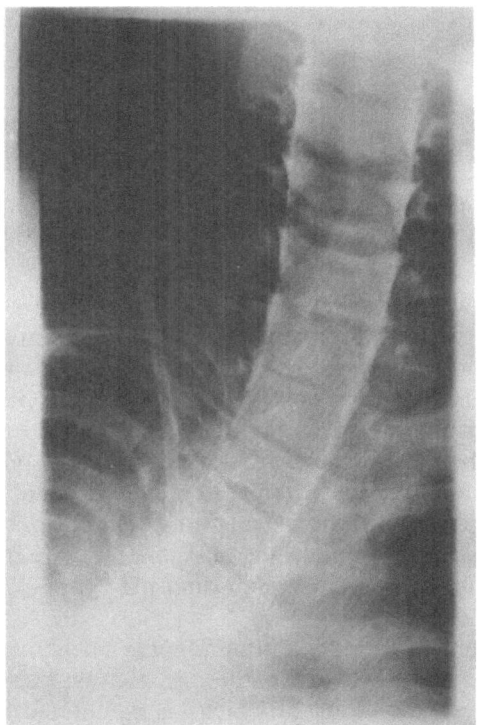

Figure 15.3B. Same case. Myelography demonstrates a widened cord.

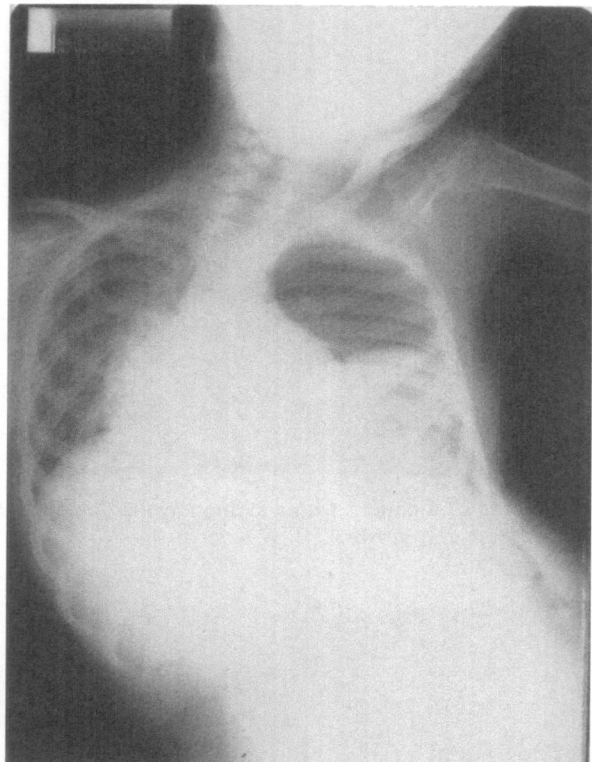

Figure 15.3C. Same case. Marked scoliosis is also present.

tiple patterns of weakness and sensory and reflex changes.[12] These do not depend only on the location and extension of the syrinx. In other words, there is not a good clinical radiological correlation. Although the radiographic appraisal of our patients was performed before MRI was introduced, we do not believe from our experience and others' that the MRI will change this point.[13] It seems, therefore, that the spinal cord does not respond in a monotonous way to the distending forces of the syrinx cavity, and edema, gliosis, and vascular changes may all play a role.

It still holds true that thermal and pain modalities are more affected than the deep sensation or proprioception, and the "cape" hyposthesia is the most common pattern.

The involvement of the lower cranial nerve in these patients is due in most instances to the associated pathology, that is, the Chiari malformation, and not to the syrinx itself, which, as mentioned before, rarely extends to the level of the medulla.

We have been interested in studying the subclinical respiratory distur-

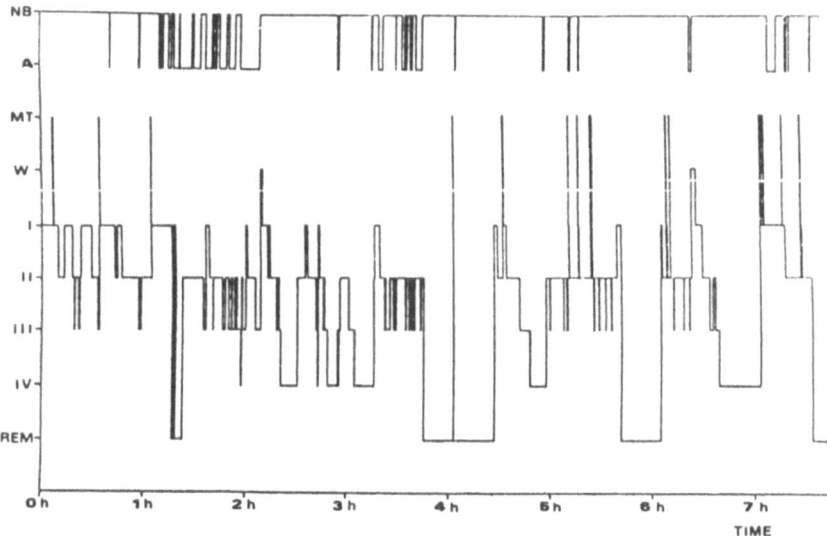

Figure 15.4. Hypnogram in a case of Chiari I malformation. NB, normal breathing; A, apnea episodes; MT, movement time; W, wakefulness time; I, stage I, NREM; II, stage II, NREM; III, stage III, NREM; IV, stage IV, NREM; REM, stage of REM sleep.

bances (Fig. 15.4) in these patients, which may become evident during sleep. In fact, sleep apnea has been described in the Chiari malformation, and it is probably one of the causes of unexplained death after posterior fossa decompression. We have found that these patients have a decreased percentage of rapid eye movement (REM), decreased number of REM cycles, and shortened REM periods. The number and duration of hypoventilation periods is significantly higher in this population of patients.

To confirm the diagnosis of syringomyelia, it is absolutely necessary to document the presence of a cavity within the spinal cord, which usually determines an enlargement of its diameter.

Myelography was initially the only technique available, and diagnosis was based on the demonstration of a dilated cord, involving predominantly the lower cervical and upper thoracic segments, which collapsed, with changes in the position of the patient.[14] This was particularly well documented with pneumomyelography and occurred in 85% of our cases. In two of these, progression of the lesion over the years was well demonstrated. In some cases, one was able to visualize the presence of contrast medium within the dilated canal. With the introduction of the computed tomography (CT) scan the diagnosis was simplified; the widened cord was easily visualized and late films obtained 6 to 12 hours after subarachnoid instillation of water-soluble contrast medium clearly depicted the central

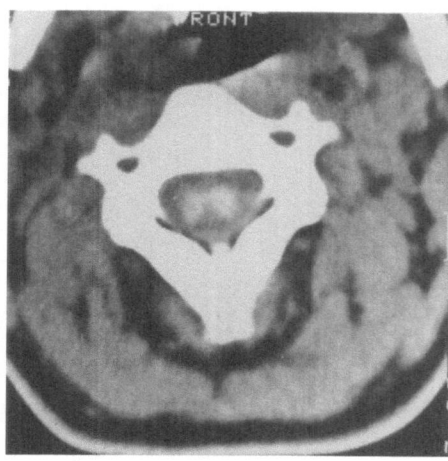

Figure 15.5. Communicating syringomyelia. The cyst is well demonstrated in this CT scan of the cervical spine obtained 6 hours after the subarachnoid instillation of metrizamide.

cavity (Fig. 15.5). It is important to emphasize, however, that the same phenomenon occurs in other conditions, such as cervical myelopathy (Fig. 15.6) or spinal cord tumors.

It should be mentioned that there may be skeletal anomalies in these patients and plain spine films should always be performed. We have encountered various congenital lesions such as occiput-C1 fusion, Klippel-Feil's syndrome, basilar impression (Fig. 15.7), fused ribs, absent vertebral pedicles, and so forth.

The diagnosis of the disorder was extremely simplified with the introduction of MRI. With this technique it became easy to demonstrate the extension of the lesion, its likely etiology, the presence of areas of edema, gliosis, or malacia, and the pulsatility of the syrinx cavity.[16,17] This technique thus helps to decide which therapeutic option should be adopted, and will probably allow to delineate better the prognosis of the individual patient. It may be important, for instance, to try to find out whether or not patients who show a pulsatile syrinx are better candidates for surgery than the ones with wide subarachnoid spaces and flat, atrophic cords. MRI will also be quite useful in following patients postoperatively. Indeed, the goal in these patients will be to reduce the size of syrinx and reestablish normal spinal fluid circulation.

When discussing the treatment of syringomyelia, one should be reminded that the natural history of the disorder is somewhat unpredictable.[18,19] We have followed several patients who have not shown any deterioration over periods of several years. There seems to be no role for

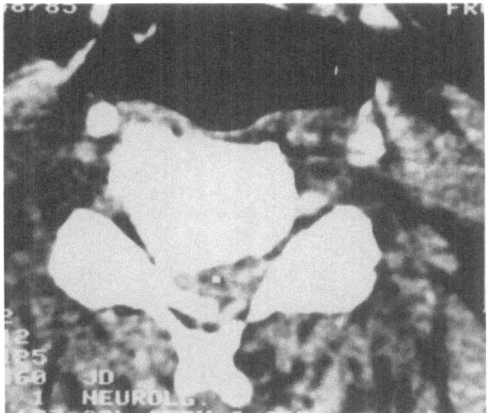

Figure 15.6. Spondylotic cervical myelopathy. **A**, CT scan demonstrates a cavity within the cord (*white square*).

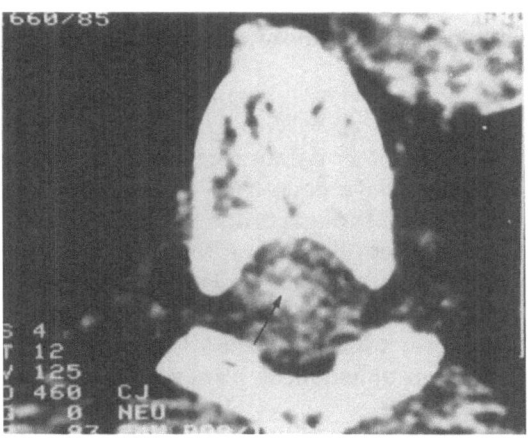

Figure 15.6B. At the thoracic level and after administration of metrizamide intrathecally the syrinx cavity is demonstrated (*arrow*).

prophylactic surgery, and one should only operate on those patients in whom neurological deterioration is clearly occurring or who complain of unbearable pain.

There are a number of therapeutic alternatives for these patients and the choice of the correct one depends mainly on the etiology of the syrinx.[12]

In the noncommunicating variety, the goal is to make the cyst communicate with the subarachnoid space or, with a free cavity, such as the peri-

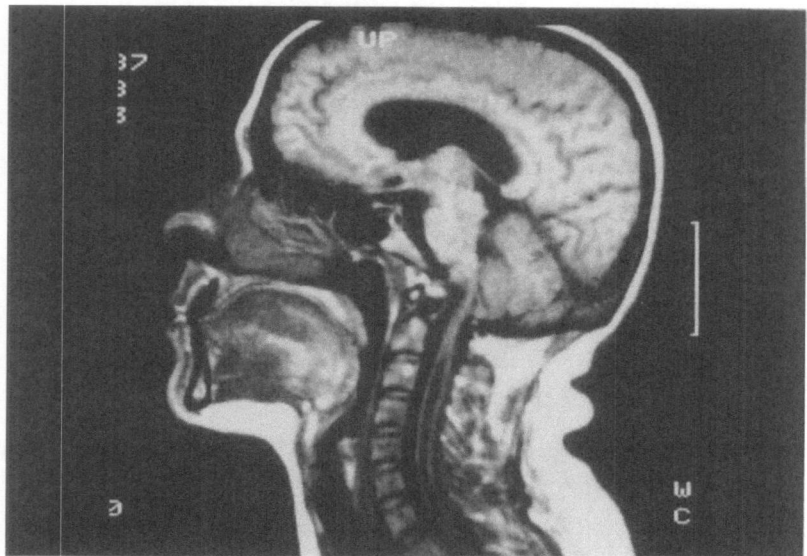

Figure 15.7. Syringomyelia secondary to a basilar impression. (TR = 600 msec; TE = 20 msec).

toneum. Simple myelotomies[20] do not seem to be as effective, although a great number of devices have been tried to keep open the communication.[21] The advantages of syringoperitoneal shunts are to create larger pressure differences, and not depend on the patency of the subarachnoid space, which is often compromised.[22,23] For the cases in whom the cavity extends all the way down to the filum terminale, Gardner proposed the section of this structure, which he called "terminal ventriculostomy".[24] The technique has been abandoned, however, because it afforded only temporary relief.[25]

In cases of the communicating type, one should address the causal pathology and only perform syringostomies or syringoperitoneal shunts if the original surgery fails. In cases of Chiari I malformation, adequate decompression of the lower occiput and the posterior arches of the upper cervical vertebrae until one goes beyond the descended tonsils is necessary.[26-28] A duroplasty should be performed but, in my opinion, there is no need, and it may indeed be dangerous to plug the obex, to perform extensive dissections of the arachnoid around the tonsils, or to open the syrinx cavity. These patients may have difficult postoperative courses, and should be watched closely for the development of autonomic disturbances or hydrocephalus.

About 10% of the patients have hydrocephalus; this has to be dealt with first and may result in significant improvement.[29]

The percutaneous aspiration of the cord first proposed by Vitek[30] and widely used by Schlesinger may be quite useful and give a long-lasting amelioration.

Radiotherapy plays no role in the treatment of this condition.

It should be mentioned that whatever the technique used, improvement or stabilization of the clinical course does not exceed 60% to 70% of the cases. A number of these patients, however, will show recurrence of symptoms. The problem is not so much what to do first, but what to do next. In patients who have already been submitted to a posterior fossa decompression it is of no use to go back. One has therefore to deal directly with the syrinx cavity. When myelotomies or shunts were the original procedures, we are forced to re-operate and try to establish a more durable communication.

References

1. Estienne C quoted by Foster JB, Hudgson P. Historical introduction. In: Barnett HJM, Foster JB, Hudgson P, eds. *Syringomyelia*. London: WB Saunders; 1973:3–10.
2. Olivier d'Angers CP. *Traité de la Moelle Épinière et de ses Maladies*. Paris: Chez Crevot, 1827.
3. Simon T. Uber Syringomyelie und Geschwulstbildung im Rückenmark. *Arch Psychiatrie Nervenkrankheiten*. 1875;5:120.
4. Chiari H. Uber Veränderungen des Kleinhirns infolge von Hydrocephalie des Grosshirns. *Deutsche Med Wochenschrift*. 1891;17:1172.
5. Gardner WJ. Hydrodynamic mechanism of syringomyelia: Its relationship to myelocele. *J Neurol Neurosurg Psychiatry*. 1965;28:247–259.
6. Gardner WJ, Abdullah AF, McCormack LJ. Varying expressions of embryonal atresia of fourth ventricle in adults. Arnold-Chiari malformation, Dandy-Walker syndrome, "arachnoid" cyst of the cerebellum and syringomyelia. *J Neurosurg*. 1957;14:591–607.
7. Sedzimir CB, Roberts JR, Occleshaw JV, Buxton PH. Gowers' syringal hemorrhage. *J Neurol Neurosurg Psychiatry*. 1974;37:312–315.
8. Barnett HJM. The epilogue. In: Barnett HJM, Foster JB, Hudgson P, eds. *Syringomyelia*. London: WB Saunders; 1973:303–313.
9. Fischer EG, Welch K, Shilltio J. Syringomyelia following communicating lumboureteral shunting for communicating hydrocephalus. *J Neurosurg*. 1977;47:96–100.
10. Rossier AB, Foo D, Shillito J, Dyro FM. Posttraumatic cervical syringomyelia. *Brain*. 1985;108:439–461.
11. Barnett HJM, Newcastle NP. Syringomyelia and tumours of the nervous system. In: Barnett HJM, Foster JB, Hudgson P, eds. *Syringomyelia*. London: WB Saunders; 1973:261–301.
12. Schlesinger EB, Antunes JL, Michelsen WJ, Louis KM. Hydromyelia: Clinical presentation and comparison of modalities of treatment. *Neurosurgery*. 1981;9:356–365.
13. Grant R, Hadley DM, MacPherson P, et al. Syringomyelia: Cyst measurement by magnetic resonance imaging and comparison with symptoms, signs and disability. *J Neurol Neurosurg Psychiatry*. 1987;50:1008–1044.
14. Heinz ER, Schlesinger EB, Potts DG. Radiologic signs of hydromyelia. *Radiology*. 1966;86:311–318.
15. Gates PC, Fox AJ, Barnett HJM. CT metrizamide myelography in syringomyelia: Sensitivity and specificity. *Neurology*. 1986;36:1245–1248.
16. Enzmann DR, O'Donohue J, Rubin JB, Shuer L, Gogen P, Silverberg G. CSF pulsations within nonneoplastic spinal cord cysts. *Am J Radiol*. 1987;149:149–157.
17. Sherman JL, Barkovich AJ, Citrin CM. The MR appearance of syringomyelia: New observations. *Am J Radiol*. 1987;148:381–391.
18. Boman K, Iivanainen M. Prognosis of syringomyelia. *Acta Neurol Scand*. 1967;43:61–68.
19. Anderson NE, Willoughby EW, Wrightson P. The natural history and influence of surgical treatment in syringomyelia. *Acta Neurol Scand*. 1985;71:472–479.

20. Abbe R, Coley WB. Syringomyelia, operation-exploration of cord, withdrawal of fluid, exhibition of patient. *J Nerv Ment Dis.* 1892;19:512.

21. Love JG, Olofson RA. Syringomyelia: A look at surgical therapy. *J Neurosurg.* 1966;24:714–718.

22. Barbaro NM, Wilson CB, Gutin PH, Edwards MSB. Surgical treatment of syringomyelia. Favorable results with syringoperitoneal shunting. *J Neurosurg.* 1984;61:531–538.

23. Suzuki M, Davis C, Symon L, Gentili F. Syringoperitoneal shunt for treatment of cord cavitation. *J Neurol Neurosurg Psychiatry.* 1985;48:620–627.

24. Gardner WJ, Bell HS, Poolos PN, Dohn DF, Steinberg M. Terminal ventriculostomy for syringomyelia. *J Neurosurg.* 1977;46:609–617.

25. Williams B, Fahy G. A critical appraisal of "terminal ventriculostomy" for the treatment of syringomyelia. *J Neurosurg.* 1983;58:188–197.

26. Rhoton Jr AL. Microsurgery of Arnold-Chiari malformation with and without hydromyelia. *J Neurosurg.* 1976;45:473–483.

27. Logue V, Edwards MR. Syringomyelia and its surgical treatment. *J Neurol Neurosurg Psychiatry.* 1981;44:273–284.

28. Williams B. A critical appraisal of posterior fossa surgery for communicating syringomyelia. *Brain.* 1978;101:223–250.

29. Krayenbühl H, Benini A. A new surgical approach in the treatment of hydromyelia and syringomyelia: The embryological basis and the first results. *J R Coll Surg Edinb.* 1971;16:147.

30. Vitek J. La ponction dorsal thérapeutique et diagnostique des cavités syringomyéliques. *Brux Med.* 1929;9:311–312.

Discussion

Spinal Stabilization in Posttraumatic Syringomyelia

Dr. Schlesinger noted that spinal fusions play an important role in the prevention of posttraumatic syringomyelia particularly after decompressive laminectomies. He believes that the incidence of posttraumatic syringomyelia would be less if more attention were paid to spinal stabilization in patients with traumatic paraplegia. He believes that the syringomyelia in these patients is due to spinal cord tethering and scar formation at the level of injury combined with local instability.

Dr. Antunes added that most of the patients in his experience are patients who have suffered thoracic spinal cord injuries and these are relatively stable after a long period of bedrest. Syrinxes are much more common in the thoracic than in the cervical spine for some reason.

Dr. Antunes: The problem of posttraumatic syringomyelia is a rather interesting one. These patients are usually seen in the large rehabilitation centers and in a recent series published by Rossier et al. the incidence was about 3%. A number of patients treated conservatively remained quite stable.

Surgical results in most patients who were operated because of progressive motor incapacity or pain were quite good. I have found no reference to the question of whether or not spinal instability contributes to the development of syringomyelia.

Management of Syringomyelia in the Soviet Centers

Dr. Livshitz indicated that they performed a drainage of the cysts with silicon tube to the subarachnoid space by microsurgical technique.

Correlation Between Pathology and the Severity of Symptoms

Dr. Kliot raised the question of the correlation between the severity of symptoms and the observed pathology in syringomyelia. He indicated that Dr. Antunes suggested that patients with gliosis in addition to their syrinxes might do worse and other patients with massive compromise of the cord experienced clinical recoveries.

Dr. Antunes responded: The pathological process involves both the white and the gray matter, and there is indeed neuronal loss. The destruction of anterior horn cells, for example, explains the atrophies of the small hand muscles. As you know there are very few good pathological studies of patients with syringomyelia. I am sure there is an element of pressure because when surgeons relieve the pressure by drainage clinical improvement is seen. The point I was trying to raise is that the pathophysiological mechanism is not simply one of pressure. There are a number of secondary changes. In the past when we observed small spinal cords on myelography and CT scanning we felt the patients would not be good surgical candidates and indeed they usually did not show significant clinical improvement. The situation was different in patients with large spinal cords and large cavities, which strongly implicated pressure as one of the mechanisms. I think that MRI would be helpful in trying to establish this correlation if it can show us gliosis. In addition, if it can show us pulsations within the cord and that these pulsations are shifted from the syringomyelic cavity to the subarachnoid space, then clinical and pathophysiological correlations can be better established.

Dr. Kliot asked if any blood flow studies or PET scans have been useful in analyzing this problem. Dr. Antunes said, No.

The Arnold–Chiari Malformation and Syringomyelia

Dr. Marin-Padilla said, I have been interested in the embryology of the occipital and cervical regions for a long time. I have always complained that radiologists and surgeons do not care much about the occipital bone—they seem concerned primarily with what is contained within the bony compartment. I have always contended that there are many cases in which the primary bony abnormalities may be the cause of these problems.

When you discussed the Arnold–Chiari malformation you never mentioned that the posterior fossa is very small; you never mentioned that the planum nuchale of the occipital bone is very small; you never mentioned that the angle of the base of the skull is very small, yet you did mention that the cervical spinal canal is very wide. What is the explanation for this and what is the explanation for the Arnold–Chiari malformation?

I produced the Arnold–Chiari malformation experimentally by creating a lesion in the paraaxial mesoderm that resulted in hypoplasia of the occipital bone. The occipital bone is a modified vertebra. It actually represents a fusion of three somites into a single bone. These somites give rise to three occipital vertebrae that are incorporated as a single bone into the occiput. Somitic abnormalities induced by vitamin A affect not only the occipital somites, but also the widening of the vertebral canal. Therefore, we are looking into something extremely primitive, occurring much earlier than the development of the brain, cerebellum, or spinal cord. When these lesions are produced in an embryo it is possible to follow their progress leading to the development of a very small posterior fossa.

When growth continues postnatally and the enlarging cerebellum is compelled to occupy this small cavity, the response is a downward herniation that leads to the obliteration of the spinal canal. I am sure some of these instances are explained by very early primary mesodermal abnormalities. In addition, if the aqueduct of Sylvius is sufficiently compressed because of the tight packing of the posterior fossa contents, then hydrocephalus will ensue, which in turn will push down the tentorium and further increase the posterior fossa pressure and the resultant herniation.

You have discussed the problem of decompression of the Arnold–Chiari malformation and stressed that the decompression requires opening of the foramen magnum. I disagree. There is no problem with the foramen magnum. The foramen is very big. It is the posterior fossa that has to be decompressed. I suggested previously that a nuchalectomy is what must be accomplished. You must decompress the posterior fossa and open it wide and laterally.

I believe that this is especially true for children with a familial incidence of spina bifida with or without meningocoeles that they will develop the Arnold–Chiari malformation, in particular, type II.

Similarly, I believe that Paget's disease, which produces a reduction of the size of the posterior fossa, can result in a secondarily induced Arnold–Chiari malformation in adults.[1]

Dr. Antunes responded, you are right as far as posterior fossa decompression is concerned, but the point we wanted to make is that you do not have to do a very wide decompression. It is not necessary to expose the dura all the way to the sinuses as we would in tumor surgery. On the other hand, if you are operating on a child with Arnold–Chiari malformation type II you probably should not go farther than the foramen magnum. I think your point about Paget's disease is interesting and may be something Dr. Bello would be interested in looking at since I do not recall ever seeing or having read about syringomyelia in Paget's disease. Last, I feel that the widening of the cervical spinal canal is a consequence of the enlarged spinal cord.

Dr. Marin-Padilla said, there is plenty of space in the canal you can actually see it in the newborn. In the newborn with Arnold–Chiari there is widening of the canal and there is no syringomyelia at that time. This is a congenital anomaly.

Dr. Leeds said we do not use the term Arnold–Chiari malformation—we use Chiari I or cerebellar ectopia and we believe its incidence is about 50%. I think it is a mesenchymal abnormality that occurs at about the time that cerebellar ectopia occurs. We do not see it in Paget's because Paget's is a delayed phenomenon. It is in the bone so there is no relationship. You will see many cases of basilar invagination because of the softness of the base of the skull in achondroplastic dwarfs as well. We have been primarily looking at the cerebellar ectopia and not at the occipital bone. The occipital bone is different from the remainder of the calvarium. It is cartilaginous bone with four endochondral ossification centers. The association of Chiari malformation and a small posterior fossa and syringomyelia does not explain to me the whole problem of syringomyelia, namely, why some occur in the thoracic spinal cord, some in the cervical cord, and why some involve the entire extent of the cord. Also, we do not understand the "segmetation" that was initially seen with the cavity injections and now with MRI.

The French have a totally different attitude. They really believe that the syringomyelic cavity is filled via the Virchow-Robins spaces. We sometimes use the term "hydrosyringomyelia" and we think the pathogenetic mechanisms are hard to distinguish.

Dr. Schlesinger added that these points are well made. There have been questions addressing the genetic and embryological aspects of syringomyelia. However, there are many adult individuals with hydromyelia who show none of the stigmata of involvement of the occipital bone or widening of the vertebral canal. Dr. Antunes and I have cases published in the literature showing isolated cysts of the spinal cord who by chance were restudied and found to have full-blown hydromyelia.

Dr. Antunes added, in other words, there are many more idiopathic instances than was initially believed. Some of them will turn out to have tumors such as astrocytomas, even 20 to 30 years later.

Dr. Schlesinger continued, there are cases that show other bony changes. They show, what I, for lack of a better term, call fish vertebrae. These are vertical vertebrae, narrow and long. I have seen these in a number of genetic disorders and it points further to the importance of familial studies and genetic trees in these cases.

Dr. Leeds added, we have noticed now that we use water-soluble dye studies in patients with hydrocephalus that there have been instances of reflux down the central canal in patients without any evidence of hydromyelia. This suggests that there is flow through a patent obex and that the central canal may participate in diminishing the pressure in the hydrocephalic situation.

Technical Aspects of Decompression

Dr. Oldfield noted if decompression only is just as successful a treatment as decompression plus obex plugging or plus syringostomy as you suggested, and has been shown in a large series from the Cleveland Clinic why would one ever want to do the latter of the two procedures, particularly if the danger is greater and the benefits are equal?

Dr. Antunes responded that he participated in a roundtable discussion with Dr. Rhoton, who suggested the importance of doing two things in the management of syringomyelia, namely, decompressing the posterior fossa and placing a silicon tube in the syringomyelic cavity. During this discussion some participants said, well I have never had one of my patients return for failure of treatment and another participant said I have your patient Mr. So and So. It made an impact on me.

Of course, the question is, should both procedures be done at a single sitting or should they be staged and more importantly are both necessary? It is difficult to keep the silicon tube patent and draining and it may require revision. In addition, there are real risks in doing cervical laminectomies in patients with syringomyelia. They can develop a very severe swan-neck deformity that is difficult to treat. I have seen at least three such instances and I would recommend that one should avoid the cervical laminectomy. Apparently, even if a limited cervical laminectomy is performed, the swan-neck deformity may occur.

Dr. Antunes: You are right. The decompression that is performed does not have to extend all the way up to the torcula, and usually it is sufficient to remove the posterior arches of C-1 and C-2. The question is quite different for patients with Chiari type II malformations. In these cases, the laminectomy may have to be extended all the way down to C3-4 or even lower. On the other hand, it may not be necessary to open the occipital bone, and it may in fact be dangerous, due to the dural venous sinuses present in these small children.

The point about Paget's disease is well taken. Curiously, I do not recall any report concerning the association of these two disorders except when the Paget's involves the spinal column.

Dr. Oldfield added, your conclusions would be supported in the traumatic area by Giovanni DeChiro and his group. They recently completed a study consisting of noninvasive methods of examining the spinal cord such as MRI. What they did was just look at patients with posttraumatic paraplegia who did not necessarily have progressive symptoms. Every one of them had a localized syringomyelia so that most of those patients do not need treatment—only the minority who develop progressive symptoms at a later date.

Dr. Marin-Padilla suggested the plausibility of reconstructing the bony contour of the posterior fossa. In other words, enlarge the posterior fossa cavity so that it can properly accommodate the enlarging cerebellum. Dr. Antunes responded that it is possible to replace the bone of the posterior fossa just as when one performs a craniotomy, but most surgical procedures involve a craniectomy with bony removal. The cervical muscles provide sufficient protection. My experience with bony replacement is that it may result in bony overgrowth into the posterior fossa with further direct cerebellar and brain stem compression.

Draining the Syrinx

Dr. Friedman asked Dr. Hecht-Nielsen about the microchannel device he mentioned that could be used to bridge cut ends of the spinal cord and about the possibility of creating little spacers, something like an H-shape that has very fine wires on the sides of the H and place these spacers in a myelotomy incision. Would that be effective in maintaining the drainage of the syrinx?

Dr. Antunes said, it is not only the problem of draining the syrinx but the problem of keeping the subarachnoid spaces open. At the present time we have used T tubes, but there is nothing more vexing than taking care of cysts in the central nervous system.

Dr. Hecht-Nielsen said, I think the issue of having microporous devices where the actual size of the pores is below the size of cells can be done, might be useful. There is no question that it is now possible to build massive arrays of tubes, each of which is well below the size of any cell so that the tubes might remain porous since cellular material could not get in them.

Dr. Holtzman asked if the flow could be unidirectional.

Dr. Hecht-Nielsen responded that that was possible, but much more difficult. The problem with unidirectional flow is keeping the valves clear of build-up of various types. That system typically works only when you have rather pure material. It might also work best if you had not only the small tubes, but also an osmotic pore material that had pores so small that you could guarantee that only water molecules could get through. That is available as well, so that it is conceivable, depending on how effectively the wall of cells that form to block flow, that permeability could be maintained. Most tubes clog because they are large enough to permit particulate debris to enter. Once again, whether it will work or not depends on the permeability of the layer of cells that does emerge to block the flow. One other thought concerns the clinical use of optical fibers that can transmit extraordinary amounts of light and power that is now becoming available although without a certain clinical usefulness. One might think of a chronic implant where one fully expects the opening created to become clogged and blocked periodically, but then without any surgery one could simply connect this chronically implanted fiber and literally blow out the clogging material every 6 months or so and continue to open the passage even though it eventually clogs again. The question regarding its clinical usefulness would be the extent to which it creates an inflammatory response.

Dr. Schlesinger added that attempts have been made using the laser to fenestrate the cord with multiple small punctures with presumably lesser possibility of a glial reaction, but I do not know the long-term follow-up of that work by Dr. Cerullo. However, as Dr. Antunes pointed out, sometimes after spinal cord punctures the patients had an inordinately long period of improvement. Undoubtedly in those patients, the spinal cord had become so attenuated and its structure such that the simple puncture allowed it to "weep" and act as an ostomy almost in perpetuity, because some of the patients did sustain their improved status.

Dr. Antunes added that there may well have been an additional factor of the venous pressure that may be reversed when the cord has become collapsed and normal circulation restored. This thought relates to a patient whose only symptoms were hemianesthesia after sneezing.

Dr. Antunes: This metameric segmentation is a very interesting phenomenon, and probably is not metameric at all. In other words, it has no developmental basis. Obviously not all segments of the cord suffer the same degree of dilatation. In fact, the C1-2 segments are usually spared. Some have suggested that this "beady" appearance just means that the cord is under pressure.

Further Thoughts on Pathophysiology and Therapy

Dr. Holtzman asked Dr. Marin-Padilla: I have noted in some of my cases of syringo-hydromyelic complex with the Chiari malformation that the cerebellar tonsils are asymmetric and different in appearance. Some patients have thick tonsils, some have thin tapered tonsils, and sometimes the tonsils look as though there may be compression and sometimes not.

Dr. Marin-Padilla responded if you look at the posterior fossa in those people you will find that it is deformed. The vertebrae may be deviated to one side or the other and the posterior fossa itself asymmetric.

Dr. Schlesinger remarked that from the surgeon's standpoint there are great variations in the posterior fossa.

Dr. Stein agreed and remarked that the idea of decompressing the entire pos-terior fossa is a very good one. Approximately 20 years ago this idea was used in Baltimore for meningomyelocele associated with Arnold–Chiari malformation. The stated purpose was to avoid the onset of hydrocephalus. This procedure was performed at the time of repair of the meningomyelocele and a wire screen was inserted to prevent the bone from reforming. A high success rate was claimed in preventing hydrocephalus but the operation fell into disrepute as a big operation in young children. Surgeons seem more willing to face the need for a shunt and re-serve the suboccipital craniectomy for later after growth had been completed. Perhaps it is an issue that should be reopened among pediatric neurosurgeons.

Dr. Marin-Padilla said that I cannot talk about all cases, but when I ex-perimentally produce the Arnold–Chiari malformation, I use only one dose of vitamin A and I can produce anencephaly, spina bifida, encephalocele, and the Arnold–Chiari depending at what time in the 8 days of gestation I give the vitamin to the mouse. I can have the entire spectrum, but in the Arnold–Chiari the pos-terior fossa is small, there is hypoplasia of the occipital bone, and it appears to me that in some cases with modern technology reconstruction of the posterior fossa is indicated.

Dr. Stein said, it would have to be done quite early.

Dr. Marin-Padilla agreed, very early.

Dr. Stein asked, can you then identify the cases where you believe it would be effective?

Dr. Marin-Padilla said, I believe it would be preventive medicine. Once you have syringomyelia there is nothing available that is totally curative. Another point about syringomyelia when there is a cavity involving the entire spinal cord it does not make sense. You must return to a time when things are simpler, such as during the embryonic period.

What I have seen is forking of the aqueduct of Sylvius. Now you can also have forking of the spinal central canal. This occurs because the longitudinal distance is reduced. There is nothing wrong with the brain in development and the ependyma continues to develop, but because there is room the spinal cord may buckle medially like an accordion. I can show you this phenomenon in embryos.

When spina bifida was originally described it was considered a focal overgrowth of the neural tube, a focal overgrowth of the ependyma. This is not a focal overgrowth. This is an accordion. Once you have those little pockets, then you have the beginning of the big problem, because the "little pockets" are going to develop into big pockets that you have termed segments. These are pockets, not segments.

Dr. Antunes said, that is correct. I did not suggest that there was any correlation with a metameric pattern. People are trying to explain that in two ways. Either because the sites with root centers have more resistance and therefore they open between the roots. The same reason is given to explain why the central canal is not enlarged at the C1-2 level, which is that there is too much decussation of fibers occurring and therefore it is more difficult for the canal to dilate. A similar reason is given for the preferential dilation of the occipital versus the frontal horns of the lateral ventricles in hydrocephalus. I personally do not believe that they have any neurological implication.

Dr. Marin-Padilla continued, what I see in the little embryo spinal central canal is a pocket and when the tissues grow and the tube has to elongate, but the bony space allotted is a little bit smaller then the tube buckles. Once you have buckles like that you have the beginning of syringomyelia, the beginning of big problems. When the cyst develops it will continue to enlarge until it creates symptoms. By that time it is already too late. Therefore, prevention is of great importance. In my opinion if you decompress the posterior fossa you may prevent syringomyelia.

The same is true of the tethered spinal cord. When you describe the tethered cord you never describe that the laminae are open, that the bones never close. Why aren't the bones closed? Because you have rachischisis. Underneath there is dural-schisis. If the dura is open the spinal cord is in contact with the subcutaneous tissues and subcutaneous fat is incorporated into the neural tissue. This is not a cord lipoma, this is subcutaneous fat. Therefore, you have a neural tube defect in the tethered cord. Originally, when neurosurgeons performed surgery they never closed the dura; subsequently they discovered that they had to close the dura. The dura must be closed to reestablish the anatomic integrity or there will be ongoing problems because the fat continues to grow.

In addition, when you talk about neural tube closure you must close the skin, the mesodermal elements, and the meninges, including the dura and arachnoid, and then you close the spine and spinal canal.

Dr. Oldfield mentioned that most of the neurosurgical procedures that Dr. Antunes was telling us about are based on the acceptance of the fact that the constriction is the mesodermally derived elements at the base of the skull. That is why we do posterior fossa and upper cervical laminectomies. The embryologists really condemned Gardener's idea of the water hammer effect, on which most of our surgical procedures are based.

Dr. John Mealey at the University of Indiana about 7 or 8 years ago reported an experiment he did in pups. He injected kaolin into the posterior fossa and subarachnoid space in newborn pups. About half of them died of acute hydrocephalus. Those that survived had radioisotope inserted in the ventricular system that could be followed down into the central canal until it ruptured into the spinal subarachnoid space.

The same thing is known for children with myelomeningoceles. The central canal is patent. George DeBoulay, who is the head of Neuroradiology at Queens Square, back in the 1960s did some cineradiographs on patients who were having ventriculography. If he pooled the contrast medium in the posterior third ventricle and looked at it in the AP direction with each pulsebeat he could see a compression of the third ventricle and in the lateral views there was a $1\frac{1}{2}$ to 2 inch tall movement of fluid through the aqueduct into the fourth ventricle with each pulse beat. This is what I think we are seeing on the MRIs presented yesterday. This is the milking effect of the expansion of the brain with each pulse beat pushing the fluid into the central canal. Therefore, pulsations themselves may have a great deal to do with the pathogenesis of syringomyelia. Perhaps when we perform a ventriculoperitoneal shunt the dampening of the pulsation is enough to relieve some of the symptoms that these patients are experiencing.

As an aside, in the past few years we have removed five or six hemangioblastomas that were associated with syringomyelia in which we have carefully avoided entering the syrinx. Clearly, by removing the tumor the syrinx has disappeared in each case. Therefore, it is not clear that mechanical drainage is required in the therapy of all syringomyelic cavities. There may be something about the movement of blood or the mass effect of the tumor that is contributing to the production of the syrinx.

Reference

1. Epstein BS, Epstein JA. The association of cerebellar tonsillar herniation with basilar impression incident to Paget's disease. *Am J Roentgenol.* 1969;107:535–542.

CHAPTER 16

Surgery of the Infected Spine and Spinal Cord Function

James E.O. Hughes, George V. DiGiacinto, and Narayan Sundaresan

The surgical treatment of spinal infections has taught us a great deal about the pathophysiology of the spinal cord. In the past 15 years at St. Luke's–Roosevelt, we have operated on 23 patients with various forms of Pott's paraplegia and done 61 anterior explorations for pyogenic infections in 57 patients (cervical 24, thoracic 14, lumbar 23). During the same period, we have done more than 250 anterior explorations of the spine for tumor. Successful surgery required adequate decompression and maintenance of bony stability. Surgical cases in our series of spinal infections presented a myriad of combinations of cord compression and spinal instability. In my discussion of the cases presented, we will point out that the blood supply of the spinal cord does not appear to be precarious. Cord infarction from the anterior transthoracic surgery does not appear to be a problem. We believe that the deleterious effects of infection arise from mechanical compression, not from "arteritis or phlebitis," and that it is rare in spinal surgery to have a vascular spinal cord complication except in the vigorous correction of scoliosis.

Infarction due to Cord Surgery

Infarction of the cord is a rare complication of transthoracic vertebrectomy.

Some surgeons had cautioned about operating on the left side from T-9 to L-2 without spinal angiography to identify the artery of Adamkiewicz. Hodgkins and Stock never mentioned it in their pioneering description of transthoracic spinal surgery in Pott's disease.[1] Kemp et al. in 1973 reported their series of 131 cases of anterior spinal decompression in infection and had no cases of cord infarction.[2] Rollin and Southwick in their chapter in Rothman and Simeone's book, *The Spine*, stated that no complications have been reported by a number of authors after unilateral resection of multiple segmental vessels in the lower thoracic spine.[3] Our group has done more than 200 transthoracic operations for tumor and infection. We take the intercostal arteries necessary to get the exposure and have never had a cord infarction attributed to ligation of intercostal arteries. The thoracic spinal cord is described as having its anterior spinal artery supplied by three major intercostal arteries. However, every intercostal artery gives off a small radicular artery, which in turn anastomoses with adjacent radicular arteries.[4] When the intercostal artery is injected, usually the radicular arteries above and below the injected artery also fill, demonstrating this anastomosis. The anastomosis is in great part intraspinal distal to the intervertebral foramen. It is important to occlude surgically the intercostal artery as proximal to the intervertebral foramen as possible. The closer one gets from the foramen to the anterior spinal artery, the more the artery is an end artery. Burrington et al. published a good review of this phenomenon in 1976.[5] Our lack of complications does not mean it cannot happen, only that it must be very rare.

Laminectomy versus Anterior Approach

Successful treatment of spinal infections is predicated on doing the correct operation. Most of the time, this is an anterior approach as the pathology is in the vertebral body. Laminectomy is reserved for the rare case of epidural empyema when the preoperative computed tomography (CT) scan shows that the posterior epidural space is filled with pus, that is, the sublaminar epidural fat is obliterated. This is rare. However, we still see patients who have been operated on for vertebral osteomyelitis with a laminectomy. As recently as 1976, a pertinent article was published in *Surgical Neurology*.[6] A patient with a large anterior mass associated with C5-6 osteomyelitis was found at C3-7 laminectomy to have a bulging cord. The authors demonstrated an anterior mass with an intraoperative real-time ultrasound. The mass was drained posteriorly but unfortunately the patient remained quadriplegic. The article purported to show the value of real-time ultrasound in such cases. The logical conclusion should have been that patients with this kind of problem should be decompressed anteriorly.

Transthoracic Approach

One of the most important contributions of the surgical treatment of spinal infections has been the development of the transthoracic approach. Although costotransversectomy had been used for many years to decompress the cord in thoracic Pott's abscesses, it does not afford the exposure that the direct transthoracic approach does. Because of the posteriorly curved rib, an anterior exposure is not obtained unless a long segment of the rib is also removed (Fig. 16.1). Hodgkins and Stock perfected transthoracic surgery in Hong Kong in the 1950s and 1960s while treating a huge

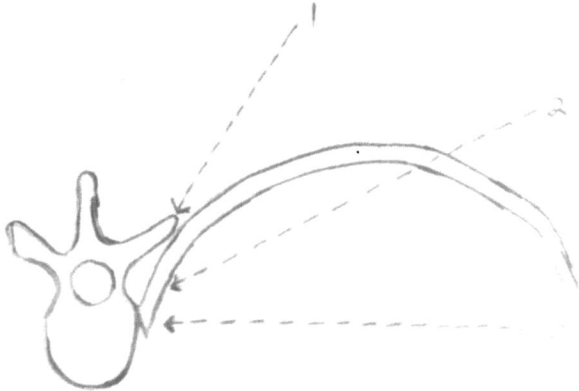

Figure 16.1. Rib resection.

caseload of patients with Pott's paraplegia.[1] Large cooperative studies in Korea and Rhodesia now question such radical surgery in all cases of Pott's disease.[7,8] Good argument can still be made in patients with cord compression. Tuli, in a study of 200 patients with Pott's paraplegia treated medically with bedrest and A.M.T., showed that only 38% of the patients responded and did not require surgery.[9] All our patients with neurological signs have made early and usually dramatic improvement after anterior decompression. We therefore feel all patients with Pott's paraplegia ought to be decompressed anteriorly.

Case 1. A 38-year-old African man illustrates this point. He presented with paraparesis, a sensory loss to pinprick at T-1 and marked weakness of all left hand intrinsic musculature. Plain rays x and myelography demonstrated cord compression from tuberculosis at C-7 to T-3 and also at T11-12. The cord compression was most marked at the upper level. Through an anterior cervical incision, we were able to remove C-7 through and including the T-3 body without splitting the sternum. A C-6–T-4 fibular strut graft was placed. Within 48 hours, the left hand strength improved and the sensory level dropped to T-11. He was given antimicrobial therapy and nursed in a Stryker frame. Two months postoperatively, his legs became increasingly weak, progressing to paraplegia. This was rapidly reversed by transthoracic decompression and anterior fusion at T11-12. Nine months postoperatively, he was dancing in a professional dance troupe.

Anterior decompression can be done after extensive laminectomy. One of our earlier cases demonstrated this.

Case 2. This 320-lb man with a chest mass after chest trauma was at first thought to have a traumatic thoracic aneurysm. Angiography ruled this out but showed some questionable destruction of T-4 and T-5. While being mobilized out of bed, he developed marked weakness in both legs. A thoracic myelogram showed a complete block at T-6. T4-T6 thoracic laminectomy for presumed metastatic cancer showed chronic inflammatory changes of the epidural tissue. His paraparesis initially improved but worsened whenever he was turned in the lateral position. Tomograms of the spine were consistent with Pott's disease. Transthoracically, three vertebrae producing a 70° gibbus were removed and interbody rib grafts were placed. Six months postoperatively, he was fully ambulatory without neurological deficit.

Case 3. A not uncommon presentation of Pott's paraplegia was seen in the following patient being worked up on the medical floor for a fever of unknown origin (FUO). Among this 43-year-old drug addict's many complaints of pain was an unappreciated midthoracic pain with bilateral radiating intercostal pain. When he complained he was getting weak, he was forced out of bed into a chair, where he was weaker each evening after all day out of bed. His paraparesis was finally recognized. A gibbus was clinically noted, myelography done, and transthoracic decompression and fusion performed. He rapidly regained full use of his legs.

It is apparent that cord compression in Pott's paraplegia is frequently due to spinal instability preoperatively and not always due to ventrally placed granuloma. This is why even before any microbial therapy, many patients with Pott's paraplegia were cured by bedrest alone.

Patients with metastatic cancer of the spine have disease in the body ventral to the cord. They are rarely unstable. My initial attempts at anterior decompression, however, were unsuccessful because of spinal instability postoperatively. Dr. Sundaresan and others have solved this problem with successful immediate stabilization of the spine with interbody Steinman pins and acrylic vertebral replacement.[10,11] Without the Steinman pins, the acrylic body will rapidly loosen. In selective cases later posterior stabilization with bone and instrumentation may be necessary.

Cord Infarction and Vasculitis

Most authors reporting clinical series of spinal infection attribute paraplegia in great part to vasculitis, either arteritis or phlebitis. Typical is the statement by Hulme and Dott in 1954, "It is generally believed that these changes are caused by thrombosis or stasis in blood vessels supplying or draining the cord".[12]

In a series of eloquent animal studies, Feldenzer et al. have questioned these theories.[13] They injected staph aureus into the posterior thoracolumbar epidural space. Histopathologic and microangiographic techniques were used. Anterior and paired posterior spinal arteries remained patent in paraplegic rabbits with mild to moderate spinal cord compression and in some cases a severe compression. In animals with severe compression, the anterior epidural venous plexus remained patent but the dorsal vein was occluded. Occlusion of the perforating arteries occurred only with extreme spinal cord compression.

From a practical treatment point of view, we have found the concept of vasculitis helpful only to withhold hope of recovery and as a reason not to operate. In some of our early nonoperated pyogenic cases, we gave up too soon because we felt the cord had infarcted. Now, whenever a patient does not improve after decompression, we restudy, looking for additional unrelieved cord compression. We invariably will find such an explanation.

Anterior Cord Syndrome

Two patients with anterior cord syndrome due to osteomyelitis demonstrated recovery of function when it was felt that the cord had infarcted in the distribution of the anterior spinal artery. In both cases decompression worked well. In one patient, the posterior cord became involved, resulting in total clinical loss of all spinal cord function for 7 months with subsequent functional recovery.

Case 4. The first patient, a 63-year-old diabetic man with staph epidermidis thoracic osteomyelitis, had been unable to move his legs for 48 hours and was in urinary retention when first seen. His legs were flaccid. Temperature and pain sensation were absent from T-6 down. He could recognize joint movement and localized touch. The cord was decompressed anteriorly. His legs remained flaccid for 2 weeks when he started to adduct his right thigh. Within 6 months, he was walking with Lostrand crutches.

Case 5. The other patient, a 39-year-old intravenous drug abuser, had had a T6-7 laminectomy in another hospital for presumed metastatic tumor. Seven days postoperatively, he stopped moving his legs. When transferred to our institution 3 weeks later, he was not able to move his legs at all. The only sensation preserved was lateralization of deep pain in his legs. Two weeks after his legs became paralyzed, we decompressed and fused the staph aureus osteomyelitis at T6-7 transthoracically. Postoperatively, he could still lateralize deep pain but nothing else. One month later, he lost the ability to localize deep pain. For 7 months he was paraplegic without any sensation below T-6. Then much to our surprise, he began to wiggle his feet. There had been no voluntary leg movements for 9 months. During this period, he had had three episodes of sepsis, acute hepatitis, multiple urinary tract infections, surgery for a sacral decubitus, and two bouts of organic psychosis lasting 2 and 3 weeks. His lower extremity function, however, continued to improve. In 24 months, he had normal lower extremity strength, intact bladder function, and normal pain, temperature, and position sensation.

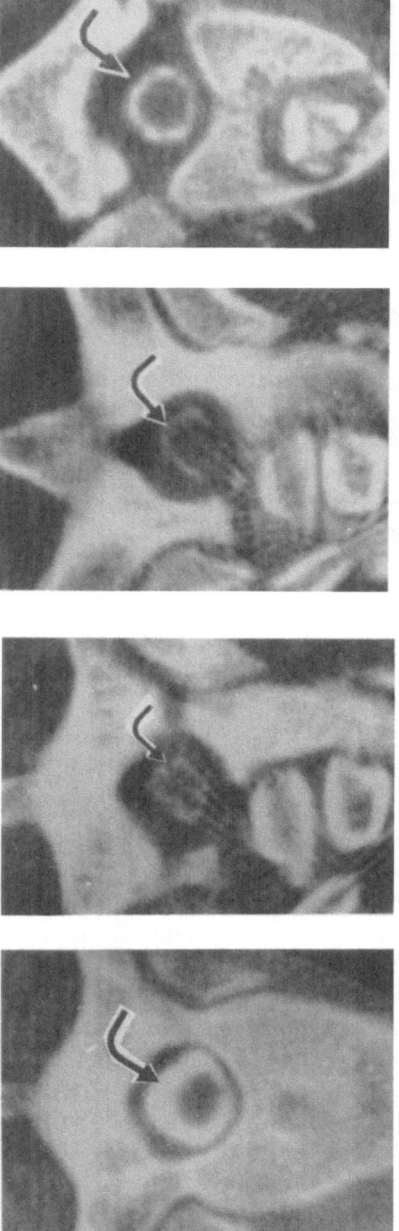

Figure 16.2. Constricting fibrous band T7-8.

As puzzling as his recovery is, we are more puzzled as to why he retained the gross posterior column function for 1 month and then lost it. If that happened now, we would have restudied him with a contrast CT. The next case suggests a possible explanation.

Case 6. This 52-year-old man with T7-8 osteomyelitis lost all voluntary movement in his lower extremities over a 72-hour period. While being rapidly worked up, he responded to a 100-mg bolus of Decadron. Just preoperatively, he was able to wiggle his left foot and adduct his thighs. He was decompressed transthoracically at T7-8 and a T6-8 rib fusion was performed. Three months postoperatively, he was able to walk in parallel bars. He suddenly developed severe proximal weakness in both legs. A myelogram/CT revealed a concentric narrowing in the subarachnoid space (Fig. 16.2). Anterior fusion was solid and there was no bony compression of the cord. At laminectomy, we found a band of constricting epidural tissue that was easily incised. Six days postoperatively, he was able to lift his legs off the bed and continued slowly to improve to independent ambulation. This was just the type of clinical deterioration that authors in the past would have attributed to vasculitis. It was clearly due to compression.

Gibbus Deformity and Spinal Cord Compression

A fixed spinal gibbus is seen in patients with either arrested or treated Pott's disease. The patient may have no neurological signs or symptoms during the active phase of the infection. Later in life, the ventral bony gibbus becomes symptomatic. Although the spine is fused, the spinal cord or cauda equina continues to move over the ventral ridge, getting constantly traumatized. We have treated four such patients.

Case 7. The first such patient we treated was admitted to the hospital twice, transiently paraplegic after falling while intoxicated. After each occasion, he was left with normal strength but increasing spasticity. On the third occasion, the paresis persisted. Studies showed a 70° thoracic gibbus. The apex was removed transthoracically and the spasticity and paresis partially receded (Fig. 16.3). Now he falls without increasing his neurological deficit.

Case 8. The second case had an 80° L2-3 gibbus. This 48-year-old woman had had a T-11–L-5 fusion at age 5 for Pott's disease. She had increasingly severe bilateral radicular pain due to cauda equina compression. We went retroperitoneally but technically were not able to remove the gibbus as the angle was too acute. It was early in our experience with translumbar spine surgery.

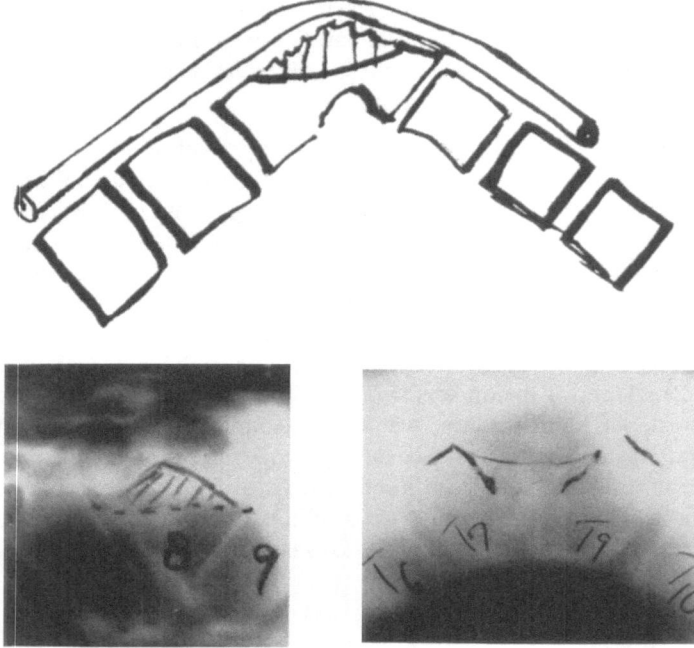

Figure 16.3. 70° thoracic gibbus.

Case 9. The third case was a 48-year-old woman who also had had a posterior lumbosacral fusion for Pott's disease at age 2. When seen, she had only minimal strength left in all muscle groups, L-2–S-1. She scooted around her apartment, sitting on a throw rug. She was incontinent of urine. We approached her gibbus posteriorly, opening the dura, retracting the roots laterally, and removing the gibbus transdurally (Fig. 16.4). Postoperatively, she became continent and was ambulatory with Lofstrand crutches (Fig. 16.5).

Case 10. Our fourth case of gibbus was a 20-year-old Tibetan woman, who at the age of 12 was quadriplegic for 30 minutes after a skating accident. She remembers that all the sensation and strength left her body. The diagnosis of Pott's disease of the cervical spine was made and she had a posterior fusion from C-2 through C-6. At the age of 19, she developed increasing weakness and spasticity of her right arm, hand, and leg. There was decreased joint position sense of her right hand and decreased pain and temperature sensation from C-8 down on the left side. Magnetic resonancy imaging (MRI) (Fig. 16.5) showed syrinx of the cervical cord plus the ventral compression at C3-4. Through a cervical laminectomy, a syrinx to peritoneal shunt was done. There was no neurological improve-

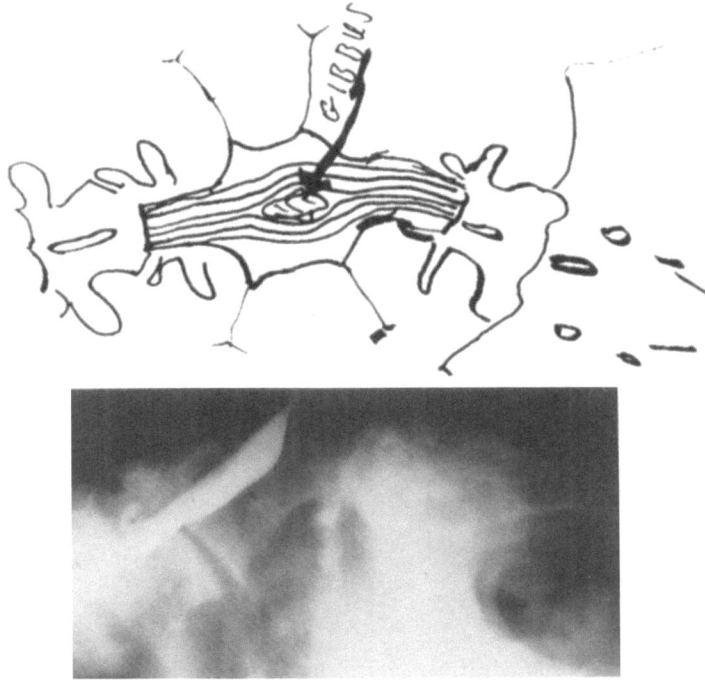

Figure 16.4. Transdural gibbus.

ment and she sought another opinion. A month before our operation, she fell twice and was transiently quadriplegic for 10 to 15 minutes. At surgery, we excised the gibbus at C3-4 anteriorly and did a C2-5 fusion. She was transiently worse postoperatively, but at 2 months is back to her preoperative status. We believe her syrinx was due to anterior cord compression like the cases discussed by Ossana et al.[14] It is too early to be sure, but we think this is another instance of the need to be certain to "make sure there is nothing compressing the cord before other more exotic etiologies are suggested."

Cervical Osteomyelitis: Root and Cord Compression

Our operative experience with cervical osteomyelitis (24 cases) has been a continuation of that reported by Dr. Henry Messer from Harlem Hospital Center in 1976.[15] Invariably, the patients present many times in the emergency room complaining of neck pain. The initial cervical spine x rays show soft-tissue swelling that frequently is missed. The patient finally presents with paresis of several cervical roots and a variable myelopathy. At

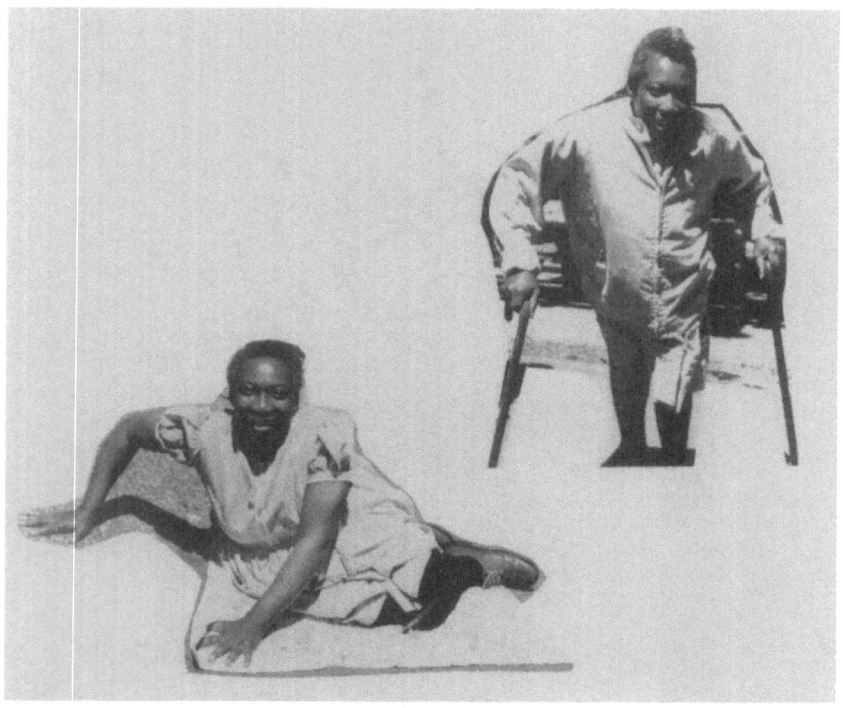

A

Figure 16.5. Ambulatory after surgery.

anterior decompression, there is significant swollen epidural granulation tissue, rare pus, and variable degrees of bone destruction. Drainage and immobilization with tongs or Halo, with or without bony fusion, usually lead to rapid improvement in upper extremity strength and lower extremity motor and sensory function. Postoperative problems are usually related to the patient not wanting to stay in tongs or Halo.

However, when the patient does not improve or plateaus at an unacceptable level, we restudy him, looking for further compression. The two following cases illustrate this.

Case 11. This 46-year-old male intravenous drug abuser with osteomyelitis involving C5-7 was just able to flex and extend his left arm and close his left hand. He could close his right hand but otherwise his right upper extremity was plegic. Lower extremity function was normal. At surgery, C6 was 60% destroyed, and C5 and C7 were 20% destroyed. There was thick epidural granulation tissue and no pus. The cord was decompressed, bone chips placed, and he was kept in tongs postoperatively. Initially, there was early improvement of his left upper extremity. However, at 1 month, his right upper extremity and hand were plegic. He was just able to move his left

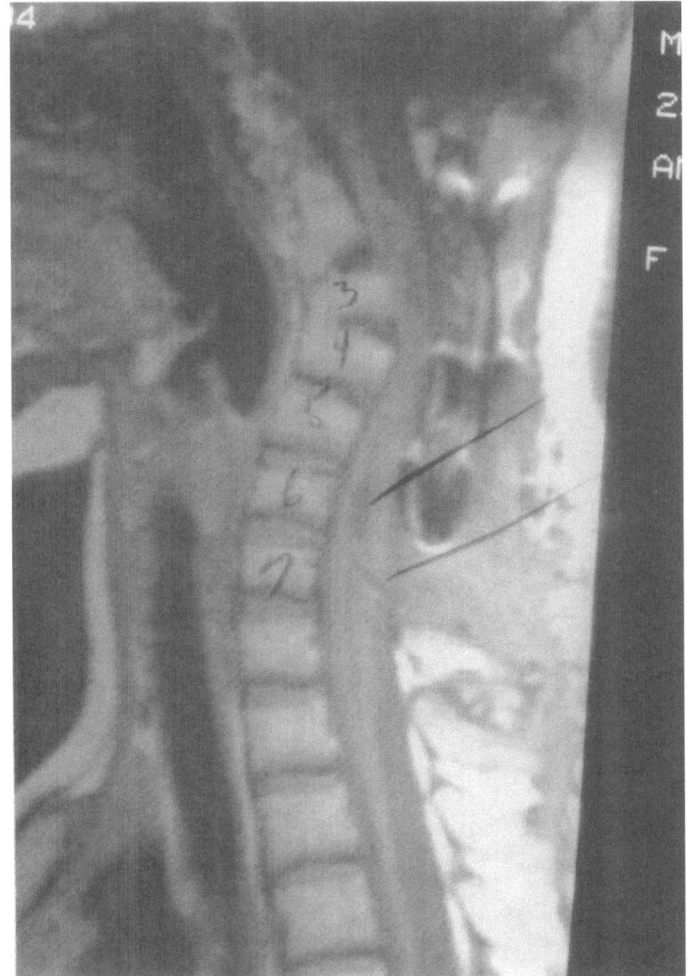

B

upper extremity. Both legs were now weak. Repeat CT myelogram showed good decompression at the operative area, C5-7, but now there was a new anterior epidural mass from C2-5, centered over more osteomyelitis at C3-4. A groove was drilled from C2 to C4 down to the dura, and widened in a wedge shape posteriorly, decompressing the very thick anterior epidural granulation tissue (Fig. 16.6). There was dramatic improvement in upper extremity and hand strength within 24 hours.

Case 12. A 61-year-old male intravenous drug abuser with osteomyelitis of C4-6 was paretic in both upper extremities and almost totally plegic in both lower extremities. On the day of surgery, all he could do was adduct his

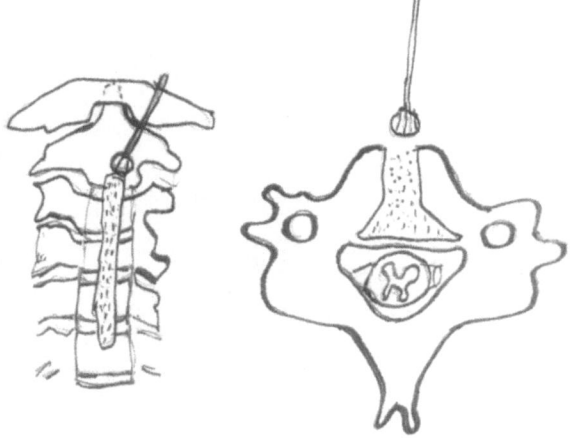

Figure 16.6. Ventral Compression C3-4.

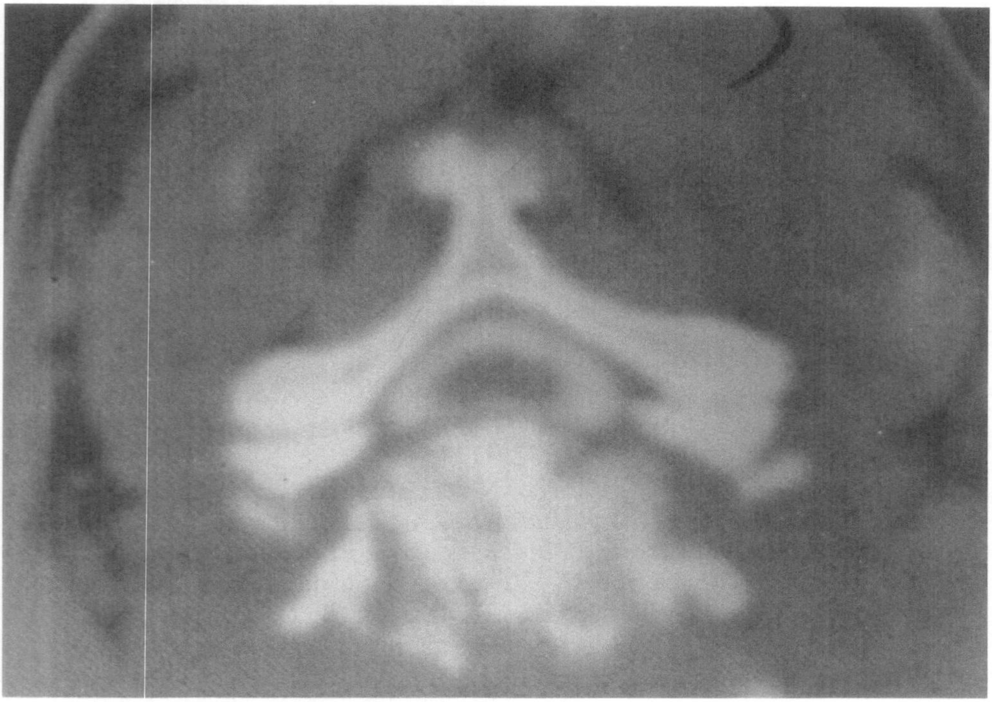

Figure 16.7. Anterior decompression.

thighs and wiggle his left foot. Myelogram showed partial blocks at C6-7 and C4-5 from a ventral mass. At anterior decompression, the C4-5, C5-6, and C6-7 discs were destroyed and the C8 vertebra moth-eaten. There was no pus but the dura was very thickened. A groove was drilled with a Midas Rex drill down to the dura from C4 through C7. An iliac crest graft was placed. There was early dramatic improvement in the quadriparesis. In about 6 weeks, he developed painful flexor spasms of both lower extremities, even though the strength had improved to 80% of normal. We restudied him and found that the fast-taking bone graft was compressing the cord at C5-6 (Fig. 16.7). At repeat operation, a new anterior groove decompression cured the flexor spasms in the lower extremities within 2 weeks. Instead of restudying these patients, we could have attributed the late deterioration to arteritis or phlebitis and not vigorously looked for a compressive lesion.

Our experience with multiple operations to decompress the spinal cord in patients with spine infection has encouraged us to be more aggressive in treating cervical and thoracic spondylosis. Myelogram/CT now usually can tell us which patient will benefit most from the anterior or posterior approach. We feel that a patient who does not improve after such surgery ought to be restudied looking for residual compression, rather than just saying the operation does not help everyone.

Conclusion

What has our surgical treatment of spinal infection taught us about spinal cord pathophysiology? One, spinal cord infarction is an exceptionally rare complication of transthoracic surgery. Two, preoperative spinal angiography is not necessary. Three, take the intercostal artery as proximal to the intercostal foramen as possible. Four, as shown experimentally by Feldenzer et al., there is not a high incidence of infarction due to arteritis or phlebitis. We are not convinced it was a factor in any of our cases. Five, cord compression due to either mass effect or instability is the overwhelming cause of cord dysfunction in patients with spinal infection, tuberculous or pyogenic. Six, syrinx due to cord compression should be decompressed and not primarily shunted. Seven, a fixed gibbus may not produce cord compression for many years and then become symptomatic. Eight, surgical decompression may relieve profound cord dysfunction in patients with pyogenic or tuberculous spine infection. One patient had complete loss of function for 7 months and walked. Many patients had complete loss of strength in arms or legs and recovered. Nine, if a patient does not respond to decompression, restudy and do not hesitate to reoperate. These concepts can be applied to all causes of cord compression, particularly spondylosis.

References

1. Hodgkins AR, Stock FE. Anterior spine fusion for the treatment of tuberculosis of the spine. *J Bone Joint Surg*. 1960;42A:295–311.
2. Kemp HBS, Jackson JW, Jeremiah J, Cook JD. Anterior fusion of the spine for infective lesions in adults. *J Bone Joint Surg*. 1973;55B:715–734.
3. Rollin MJ, Southwick WO. Surgical approaches to the spine in: Rothman, Simeone, eds. *The Spine*. Philadelphia: WB. Saunders; 1982.
4. Lazorthes G, Gonage A, Zadeh JU, Santini JJ, Lazorthes Y, Burdin P. Arterial vascularization of the spinal cord: Recent studies of the anastomotic substitution pathways. *J Neurosurg*. 1970;35:253–262.
5. Burrington JD, Brown C, Wayne ER, Odom J. Anterior approach to the thoraco-lumbar spine, technical considerations. *Arch Surg*. 1976;111:456–463.
6. Feldenzer JA, Waters DC, Knake JE, Hoff JT. Anterior epidural abscess: The use of intraoperative spinal angiography. *Surg Neurol*. 1986;25:105–108.
7. Medical Research Council Working Party on Tuberculosis of the Spine. A controlled trial of ambulant outpatient treatment and inpatient rest in bed in the management of tuberculosis of the spine in young Korean patients on standard chemotherapy, a study in Misan, Korea. *J Bone Joint Surg*. 1973;55B:678–697.
8. Medical Research Council Working Party on Tuberculosis of the Spine. A controlled trial of debridement and ambulatory treatment in the management of tuberculosis of the spine in patients on standard chemotherapy, a study in Bulawayo, Rhodesia. *J Trop Med Hyg*. 1974;77:72–92.
9. Tuli SM. Results of treatment of spinal tuberculosis by "middle path" regime. *J Bone Joint Surg*. 1975;57B:13–23.
10. Sundaresan N, Galicich JH, Lane JM, Bains M, McCormack P. Treatment of neoplastic epidural cord compression by vertebral body resection and stabilization. *J Neurosurg*. 1985;63:676–684.
11. Dunn EJ. The role of methyl methacrylate in stabilization and replacement of the cervical spine. *Spine*. 1977;2:15–24.
12. Hulme A, Dott NM. Spinal epidural abscess. *Br Med J*. 1954;1:64–68.
13. Feldenzer JA, McKeever PE, Schlaberg D, Campbell JA, Hoff JT. The pathogenesis of spinal epidural abscess: Microangiographic studies in an experimental model. *J Neurosurg*. 1988;69:110–114.
14. Ossana AM, Harkey LJ, Middletown TH, Smith RS, Fox JL. Myelopathic cervical spondylotic lesions demonstrated by magnetic resonance imaging. *J Neurosurg*. 1988;68:217–222.
15. Messer HD, Litvinoff J. Chondro-osteomyelitis of the cervical spine associated with parenteral drug use. *Arch Neurol*. 1976;33:571–576.

Index